Geriatric Anesthesia

Editors

ELIZABETH L. WHITLOCK
ROBERT A. WHITTINGTON

ANESTHESIOLOGY CLINICS

www.anesthesiology.theclinics.com

Consulting Editor
LEE A. FLEISHER

September 2019 • Volume 37 • Number 3

ELSEVIER

1600 John F. Kennedy Boulevard • Suite 1800 • Philadelphia, Pennsylvania, 19103-2899

http://www.theclinics.com

ANESTHESIOLOGY CLINICS Volume 37, Number 3
September 2019 ISSN 1932-2275, ISBN-13: 978-0-323-68221-3

Editor: Colleen Dietzler
Developmental Editor: Kristen Helm

Anesthesiology Clinics (ISSN 1932-2275) is published quarterly by Elsevier Inc., 360 Park Avenue South, New York, NY 10010-1710. Months of issue are March, June, September, and December. Periodicals postage paid at New York, NY and at additional mailing offices. Subscription prices are $100.00 per year (US student/resident), $360.00 per year (US individuals), $446.00 per year (Canadian individuals), $693.00 per year (US institutions), $876.00 per year (Canadian institutions), $225.00 per year (Canadian and foreign student/resident), $469.00 per year (foreign individuals), and $876.00 per year (foreign institutions). To receive student and resident rate, orders must be accompanied by name of affiliated institution, date of term, and the *signature* of program/residency coordinator on institutions letterhead. Orders will be billed at individual rate until proof of status is received. Foreign air speed delivery is included in all *Clinics'* subscription prices. All prices are subject to change without notice. POSTMASTER: Send address changes to *Anesthesiology Clinics,* Elsevier Health Sciences Division, Subscription Customer Service, 3251 Riverport Lane, Maryland Heights, MO 63043. Customer Service (orders, claims, online, change of address): Elsevier Health Sciences Division, Subscription Customer Service, 3251 Riverport Lane, Maryland Heights, MO 63043. **Tel:1-800-654-2452 (U.S. and Canada); 314-447-8871 (outside U.S. and Canada). Fax: 314-447-8029. E-mail: journalscustomerservice-usa@elsevier.com (for print support); journalsonlinesupport-usa@elsevier.com (for online support).**

Reprints. For copies of 100 or more of articles in this publication, please contact the Commercial Reprints Department, Elsevier Inc., 360 Park Avenue South, New York, NY 10010-1710. Tel.: 212-633-3874; Fax: 212-633-3820; E-mail: reprints@elsevier.com.

Anesthesiology Clinics, is also published in Spanish by McGraw-Hill Inter-americana Editores S. A., P.O. Box 5-237, 06500 Mexico D. F., Mexico.

Anesthesiology Clinics, is covered in *MEDLINE/PubMed (Index Medicus), Current Contents/Clinical Medicine, Excerpta Medica, ISI/BIOMED*, and *Chemical Abstracts*.

Contributors

CONSULTING EDITOR

LEE A. FLEISHER, MD
Robert D. Dripps Professor and Chair of Anesthesiology and Critical Care, Professor of Medicine, Perelman School of Medicine, University of Pennsylvania, Philadelphia, Pennsylvania, USA

EDITORS

ELIZABETH L. WHITLOCK, MD, MSc
Assistant Professor, Department of Anesthesia and Perioperative Care, University of California, San Francisco, San Francisco, California, USA

ROBERT A. WHITTINGTON, MD
Professor of Anesthesiology at CUMC, Department of Anesthesiology, Columbia University Irving Medical Center, New York, New York, USA

AUTHORS

BRIAN F.S. ALLEN, MD
Assistant Professor of Anesthesiology, Program Director, Regional and Acute Pain Medicine Fellowship, Director, Regional and Acute Pain Medicine Service, Division of Multispecialty Anesthesiology, Department of Anesthesiology, Vanderbilt University Medical Center, Nashville, Tennessee, USA

FAHAD ALAM, MD, MHSc, FRCPC
Department of Anesthesia, University of Toronto, Department of Anesthesia, Sunnybrook Health Sciences Centre, Toronto, Ontario, Canada

TATE M. ANDRES, MD
Resident, Department of Anesthesiology, Vanderbilt University Medical Center, Nashville, Tennessee, USA

SYLVIE AUCOIN, MD, FRCPC
Department of Anesthesiology and Pain Medicine, The Ottawa Hospital, University of Ottawa, Ottawa, Ontario, Canada

SINZIANA AVRAMESCU, MD, FRCPC, PhD
Department of Anesthesia, University of Toronto, Department of Anesthesia, Sunnybrook Health Sciences Centre, Department of Anesthesia, Humber River Hospital, Toronto, Ontario, Canada

SHEILA RYAN BARNETT, MD, FASA
Vice-Chair of Perioperative Medicine, Associate Professor of Anesthesia, Department of Anesthesia, Critical Care and Pain Medicine, Harvard Medical School, Beth Israel Deaconess Medical Center, Boston, Massachusetts, USA

MATTHIAS BEHRENDS, MD
Department of Anesthesia and Perioperative Care, University of California, San Francisco, San Francisco, California, USA

JAUME BORRELL-VEGA, MD
Department of Anesthesiology – Clinical Research, The Ohio State University Wexner Medical Center, Columbus, Ohio, USA

STEPHEN CHOI, MD, MSc, FRCPC
Department of Anesthesia, University of Toronto, Department of Anesthesia, Sunnybrook Health Sciences Centre, Toronto, Ontario, Canada

PHILIPPE DESMARAIS, MD, MHSc, FRCPC
Cognitive and Movement Disorders Clinic, L.C. Campbell Cognitive Neurology Research Unit, Sunnybrook Health Sciences Centre, Hurvitz Brain Sciences Program, Sunnybrook Research Institute, University of Toronto, Toronto, Ontario, Canada

ANNE L. DONOVAN, MD
Associate Clinical Professor, Department of Anesthesia and Perioperative Care, Division of Critical Care Medicine, University of California, San Francisco, San Francisco, California, USA

ALAN G. ESPARZA GUTIERREZ, BS
Department of Anesthesiology – Clinical Research, The Ohio State University Wexner Medical Center, Columbus, Ohio, USA

EMILY FINLAYSON, MD, MS
Departments of Surgery and Medicine, Phillip R. Lee Institute for Health Policy Studies, University of California, San Francisco, San Francisco, California, USA

ALLEN N. GUSTIN Jr, MD, FCCP, FASA
Professor of Anesthesiology, Stritch School of Medicine, Anesthesiology, Critical Care Medicine, Hospice/Palliative Medicine, Department of Anesthesiology and Perioperative Medicine, Loyola University Medical Center, Maywood, Illinois, USA

KAVEH HEMATI, MD
Resident Physician, Department of Anesthesia and Perioperative Care, University of California, San Francisco, San Francisco, California, USA

NATHAN HERRMANN, MD, FRCPC
Department of Psychiatry, University of Toronto, Sunnybrook Health Sciences Centre, Toronto, Ontario, Canada

MAY HUA, MD, MSc
Assistant Professor of Anesthesiology (in Epidemiology), Department of Anesthesiology, Columbia University Medical Center, New York, New York, USA

CHRISTOPHER G. HUGHES, MD
Associate Professor, Department of Anesthesiology, Division of Anesthesiology Critical Care Medicine, Vanderbilt University School of Medicine, Nashville, Tennessee, USA

MICHELLE L. HUMEIDAN, MD, PhD
Assistant Professor, Department of Anesthesiology, The Ohio State University Wexner Medical Center, Columbus, Ohio, USA

STANLEY G. JABLONSKI, MD
Resident, Department of Anesthesiology, Perioperative and Pain Medicine, Brigham and Women's Hospital, Boston, Massachusetts, USA

JENNIFER ANNE KAPLAN, MD, MAS
Department of Surgery, University of Minnesota, Minneapolis, Minnesota, USA

KASHIF T. KHAN, MD, SM
Fellow Physician, Department of Anesthesia and Perioperative Care, Division of Critical Care Medicine, University of California, San Francisco, San Francisco, California, USA

MICHAEL C. LEWIS, MD, FASA
Joseph L. Ponka Chair, Department of Anesthesiology, Pain Management and Perioperative Medicine, Henry Ford Health System, Detroit, Michigan, USA

MATTHEW D. McEVOY, MD
Professor of Anesthesiology, Vice-Chair for Educational Affairs, Director, Perioperative Consult Service, Division of Multispecialty Anesthesiology, Department of Anesthesiology, Vanderbilt University Medical Center, Nashville, Tennessee, USA

TRACY McGRANE, MD, MPH
Assistant Professor, Department of Anesthesiology, Division of Anesthesiology Critical Care Medicine, Vanderbilt University Medical Center, Nashville, Tennessee, USA

DANIEL I. McISAAC, MD, MPH, FRCPC
Department of Anesthesiology and Pain Medicine, The Ottawa Hospital, Ottawa Hospital Research Institute, School of Epidemiology and Public Health, University of Ottawa, Ottawa, Ontario, Canada

AARON MITTEL, MD
Assistant Professor, Department of Anesthesiology, Columbia University Medical Center, New York, New York, USA

PRATIK P. PANDHARIPANDE, MD
Professor, Department of Anesthesiology, Division of Anesthesiology Critical Care Medicine, Vanderbilt University School of Medicine, Nashville, Tennessee, USA

JAY RAJAN, MD
Department of Anesthesia and Perioperative Care, University of California, San Francisco, San Francisco, California, USA

KIMBERLY F. RENGEL, MD
Critical Care Fellow, Department of Anesthesiology, Division of Anesthesiology Critical Care Medicine, Vanderbilt University School of Medicine, Nashville, Tennessee, USA

JOSIANNA SCHWAN, MD
Resident Physician, Department of Anesthesiology, Perioperative and Pain Medicine, Stanford University School of Medicine, Stanford, California, USA

JOSEPH SCLAFANI, MD
Department of Anesthesiology, Perioperative and Pain Medicine, Stanford University School of Medicine, Stanford, California, USA

VICTORIA TANG, MD, MAS
Division of Geriatric Medicine, University of California, San Francisco, San Francisco Veterans Affairs Medical Center, San Francisco, California, USA

VIVIANNE L. TAWFIK, MD, PhD
Assistant Professor, Department of Anesthesiology, Perioperative and Pain Medicine, Stanford University School of Medicine, Stanford, California, USA

RICHARD D. URMAN, MD, MBA
Associate Professor of Anaesthesia, Department of Anesthesiology, Perioperative and Pain Medicine, Brigham and Women's Hospital, Boston, Massachusetts, USA

NICHOLAS S. YELDO, MD
Director, Educational Programs, Program Director, Anesthesiology Residency, Henry Ford Health System, Detroit, Michigan, USA

Contents

The population of older adults is rapidly growing. With the continued advancement of medical and surgical interventions, the average age of this population will continue to increase. Nearly one-third of surgical procedures are performed in older adults. Physiologic changes, multiple comorbidities, frailty, and postoperative cognitive dysfunction affect an elderly patient's postoperative recovery. Anesthesia providers can play a key role in creating perioperative geriatric pathways. The perioperative care of a geriatric patient is associated with unique and anesthetic risks. Perioperative care must be tailored to individual patients to reduce perioperative complications in this important, vulnerable population.

The decision to offer surgery to an older adult with medical comorbidities involves candid conversations between the surgeon, patient, and caregivers. Tools are available to physicians that facilitate patient empowerment. Beyond short-term risks, the conversation should include the potential for institutional discharge, functional and cognitive decline, and longer term mortality.

Older patients undergoing surgery have reduced physiologic reserve caused by the combined impact of physiologic age-related changes and the increased burden of comorbid conditions. The preoperative assessment of older patients is directed at evaluating the patient's functional reserve and identifying opportunities to minimize any potential for complications. In addition to a standard preoperative evaluation that includes cardiac risk and a systematic review of systems, the evaluation should be supplemented with a review of geriatric syndromes. Age-based laboratory testing protocols can lead to unnecessary testing, and all testing should be requested if indicated by underlying disease and surgical risk.

Multidisciplinary perioperative care aligned with goals of care is most likely to achieve optimal patient and health system outcomes; however, substantial knowledge gaps exist in emergency general surgery for older people. Anesthesiologists are uniquely positioned to address these knowledge gaps, including optimizing goal-directed intraoperative care, appropriate provision of acute postoperative monitoring, and integration of principles of geriatric medicine in perioperative care.

The management of acute pain in older adults (age 65 or greater) requires special attention due to various physiologic, cognitive, functional, and social issues that may change with aging. Especially in the postoperative setting, there are significant complications that can occur if pain is not treated adequately for elderly patients. In this article, the authors describe these changes in detail and discuss how pain should be assessed appropriately in older patients. In addition, the authors detail the unique risks and benefits of several mainstream analgesic medications as well as interventional treatments for elderly patients. The authors' goal is to provide recommendations for health care providers on appropriately recognizing and treating pain in a safe, effective manner for aging patients.

Postoperative delirium and postoperative cognitive dysfunction (POCD) occur commonly in older adults after surgery and are frequently underrecognized. Delirium has been associated with worse outcomes, and both delirium and cognitive dysfunction increase the risk of long-term cognitive decline. Although the pathophysiology of delirium and POCD have not been clearly defined, risk factors for both include increasing age, lower levels of education, and baseline cognitive impairment. In addition, developing delirium increases the risk of POCD. This article examines interventions that may reduce the risk of developing delirium and POCD and improve long-term recovery and outcomes in the vulnerable older population.

Geriatric admissions to the intensive care unit (ICU) are common and require unique considerations for ICU clinicians. Admission to the ICU should be considered on an individual-patient basis. It is reasonable to consider a "trial of critical care" for many patients, even those who have uncertain chances of meaningful recovery. Quality of life and functional independence are especially important to older adults, and these outcomes should be considered when weighing the risks and benefits of admission or continuing ICU care.

ANESTHESIOLOGY CLINICS

THE CLINICS ARE AVAILABLE ONLINE!
Access your subscription at:
www.theclinics.com

Foreword

Geriatric Anesthesia: Ensuring the Best Perioperative Care for Older Adults

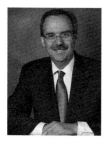

Lee A. Fleisher, MD
Consulting Editor

With advances in care of chronic diseases and cancer treatments, there are a growing number of individuals who would be considered both older adults and the very old. These individuals are at great risk of cardiopulmonary, neurologic, and other complications after surgery. It is becoming increasingly clear that those at greatest risk are frail and that surgery may not lead to any improvement in their lives. In addition, optimization or preparation of older adults before surgery may be the best approach to ensuring the best outcome after surgery. In this issue of *Anesthesiology Clinics*, innovations in the optimal care for older adults are discussed.

In order to bring together a state-of-the-art issue, 2 leaders in geriatric anesthesia were chosen. Elizabeth L. Whitlock, MD, MSc is Assistant Professor of Anesthesia and Perioperative Care at the University of California, San Francisco and focuses on clinical and patient-oriented research. Her research centers on understanding cognitive change over time in the elderly, particularly as it relates to surgery and anesthesia, using population-based data sources, and is funded by the National Institutes of Health. Robert A. Whittington, MD is Professor of Anesthesiology at Columbia University and has a funded basic science laboratory. The Whittington Lab studies the impact of surgery and anesthesia on the progression of Alzheimer disease pathologic condition and its related cognitive decline. Together, they have assembled a

Anesthesiology Clin 37 (2019) xiii–xiv
https://doi.org/10.1016/j.anclin.2019.05.004
1932-2275/19/© 2019 Published by Elsevier Inc.

diverse group of authors and articles, which include novel topics, such as decision making and palliative care.

Lee A. Fleisher, MD
Perelman School of Medicine
University of Pennsylvania
3400 Spruce Street, Dulles 680
Philadelphia, PA 19104, USA

E-mail address:
Lee.Fleisher@uphs.upenn.edu

Preface

Aging Gracefully: The Evolution of Perioperative Care for Older Adults

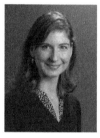 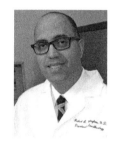

Elizabeth L. Whitlock, MD, MSc   Robert A. Whittington, MD
Editors

The philosophy and reality of perioperative care for older adults have both undergone a rapid and fascinating evolution over the last decade. It is time to move past the fear around a "silver tsunami" overwhelming clinical resources; anesthesiologists and perioperative care providers, in general, are beginning to take a more open view toward whole-patient care, whether the recipient is older or not. This issue of *Anesthesiology Clinics* is meant to update the anesthesia provider who cares for older adults with the rapidly evolving science around how to best support this vulnerable population, and to explore new ways of thinking about the care we provide to older adults.

Concepts that started in the geriatrics and palliative care fields, such as advanced care planning and shared decision making, are now found on equal footing as the ever-important physiology and pharmacology of aging adults. Shared decision making is relatively new to the anesthesiology literature and yet offers a way to frame difficult decisions facing a care provider and patient in the perioperative care setting, even in urgent or acute situations. Similarly, as these issues often challenge caregivers in the intensive care unit, the article on critical care focuses on how to improve care alignment, which appropriately holds an ever-increasing role as we learn more about the (unfortunately high) prevalence of goal-misaligned care at the end of life.

Recognizing the importance of multidisciplinary opinions in selecting the best approach, which may or may not include surgical interventions, we include articles co-authored by surgeons and neurologists, as well as an article focusing on an inherently multimodal approach: prehabilitation. Just as older adults are not well served by considering their medical problems in isolation, as with an approach that ignores the potential benefits offered by multidisciplinary evaluation and treatment, many perioperative concerns, such as delirium, frailty, and cognitive and functional decline, are also

Anesthesiology Clin 37 (2019) xv–xvi
https://doi.org/10.1016/j.anclin.2019.05.003
1932-2275/19/© 2019 Published by Elsevier Inc.

anesthesiology.theclinics.com

not well served by an isolated organ systems–based approach. These "geriatric syndromes" are not our typical fodder, impacting multiple physiological pathways in intersecting and complex ways, and yet they resonate throughout this issue. Frailty, for example, is discussed extensively in the context of geriatric physiology but also proves a highly relevant consideration for emergency surgery, prehabilitation, and preoperative assessment. Brain health, delirium and postoperative cognitive change, has recently received attention in the popular media and by our own specialty societies as an issue of tremendous importance to older adults wishing to maintain cognitive fitness well into their later years. This is also not an area that respects specialty barriers. Contributions from neurologists, psychiatrists, immunologists, and others have joined anesthesiologists in pressing forward to define, treat, and prevent these unfortunately common neurologic sequelae.

The field of geriatrics has emphasized that framing the aging of our population as a "silver tsunami" lends negativity to the tremendous opportunities presented by the care of older adults. As anesthesiologists, we are uniquely positioned on the "front lines" of critical moments in the health of older adults. We are empowered to evolve care from one size fits all to an approach that considers physiology *and* psychology, techniques *and* philosophy as well as disease *within* the context of a human with decades of life experience, opinions, preferences, and goals. This issue is intended to help us all understand how to do this, compassionately and thoughtfully, for every patient.

Elizabeth L. Whitlock, MD, MSc
Department of Anesthesia &
Perioperative Care
University of California, San Francisco
500 Parnassus Avenue
Campus Box 0648
San Francisco, CA 94143, USA

Robert A. Whittington, MD
Department of Anesthesiology
Columbia University Irving Medical Center
622 West 168th Street PH5-546
New York, NY 10032, USA

E-mail addresses:
elizabeth.whitlock@ucsf.edu (E.L. Whitlock)
raw9@cumc.columbia.edu (R.A. Whittington)

The Growing Challenge of the Older Surgical Population

Stanley G. Jablonski, MD, Richard D. Urman, MD, MBA*

KEYWORDS

- Frailty • Postoperative • Cognitive • Elderly • Surgery • Anesthesia

KEY POINTS

- The elderly population, defined as greater than 65 year old, continues to grow and in 2016 accounted for 33% of the population undergoing surgical procedures.
- Older adults have a higher incidence of comorbidities and disease burden, which can lead to increases in surgical complications.
- There are unique considerations for the care of this population, prompted by common physiologic and neurologic changes, that may benefit from increased preoperative planning and optimization.

INTRODUCTION

As medical interventions and social conditions continue to improve, the life expectancy of the US population has dramatically increased in the last century. The life expectancy of newly born American children is nearly double that of children born over the last century and around triple that of humans over the course of history.[1]

Although it is clear that the life expectancy is continuing to increase, the definition of "elderly" remains static, generally defined as an age of greater than 65 years. This is further classified as the chronologic age (in contrast with physiologic age, which takes into account the general health of the patient).[2] The chronologic age cutoff was initially developed in the 19th century around the development of socialist economic ideals. In that era, only 4% of the population was older than age 65. However, 13.0% of Americans currently fall into this age range, a group that is growing at a faster rate than the total US population.[1,3] The 2010 US Census documented a 15% increase in people greater than 65 years of age since the 2000 Census. Perhaps a better demonstration of the increase in the elderly population can be seen in the age group greater than

Disclosure Statement: Nothing to disclose.
Department of Anesthesiology, Perioperative and Pain Medicine, Brigham and Women's Hospital, 75 Francis Street, Boston, MA 02115, USA
* Corresponding author.
E-mail address: rurman@bwh.harvard.edu

Anesthesiology Clin 37 (2019) 401–409
https://doi.org/10.1016/j.anclin.2019.04.001
1932-2275/19/© 2019 Elsevier Inc. All rights reserved.

anesthesiology.theclinics.com

85 years of age. Between 2000 and 2010, there was a nearly 30% increase in the number of Americans greater than 85 years of age. In fact, in 2000, only 1.5% of the population was greater than 85 years of age, whereas in 2010, 12% of the population falls into this age range.[3] With advancements in medical care and social interventions, it is projected that the number of people over the age of 85 will continue to increase. However, the presently accepted definition of older adults, when an age cutoff is needed, is greater than 65 years of age (**Fig. 1**).[3]

The population of older adults is likely to continue to grow, according to the Administration on Aging. In 2016, there were an estimated 49.2 million elderly Americans, a number predicted to double to 98 million by 2060.[1] This future growth particularly applies to racial and ethnic elderly minorities, which are anticipated to grow by 89% between of 2016 and 2030, as compared with the Caucasian population, which is anticipated to grow by 39%.[1]

The increasing prevalence of older adults has a significant impact on social structure and health care. For instance, in the United States, older adults are eligible for government-run supportive programs such as Medicare and Social Security. These programs have been strained financially over the recent years and with the continued growth of the elderly population will likely continue to be strained; they remain the target of active policy work to maintain benefits for older adults while being mindful of competing funding priorities.

IMPLICATIONS FOR ANESTHESIA

The impact of the aging population is significant owing to disease incidence and burden, along with the apparent increased financial burden on social services, including health care. It is widely accepted that people of different ages have different health care needs and the outcomes of surgery and anesthesia can be influenced by age. Unsurprisingly, as the percentage of the population greater than 65 years of age

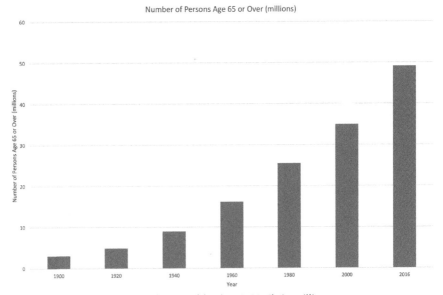

Fig. 1. Number of persons aged 65 or older (1900–2016), in millions.

continues to grow, there is an increased number of older adults undergoing surgical operations requiring anesthesia.[4] Even though the population greater than 65 years of age is currently about 12% of the total population, these individuals undergo about one-third of the annual surgical procedures.[4] There are several implications of surgical and anesthesia care in older adults, including an overall increase in mortality (primarily for patients >80 years of age) and an increase in the frequency of major and minor complications.[5]

Areas of special concern in the older adult population are multimorbidity, frailty, and cognitive impairment, which have (outside the operating room) prompted the development of the subspecialty of geriatrics. Perhaps as appreciation for the dynamic changes of aging grows, new geriatric anesthesia fellowships will gain popularity. According to the Accreditation Council for Graduate Medical Education (ACGME) 2019 fellowship website, there are no ACGME-accredited geriatric anesthesia fellowship programs; however, it is possible that anesthesia programs may begin to offer non–ACGME-accredited geriatric anesthesia fellowships in the near future.[6] Special concerns that arise in the care of the older adult may benefit from patient-specific optimization, including prehabilitation and the development of perioperative clinical pathways, further discussed in Drs Jaume Borrell-Vega and colleagues' article, "Multimodal Prehabilitation Programs for Older Surgical Patients," in this issue. For example, Enhanced Recovery After Surgery pathways aim to standardize care and are both patient centered and procedure specific.[7]

Physiologic Changes in the Geriatric Population

As the body ages, there are several important physiologic changes that can affect anesthetic delivery. There are several presumed mechanisms leading to normal physiologic aging, which include oxidative stress, mitochondrial dysfunction, telomere shortening, and several other genetic mechanisms.[8] The results of these changes affect nearly all organ systems, including the cardiovascular, pulmonary, neurologic, renal, and hepatic systems.

From a cardiovascular standpoint, blood vessels lose distensibility, which can lead to an overall increase in systolic blood pressure and there can be a stiffening of the left ventricle, which can make the geriatric patients susceptible to volume overload.[9] In the aging pulmonary system, there is a decrease in forced expiratory volume, an increase in closing volume, and increased physiologic shunting, which can lead to increased risks of pulmonary complications including pneumonia and atelectasis in the postoperative period.[10] These important physiologic changes are further discussed in Drs Kashif T. Khan and colleagues' article, "Geriatric Physiology and the Frailty Syndrome," in this issue. Furthermore, changes in the renal and hepatic systems lead to overall changes in the pharmacokinetics of drug metabolism. The elderly patient has increased adipose tissue while also having decreased total body water and muscle mass, which affects the creatinine clearance and glomerular filtration rate, and thus changes how the geriatric body metabolizes and clears drugs.[11] The article on "Geriatric Pharmacology: An Update" by Drs Tate M. Andres and colleagues, in this issue, is devoted to the changes in pharmacokinetics and pharmacodynamics relevant to caring for an older adult population.

Medical Comorbidities

It is widely accepted that the older adults have proportionally the highest number of medical comorbidities. In fact, patients over the age of 65 have, on average, 3 to 4 more medical comorbidities than a younger patient.[12] Even without specific medical comorbidities, there is a decrease in both basal and maximal function of all organ systems in the geriatric population, meaning that individual organ systems in the geriatric patient have less functional reserve and a decreased ability to compensate for physiologic stressors such as surgery.[13] This combination may lead to increased surgical complication rates and challenging anesthetic management; hence, careful planning and communication among health care providers needs to take place before surgery. The development and expansion of preoperative evaluation clinics is one way in which patient optimization is being addressed, and is further discussed in Dr Sheila Ryan Barnett's article, "Preoperative Assessment of Older Adults," in this issue. Identifying and optimizing the modifiable risk factors before an operation improves surgical outcomes and increases patient and family satisfaction.[14]

In addition, a preoperative evaluation provides the anesthetic provider with an opportunity to evaluate the medication regimen of the patient. Polypharmacy is a major issue for older adults, because multiple medical comorbidities can result in a large number of medications per patient, potentially prescribed by disparate specialist providers. Although there are no criteria to define polypharmacy, medication reactions, side effects, and compounding effects of medications are a concern for both the gerontologist and the anesthesiologist alike.[15] Older adults exposed to polypharmacy in the preoperative setting have decreased rates of postoperative survival along with increased rates of complications and increased resource use.[16] Certain home medication regimens must be altered in the perioperative period to allow for safe induction, maintenance, and emergence from anesthesia. For example, patients on anticoagulation therapy for atrial fibrillation would be required to hold their anticoagulation to qualify for spinal anesthesia for a joint replacement; if anticoagulation is deemed to be vital in the perioperative period, an alternative anesthetic technique must be considered. Alternatively, angiotensin-converting enzyme inhibitors or angiotensin receptor blockers should possibly be held on the day of surgery to avoid refractory hypotension; this is particularly important for the elderly patients who have decreased vascular compliance owing to age-related changes.[17] Preoperative evaluation allows for a multidisciplinary approach to the elderly patient, affording an opportunity to discuss medication regimens and anesthetic options with patients, their subspecialty providers, and their families.

Not only can anesthesiologists optimize the geriatric patient's medical conditions, they can tailor the anesthetic regimen to help prevent complications and unwanted side effects. Older adults are more susceptible to cognitive changes from sedating medications such as benzodiazepines and opioids and, when administered with other medications, can lead to a higher likelihood of postoperative delirium.[11] Accordingly, these medications should be used judiciously in the perioperative period. Regional anesthetic techniques are helpful in decreasing the amount of opioids required to control pain, and in certain cases can be used as the primary anesthetic for the operation, avoiding the side effects of general anesthesia.[18] Special concerns regarding the management of acute pain in an older population are discussed in Drs Jay Rajan and Matthias Behrends' article, "Acute Pain in Older Adults: Recommendations for Assessment and Treatment," in this issue.

Frailty

Frailty is defined as an age-related decrease in physiologic reserve resulting in increased susceptibility to environmental stressors.[19] It is commonly assessed using 2 methods, the Frailty Phenotype[20] and the Frailty Index.[21] The 5 criteria considered in the Frailty Phenotype, which may variably be referred to as the Physical Frailty

Phenotype or Fried Index, are shrinking (unintentional weight loss >10 lbs in 1 year), weakness (measured by grip strength), exhaustion, slowness (measured by walking time), and low physical activity (measured by the Minnesota Leisure Time Activity Questionnaire). The Frailty Index, also referred to as the Deficit Accumulation Model of Frailty or the Rockwood index, is a more quantitative metric to measure the degree of frailty based on number of accumulated deficits (which may include symptoms and disabilities, laboratory values, and comorbid disease).

The prevalence of frailty increases with age; 4% of population between 59 to 65 years of age are frail, and 26% of patients over the age of 85 have been shown to be frail.[22] Frailty has important implications for perioperative complications. Even for minor procedures, the postoperative complication incidence was 11.4% in frail patients compared with 3.9% in nonfrail patients.[23] These values are exacerbated for major procedures, with a staggering 43.5% incidence of postoperative complications in frail patients compared with 19.5% in nonfrail patients. The higher level of postoperative complications in the frail patient increased hospital length of stay approximately 3.5 days longer than that of the nonfrail patient. Similarly, after a major procedure, there is a 42.1% chance the frail patient will require placement in an assisted or skilled living facility versus a 2.9% chance in the nonfrail patient.[23] There is also an increase in mortality in the frail patient.[22] It has also been shown that emergency general surgery in frail patients is associated with significant increases in mortality, admissions to the intensive care unit, and length of stay.[24] This is further discussed in Drs Sylvie Aucoin and Daniel I. McIsaac's article, "Emergency General Surgery in Older Adults: A Review," in this issue. The importance of frailty to perioperative management is addressed specifically in Dr Kashif T. Khan and colleagues' article on "Geriatric Physiology and the Frailty Syndrome," in this issue, but permeates this issue as a theme of major importance to caring for older patients. With clear evidence of increased postoperative complications and ever-increasing surgical volume in this population, the importance of anesthetic optimization for the aging population cannot be overemphasized.

Perioperative Neurocognitive Disorders

Two other main areas of concern in older adults undergoing anesthesia are postoperative delirium and major or minor neurocognitive disorder, which are discussed in detail in Drs Kimberly F. Rengel and colleagues' article, "Special Considerations for the Aging Brain and Perioperative Neurocognitive Dysfunction," in this issue. The effects of anesthesia on the brain have been studied extensively over the years and there have been significant nomenclature changes with the new discoveries. According to the fifth edition of the *Diagnostic and Statistical Manual for Mental Disorders* and the National Institute for Aging and the Alzheimer Association, the overarching terminology for perioperative cognitive changes is now perioperative neurocognitive disorders (PND).[25,26] Postoperative delirium is defined as an acute, often fluctuating, disturbance in attention, awareness, and cognition that may occur hours to days after anesthesia and surgery. In contrast, cognitive decline within 1 week to 30 days is defined as delayed neurocognitive recovery, and cognitive change occurring up to a year after surgery is defined as postoperative neurocognitive disorder.[25] Notably, this is a change from "postoperative cognitive dysfunction", which was the old nomenclature used to describe cognitive changes after anesthesia and surgery.

Although the etiology underlying PND is not entirely clear, some hypothesized mechanisms include direct anesthetic toxicity, neuroinflammation, or an unmasking of underlying dementing illness.[27] PND occurs in 10% to 40% of the surgical population older than 60 years of age, making it the most common postoperative complication in this age range.[28] There are currently no definitive preventative measures to decrease the incidence of PND at this time, but there are many recommendations that may help.[29] Older adults should be screened for preoperative cognitive impairment, which can help to identify high-risk patients.[30] In some cases, a geriatric consultation preoperatively can help in medication management and general postoperative recommendations.[31] Intraoperatively, the use of electroencephalographic monitoring may help to decrease PND rates in older adults,[28] although the data are mixed. Finally, in the postoperative patient, the Confusion Assessment Method criteria are recommended to diagnose delirium, and reversible etiologies should be treated, while reserving antipsychotic medications for unresolved agitation.[31] Given the increased volume of elderly patients undergoing surgery, further understanding of PND is of utmost importance.

SHARED DECISION MAKING AND END-OF-LIFE CARE

One area that is particularly important to emphasize in the geriatric population is end-of-life care. This area is often overlooked because it can be a sensitive issue, yet it remains extremely important to have a good understanding of the patient's current medical condition and prognosis to determine the most appropriate care for that individual.[17,32] Older adults are more likely to have diminished decision-making capacity, making issues like informed consent, code status, and health care proxy documents even more important.

There are many tools that can be used to assess mental capacity and assist in determining if a geriatric patient has competence, that is, the legal capability of making informed decisions. To be deemed competent to make a choice, the patient must be able to communicate the choice (or choices), have insight and judgment to evaluate the choice, understand the risks and benefits of that choice, and come to a reasonable decision.[33] Physicians are more focused on determining capacity, which is functionally the same as competence but is not the accepted legal terminology. Capacity is often not a clear-cut issue and must be evaluated with a tool such as the Mini-Mental Status Exam. When a patient is deemed to not have capacity, the existence of the advanced care directive and the health care proxy documentation becomes extremely important. In the event there is no health care proxy document on file, the next of kin becomes the decision maker for the patient. They can assist in making medical decisions a patient would have desired if the patient had the capacity to make those decisions alone. This situation, however, is not perfect, because a surrogate decision maker may incorrectly predict the patient's preference nearly one-third of the time.[34]

Another important factor of end-of-life care that significantly impacts the health care system is the cost. According to Rice and Fineman,[35] the geriatric population makes up about 31% of the federal health care expenditures. This includes costs from long postoperative admissions or admissions to long-term nursing care facilities after surgery. The medical expenditures are even higher in the last year of life. Caring for a geriatric patient in their last year of life will amount to nearly 4 times as much medical expense as for a geriatric patient who is not in their last year of life.[35] In the era of bundled and pay-for-performance payments, these are important considerations as end-of-life care increases medical expenditure, while it does not necessarily improve long-term patient outcomes.

The many complex issues in participating in, managing, or observing an older adult's end-of-life care, particularly as it relates to the perioperative environment and in the intensive care unit as well, are discussed in several articles in this issue.

Ethical challenges are addressed in Drs Michael C. Lewis and Nicholas S. Yeldo's article, "The Ethics of Surgery at End of Life," in this issue; the role of the shared decision-making framework in aligning treatment with patient preferences and goals is discussed in Dr Allen N. Gustin's article, "Shared Decision Making," in this issue. Finally, because many older adults undergo intensive care in the last months or days of life, special concerns of the geriatric patient—and of end-of-life and palliative care in the intensive care unit—are addressed in Drs Aaron Mittel and May Hua's article, "Supporting the Geriatric Critical Care Patient: Decision-Making, Understanding Outcomes, and the Role of Palliative Care," in this issue.

SUMMARY

The population of older adults is rapidly growing in the United States and around the world. With the continued advancement of medical and surgical interventions, the average age of this population will continue to increase. Anesthesia providers can play a key role in creating perioperative geriatric pathways, facilitating shared decision making, and working with the other members of the health care system to decrease costs while improving short- and long-term patient outcomes. The perioperative care of a geriatric patient is associated with unique and considerable anesthetic risks. Ideally, anesthetic delivery can be tailored to individual patients to decrease perioperative complications.

REFERENCES

1. Administration of Aging. 2017 profile of older Americans: Washington DC: US department of health and human services 2018. Available at: Https://acl.Gov/sites/default/files/aging%20and%20disability%20in%20america/2017olderamericans profile.Pdf. Accessed October 29, 2018.
2. Shrivastava SR, Shrivastava PS, Ramasamy J. Health-care of elderly: determinants, needs and services. Int J Prev Med 2013;4(10):1224–5.
3. Werner CA. The older population 2010. US census report number c2010br-09 2011. Available at: https://www.census.gov/library/publications/2011/dec/c2010br-09.html. Accessed May 20, 2018.
4. Klopfenstein CE, Herrmann FR, Michel JP, et al. The influence of an aging surgical population on the anesthesia workload: a ten-year survey. Anesth Analg 1998;86(6):1165–70.
5. Deiner S, Silverstein JH. Long-term outcomes in elderly surgical patients. Mt Sinai J Med 2012;79(1):95–106.
6. Association of American Medical Colleges. ERAS 2019 participating specialties and programs. Available at: Https://services.Aamc.Org/eras/erasstats/par/. Accessed November 17, 2018.
7. Forsmo HM, Erichsen C, Rasdal A, et al. Enhanced recovery after colorectal surgery (ERAS) in elderly patients is feasible and achieves similar results as in younger patients. Gerontol Geriatr Med 2017;3. 2333721417706299.
8. McLean AJ, Le Couteur DG. Aging biology and geriatric clinical pharmacology. Pharmacol Rev 2004;56(2):163–84.
9. Lakatta EG. Age-associated cardiovascular changes in health: impact on cardiovascular disease in older persons. Heart Fail Rev 2002;7(1):29–49.
10. Sprung J, Gajic O, Warner DO. Review article: age related alterations in respiratory function - anesthetic considerations. Can J Anaesth 2006;53(12):1244–57.
11. Rivera R, Antognini JF. Perioperative drug therapy in elderly patients. Anesthesiology 2009;110(5):1176–81.

12. Bettelli G. Preoperative evaluation in geriatric surgery: comorbidity, functional status and pharmacological history. Minerva Anestesiol 2011;77(6):637–46.
13. Cook DJ, Rooke GA. Priorities in perioperative geriatrics. Anesth Analg 2003; 96(6):1823–36.
14. Chun A. Medical and preoperative evaluation of the older adult. Otolaryngol Clin North Am 2018;51(4):835–46.
15. Masnoon N, Shakib S, Kalisch-Ellett L, et al. What is polypharmacy? A systematic review of definitions. BMC Geriatr 2017;17(1):230.
16. McIsaac DI, Wong CA, Bryson GL, et al. Association of polypharmacy with survival, complications, and healthcare resource use after elective noncardiac surgery: a population-based cohort study. Anesthesiology 2018;128(6):1140–50.
17. Hollmann C, Fernandes NL, Biccard BM. A systematic review of outcomes associated with withholding or continuing angiotensin-converting enzyme inhibitors and angiotensin receptor blockers before noncardiac surgery. Anesth Analg 2018;127(3):678–87.
18. New York School of Regional Anesthesia. Perioperative regional anesthesia in the elderly. Continuing medical education, NYSORA. 2018. Available at: https://www. Nysora.Com/perioperative-regional-anesthesiain-elderly. Accessed October 20, 2018.
19. Alvarez-Nebreda ML, Bentov N, Urman RD, et al. Recommendations for preoperative management of frailty from the society for perioperative assessment and quality improvement (SPAQI). J Clin Anesth 2018;47:33–42.
20. Fried LP, Tangen CM, Walston J, et al. Frailty in older adults: evidence for a phenotype. J Gerontol A Biol Sci Med Sci 2001;56(3):M146–56.
21. Rockwood K, Mitnitski A. Frailty in relation to the accumulation of deficits. J Gerontol A Biol Sci Med Sci 2007;62(7):722–7.
22. Lin HS, McBride RL, Hubbard RE. Frailty and anesthesia - risks during and post-surgery. Local Reg Anesth 2018;11:61–73.
23. Makary MA, Segev DL, Pronovost PJ, et al. Frailty as a predictor of surgical outcomes in older patients. J Am Coll Surg 2010;210(6):901–8.
24. McIsaac DI, Moloo H, Bryson GL, et al. The association of frailty with outcomes and resource use after emergency general surgery: a population-based cohort study. Anesth Analg 2017;124(5):1653–61.
25. Evered L, Silbert B, Knopman DS, et al, Nomenclature Consensus Working Group. Recommendations for the nomenclature of cognitive change associated with anaesthesia and surgery-20181. J Alzheimers Dis 2018;66(1):1–10.
26. Evered LA, Silbert BS. Postoperative cognitive dysfunction and noncardiac surgery. Anesth Analg 2018;127(2):496–505.
27. Fu H, Fan L, Wang T. Perioperative neurocognition in elderly patients. Curr Opin Anaesthesiol 2018;31(1):24–9.
28. Berger M, Schenning KJ, Brown CHT, et al. Best practices for postoperative brain health: recommendations from the fifth international perioperative neurotoxicity working group. Anesth Analg 2018;127(6):1406–13.
29. Mohanty S, Rosenthal RA, Russell MM, et al. Optimal perioperative management of the geriatric patient: a best practices guideline from the American College of Surgeons NSQIP and the American Geriatrics Society. J Am Coll Surg 2016; 222(5):930–47.
30. Culley DJ, Flaherty D, Fahey MC, et al. Poor performance on a preoperative cognitive screening test predicts postoperative complications in older orthopedic surgical patients. Anesthesiology 2017;127(5):765–74.

31. Marcantonio ER. Delirium in hospitalized older adults. N Engl J Med 2017; 377(15):1456–66.
32. Brovman EY, Walsh EC, Burton BN, et al. Postoperative outcomes in patients with a do-not-resuscitate (DNR) order undergoing elective procedures. J Clin Anesth 2018;48:81–8.
33. Appelbaum PS, Grisso T. Assessing patients' capacities to consent to treatment. N Engl J Med 1988;319(25):1635–8.
34. Shalowitz DI, Garrett-Mayer E, Wendler D. The accuracy of surrogate decision makers: a systematic review. Arch Intern Med 2006;166(5):493–7.
35. Rice DP, Fineman N. Economic implications of increased longevity in the United States. Annu Rev Public Health 2004;25:457–73.

How Did We Get Here? A Broader View of the Postoperative Period

Jennifer Anne Kaplan, MD, MAS[a], Victoria Tang, MD, MAS[b],
Emily Finlayson, MD, MS[c,d],*

KEYWORDS

- Frail older adult • Elderly • Postoperative care • Patient readmission
- Cognitive reserve • Mortality

KEY POINTS

- In-hospital delirium negatively impacts long-term functional recovery and cognitive function.
- Institutional discharge is associated with postoperative complications as well as higher mortality.
- The authors recommend that surgeons adopt a shared decision-making process when discussing surgical options with older adults as opposed to the traditional model of informed consent.

INTRODUCTION

As more older adults with medical multiple chronic conditions present with surgical problems and diseases, it is essential to understand the impact of vulnerabilities on long-term postoperative outcomes and recovery. More than half of operations

Disclosure Statement: E. Finlayson receives funding from the National Institute on Aging (R01AG04425, R21AG054208, P30AG44281) of the National Institutes of Health and the Patient Centered Outcomes Research Institute (1502-27462), and is a founding shareholder of Ooney, Inc. The other authors do not have any commercial or financial conflicts of interests. There are no funding sources for this article.
[a] Department of Surgery, University of Minnesota, 420 Delaware Street, PWB 11-145E, MMC 195, Minneapolis, MN 55455, USA; [b] Division of Geriatric Medicine, University of California, San Francisco, San Francisco Veterans Affairs Medical Center, 4150 Clement Street 181(G), San Francisco, CA 94121, USA; [c] Department of Surgery, Phillip R. Lee Institute for Health Policy Studies, University of California, San Francisco, 3333 California Street, Suite 265, San Francisco, CA 94115, USA; [d] Department of Medicine, Phillip R. Lee Institute for Health Policy Studies, University of California, San Francisco, 3333 California Street, Suite 265, San Francisco, CA 94115, USA
* Corresponding author. Department of Surgery, Phillip R. Lee Institute for Health Policy Studies, University of California, San Francisco, 3333 California Street, Suite 265, San Francisco, CA 94115.
E-mail address: Emily.Finlayson@ucsf.edu

Anesthesiology Clin 37 (2019) 411–422
https://doi.org/10.1016/j.anclin.2019.04.002

performed in the United States are on patients over 65 years of age.[1] A study of elderly Medicare beneficiaries who died in 2008 demonstrated that one-third underwent an inpatient procedure during the last year of life and 18% underwent a procedure during the last month of life.[2] Whether for an elective or emergent procedure, surgeons and patients must go through a thorough decision-making process to ensure that the risks and benefits of surgery are understood and that the proposed operation and its sequelae are in line with the patient's values and goals. There is a need to move beyond the traditional surgical informed consent model to one of shared decision making to ensure that we avoid nonbeneficial therapy, conflict between patient and provider when expectations are not met, and posttreatment regret. This articles focuses on how to understand and improve preoperative conversations as well as long-term surgical outcomes to better inform high-risk patients as they consider surgery.

SPECIFIC CIRCUMSTANCES
Malignant Small Bowel Obstruction

A common difficult clinical scenario among high-risk older adults is a small bowel obstruction associated with an abdominal malignancy. These malignant bowel obstructions are present in up to 51% of patients with ovarian cancer and 28% of gastrointestinal cancers.[3] Treatment options include supportive care, venting gastrostomy tube (VGT), and exploratory laparotomy with lysis of adhesions and possible bowel resection or bypass. Lilley and colleagues[3] studied the clinical outcomes patients over age 65 with stage IV ovarian or pancreatic cancer hospitalized with malignant bowel obstruction using the National Cancer Institute Surveillance, Epidemiology, and End Results registry and Medicare Claims data. The overall median survival for their cohort was 76 days (interquartile range [IQR], 26–319 days), which was shortest after VGT (median, 38 days; IQR, 23–69 days) than after medical management (median, 72 days; IQR, 23–312 days) or surgery (median, 128 days; IQR, 42–483 days). VGT however, was also associated with a lower intensity of health care use (ie, intensive care unit admissions, readmission, in-hospital deaths) along with increased use of hospice. The increased survival in the surgery group was likely related to patient selection; surgery was associated with a decreased risk of readmission, but a higher risk of admission to an intensive care unit. Interestingly, palliative care was consulted in less than 5% of admissions. This study illustrates that although malignant bowel obstruction is a terminal process, interventions can decrease hospital readmissions at the end of life and that a VGT may be preferable over conservative management.

Hip Fractures

Hip fractures occur commonly among frail older adults, especially nursing home residents, and are associated high mortality and functional dependence.[4] Neuman and colleagues[4] looked at more than 60,000 nursing home residents who were hospitalized with hip fractures using Medicare claims and the Nursing Home Minimum Data Set. The majority of patients underwent operative intervention with 11.8% undergoing nonoperative management. At 180 days after their hospital admission, 53% had died or had a new total disability. Characteristics most associated with mortality after fracture were age greater than 90 years (vs ≤75 years; hazard ratio, 2.17; 95% confidence interval [CI], 2.09–2.26), nonoperative management (vs internal fixation; hazard ratio, 2.08; 95% CI, 2.01–2.15), and a Charleston Comorbidity Index of 5 or greater (vs 0; hazard ratio, 1.66; 95% CI, 1.58–1.73). For patients who were independent or required minimal assistance at baseline, only 20% returned to this baseline after their fracture.

These findings suggest that even though the nursing home residents represent a particular high-risk population, they still often do better with operative as opposed to nonoperative management for hip fracture, when it comes to mortality and total locomotive disability.

Tang and colleagues[5] used Medicare Claims data to study functional recovery in older adults after hip fractures. They identified 733 patients with a mean age of 84 years, 10% of whom lived in a nursing home at the time of hospitalization. At a mean follow-up of 1 year, 31% of this cohort returned to prefracture mobility after operative repair of their fracture. Of those who were functionally independent preoperatively, only 36% returned to their functional baseline. Advanced age, dementia, and the presence of medical comorbidities contributed to decreased functional recovery. It is essential to disclose realistic expected outcomes to patients and their families to ensure goal-concordant surgical decision making.

Preoperative Do Not Resuscitate Orders

Patients who present to the hospital with a life-threatening but surgically correctable problem and a preexisting do not resuscitate order (DNR) pose a particular difficulty for patients and physicians as they balance the acute issue with the patient's long-term goals. Using the American College of Surgeons National Surgical Quality Improvement Program, Kazaure and colleagues[6] compared postoperative outcomes of age- and procedure-matched patients who either had or did not have a preexisting DNR status. Patients in the DNR group were less likely to be functionally independent (42.2% vs 71.7%; $P<.001$), more likely to be coming from a long-term care facility (22.2% vs 7.2%; $P<.001$), and more likely to undergo emergent surgery (34.6% vs 24.1%; $P<.001$). Patients with a DNR order had higher rates of complications (31% vs 26.4%; $P<.001$) and, on multivariate analysis, DNR status was an independent predictor of mortality (adjusted odds ratio, 2.2; 95% CI, 1.8–2.8; $P<.001$). The overall 30-day mortality for patients with a DNR order was 23.1% versus 8.4% for those without a DNR order, a finding that is worth sharing with patients who hope to prolong their life with an operation.

Scarborough and colleagues[7] used the American College of Surgeons National Surgical Quality Improvement Program database to study patients with a preexisting DNR status undergoing emergency general surgery to study the impact of DNR status on failure to rescue, or death after 1 or more complications. Compared with patients without a DNR order, there was no difference in postoperative complications (42.1% vs 40.2%, $P = .38$); however, mortality was higher (36.9% vs 22.3%; $P<.0001$), as was mortality after at least 1 complication (56.7% vs 41.4%; $P = .001$). The authors concluded that their observed failure to rescue may have represented an unwillingness to pursue aggressive treatment in the setting of a postoperative complication despite aggressive preoperative management. This may reflect care that was in line with a patient's overall goal of wanting to prolong life with an emergent operation, but when complications arose, returning to their DNR status. This work further emphasizes the importance of realistic preoperative conversations about the procedure itself as well as treatment of complications.

LONG-TERM POSTOPERATIVE OUTCOMES
Functional Decline

A key consideration for older adults undergoing surgery is whether they will suffer functional decline as a result and the duration of this potential decline. Finlayson and colleagues[8] addressed this issue using the Medicare Inpatient File and the

Minimum Data Set for Nursing Homes, which included 6822 nursing home residents aged 65 years and older (mean age, 82 years) who underwent surgery for colon cancer. The majority (64%) of this cohort had urgent or emergent surgery suggesting that they underwent surgery owing to a cancer-related complication. Among those who survived their operation and hospitalization, one-half had functional decline (2-point increase in the Minimum Data Set–Activities of Daily Living) at 6, 9, and 12 months. The greatest decrease in functional decline was during the first 3 months postoperatively (62% of the surviving cohort). Preoperative functional decline predicted postoperative worsening and worst decline in functional status occurred in those who were most independent preoperatively.

Peripheral arterial disease is a common comorbidity among nursing home residents and revascularization procedures may be offered to improve functional status.[9] Oresanya and colleagues[9] used Medicare claims data to determine survival and functional outcome of 10,784 nursing home residents who underwent revascularization procedures during a 3-year period. At 1 year after surgery, 51% of the cohort had died, 28% were nonambulatory, and 32% had a decrease in their functional status from baseline. Of those who were nonambulatory at baseline, 89% had died or were nonambulatory at 1 year. Of those who were functionally independent at baseline, 63% had died or were nonambulatory at 1 year. Risks factors for death or nonambulatory status included age 80 or older at the time of surgery, preoperative cognitive or functional decline, and medical comorbidities.

Postoperative delirium occurs in 11% to 53% of older patients and is associated with delayed functional recovery.[10] Using a prospective cohort of patients 70 years and older undergoing elective surgery, all of whom were screened for delirium, Hshieh and colleagues[10] studied functional recovery over 18 months postoperatively. Of the 566 included patients, 24% developed postoperative delirium and these patients tended to have a lower functional status at baseline. The entire cohort had a decline in physical function from baseline at 1 month postoperatively, with the delirium group showing a greater decline and less recovery over the subsequent month. When looking at the 18-month postoperative time period, patients who had in-hospital delirium had less functional recovery from the 1-month nadir at every time point. It should be noted that all patients, regardless of delirium status, had improvements in function to above their baseline by 18 months after surgery.

In a prospective study of patients aged 65 and older undergoing elective general and thoracic surgery, Kwon and colleagues[11] determined functional trajectories over 1 year using both questionnaires and objective measures of physical performance. Overall, 28% of patients showed a significant decrease in function at 1 year postoperatively, with 40% of patients of patients undergoing hepatobiliary operations continuing to show diminished physical function at 1 year. In multivariate analysis, a cancer diagnosis was associated with 2.6 times the odds of functional decline at 1 year (95% CI, 1.14–5.96).

Older patients should be counseled that they will likely suffer some degree of functional decline in the first few months after surgery, and although most will fully recover, those who are over 80 years of age, those with significant medical comorbidities, and those who suffer from in-hospital delirium may face long-term impairments.

Cognitive Impairment

How surgery and postoperative delirium potentially affect cognitive status is another key element in preoperative conversations with older patients and their families and is covered in more detail in Allen N. Gustin's article, "Shared Decision Making," in this issue. Saczynski and colleagues[12] prospectively studied the impact of postoperative delirium on cognitive trajectories after cardiac surgery as measured by performance on the Mini-Mental State Examination. After adjustment for baseline factors, patients with postoperative delirium had lower Mini-Mental State Examination scores at month after surgery but not at 6 months or 1 year. At 6 months postoperatively, 40% of patients with postoperative delirium had not returned to their baseline cognitive status compared with 24% of patients who did not develop delirium (P = .01). At 12 months postoperatively, 31% of patients with delirium had not returned to their baseline versus 20% who did not have delirium (P = .055). Although it is unclear whether postoperative delirium is a causative factor or simply a harbinger of impending cognitive decline, patients and caregivers should be informed of this association.

A prospective cohort of adults 70 and older without dementia undergoing noncardiac elective surgery found that declines in general cognitive performance at 3 years postoperatively directly correlated with the severity of in-hospital delirium.[13] This study found no change in cognitive performance for patients who did not have in-hospital delirium, reinforcing the motivation to develop delirium prevention measures and establish methods to prevent cognitive decline. O' Brien and colleagues[14] argue that routine neurocognitive testing should occur preoperatively to capture those at highest risk for delirium and subsequent postoperative cognitive dysfunction (**Fig. 1**); however, whether hospitals could support this practice and whether it is an appropriate use of resources has yet to be proven.

Mortality

Patients with geriatric vulnerabilities are typically counseled about their short-term risks of mortality; however, physicians must also understand and communicate longer term mortality risk. In their 2012 study of colon cancer surgery in nursing home residents, Finlayson and colleagues[8] described a 53% mortality rate at 1 year. Age, preoperative functional decline, and Charleston Comorbidity Index were significant predictors. Using a cohort of adults over 50 years of age from the Veterans Administration undergoing elective operations with planned intensive care unit admissions, Moskowitz and colleagues[15] found a 44% in-hospital delirium rate and on multivariate analysis, determined that patients with delirium suffered a 7-fold higher 5-year mortality rate as compared with those who did not develop delirium.

To address the increased mortality associated with frailty, the Nebraska-Western Iowa Health Care System Veterans Affairs surgical service introduced a frailty screening initiative that served to both flag at-risk patients and review preoperative decision making.[16] Of 9153 patients, 6.8% to 11.1% qualified as frail based on a score of 21 or greater on the Risk Analysis Index, which includes age, cancer status, activities of daily living, specific comorbidities, weight loss, appetite change, and cognitive decline.[17] After the frailty screening initiative went into effect, overall mortality decreased from 1.6% to 0.7% (P<.001) and mortality among frail patients dropped from 12.2% to 3.8% (P<.001). The frailty screening initiative was also associated with improved survival at 180 and 365 days postoperatively. This improvement in outcomes was attributed to both better patient selection for surgery and greater attention to the perioperative management of patients identified as frail.

Readmission and Institutional Discharge

Many patients with geriatric vulnerabilities and medical comorbidities are unable to return home after a hospitalization, and the potential need for institutional discharge is

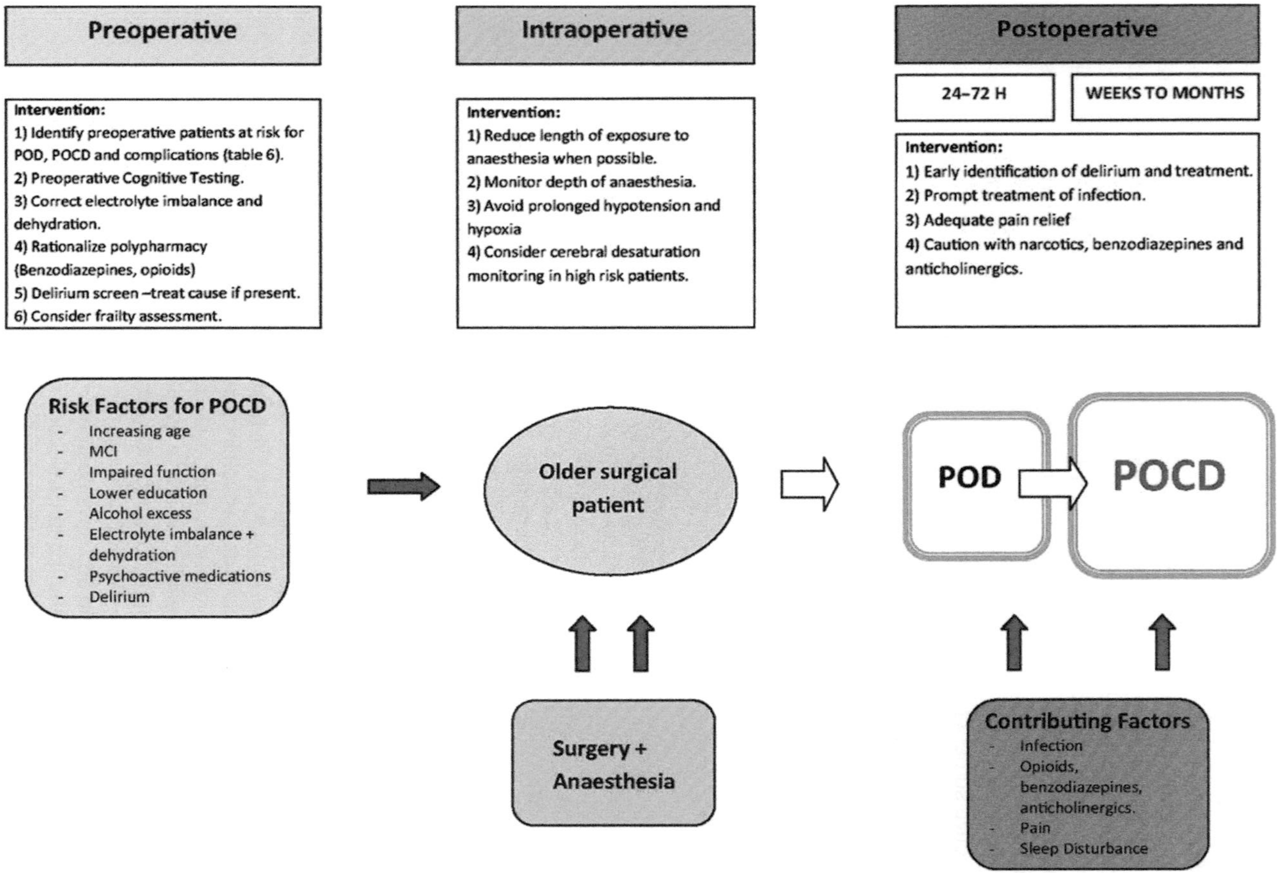

Fig. 1. Diagram demonstrating timeline of postoperative cognitive dysfunction (POCD) and possible intervention strategies. MCL, mild cognitive impairment; POD, postoperative delirium. (*From* O'Brien H, Mohan H, Hare CO, et al. Mind over matter? The hidden epidemic of cognitive dysfunction in the older surgical patient. Ann Surg 2017;265(4):677–691; with permission.)

now being discussed in the preoperative setting. Less frequently discussed is the risk of readmission, which can then compound the previously discussed postoperative cognitive and functional decline.

Legner and colleagues[18] studied the Washington State Comprehensive Hospital Abstract Reporting System for adults 65 and older who underwent abdominal or pelvic surgery and of 89,405 patients, 11% were discharged to an institutional care facility (ICF; 80% of these to a skilled nursing facility). Discharge to an ICF correlated with advancing age and postoperative complications. Those discharged to ICFs also had higher mortality than those who were discharged home at 30 days (4.3% vs 0.4%), 90 days (12.6% vs 1.4%), and 1 year (22.2% vs 5.9%). Of those who died after intermediate care facilities discharge, 53.7% died at the facility and 31% in a subsequent hospital admission. This study reinforces the need for adequate preoperative counseling and planning on the part of patients and their families.

Yeo and colleagues[19] used the National Surgical Quality Improvement Program database to study 30-day readmissions after colon and rectal cancer surgery for adults over the age of 65. For patients aged 65 to 74, chemotherapy was the most important risk factor with a rate of 20% versus 11% in those who did not undergo chemotherapy. The same was true for patients aged 75 to 84 years (23% vs 9%). For patients over the age of 85, being underweight was the most important with a 30-day readmission rate of 30% in that cohort. When Robinson and colleagues[1] studied 30-day readmission as it related to severity of frailty, they found a 4% rate in the nonfrail, 15% in the prefrail, and 32% in the frail patients.

HAVING THE CONVERSATION
Pitfalls, Solutions, and Buy-in

In a review of communication challenges between providers, elderly patients with acute surgical problems, their families, and their decision makers, Cooper and colleagues[20] discuss how decisions can be reached that are at odds with patient values and how as a system we can improve (**Fig. 2**). Multiple factors contribute to gaps in communication. Surgeons may find it difficult to prognosticate during emergencies and may not always have sufficient training on how to communicate effectively around death and dying while processing emotional signals from the patient and their family. Patients may be balancing religious factors and may not fully comprehend their prognosis. Surrogate decision makers may not truly grasp a patient's desires for end-of-life care and their understanding of what is in the best interest of the patient may be biased toward their own preferences instead of grounded in medical understanding. In addition to these individual factors, structural factors also play into misunderstanding and flawed decision making. These factors can include a lack of tools to better understand uncertainty and the fact that the physician and patient may have met for the first time just before an emergency operation and will not have had time to establish trust. Even if a patient has an advanced directive, it is not always clear how to apply it in a potentially reversible surgical emergency. Finally, despite an informed consent process, the surgeon may assume that a patient buys in to the downstream procedures and critical care associated with complications, whereas a patient may only be focusing on getting through the operation.

Cooper and colleagues[20] provide 3 solutions to address these pitfalls. First, surgeons should engage patients in advanced care planning during their preoperative visit, which includes filling out an advance directive, choosing a health care proxy, and ensuring both of these are documented in the medical record. As laid out in the

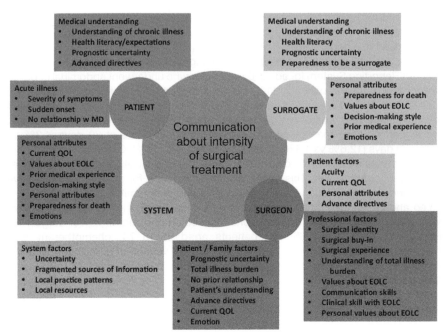

Fig. 2. Typography of communication about the intensity of surgical treatment. EOLC, end-of-life care; MD, medical doctor; QOL, quality of life. (*From* Cooper Z, Courtwright A, Karlage A, et al. Pitfalls in communication that lead to nonbeneficial emergency surgery in elderly patients with serious illness: description of the problem and elements of a solution. Ann Surg 2014;260(6):949–57; with permission.)

preoperative assessment recommendations from the American College of Surgeons and American Geriatric Society, surgeons "should understand the patient's preferences and expectations" with regard to possible outcomes and should reassess these preferences during care transitions.[21] Second, both surgeons and surgical residents should participate in formal education in palliative care and end-of-life care discussions. Third, surgeons should engage in a structured conversation with patients so as to ensure treatment is in line with patient goals and expectations. Elements of this conversation include the following:

1. Clarifying the patient's understanding and expectations for recovery.
2. Identifying the patient's priorities and goals for treatment.
3. Determining health states that the patient would find unacceptable.
4. Recommending palliative treatment alongside life-prolonging treatment as best aligned with the individual patient's goals and wishes.
5. Affirming the clinician's commitment to the patient's well-being.
6. Acknowledging the limits of prognostic information and the emotional distress uncertainty can cause.[20]

By following these recommendations, surgeons and patients can participate in shared decision making and avoid operations that are unlikely to allow them to achieve their overall health goals.

Nabozny and colleagues[22] addressed the concept of surgical buy-in between surgeons and patients through a series of structured interviews and recorded conversations. As mentioned previously, buy-in refers to a surgeon's unspoken assumption that a patient who consents to a given operation also consents to additional downstream interventions. From recordings from 43 patient–surgeon preoperative discussions, there were very few instances where a surgeon asked about an advance directive, DNR status, or unacceptable health states. Despite this, patients and their families reported feeling that their surgeon understood their preferences in the event of a serious complication. This came from an assumption that the surgeon "shared their values" and had the "expertise" to make the right decision. Preoperative patient interviews were also notable for a range of acceptable postoperative treatment, from giving their surgeon full reign to make decisions, to not wanting to consider complications or how they should be managed, to expecting a collaboration with their surgeon where shared decisions could be made in the event of a complication. Most patients were quick to assert that they would not want to be in a vegetative state, but assumed that this outcome would be clear in any decision-making process. Patients in this study also tended to discount the importance of discussing their advance directive with their surgeon, assuming it would be on file and clear to any treating doctor. Because patients and surgeons had not fully discussed these expectations, there were instances of conflict in cases where patients received unwanted resuscitation or families had to make the decision to withdraw care, which they were unprepared for. This work emphasizes the importance of preoperative conversations, the danger that can come with assumption of preferences, and that it is acceptable to reestablish goals and expectations with patients and families when complications arise.

Future Directions and Tools

The best case/worst case structure is one tool designed to facilitate conversations around life-or-death surgical decisions between surgeons and patients.[23] Surgeons give a granular and detailed narrative of what the expected outcomes of each care plan option—both surgical and nonsurgical—would look like for particular patients, based on their overall risk and make a simple hand-drawn visual aid (**Fig. 3**).[24] Patients felt that this allowed them to better understand the trade-offs of various treatment options in a way that standard risk and benefit conversations did not. After focused training with the best case/worse case framework, surgeons were able to describe 2 different treatment strategies in the context of their patient and involve the patient in the conversation, accounting for their values and preferences.[25] This tool differs from traditional decision aids because it moves away from exact numeric risk toward a personalized narrative of what is likely to happen if they were to pursue a surgical versus nonsurgical option.[26] This tool has not been studied outside of the institution where it was created and outcomes beyond decision making have not been studied.

Research is currently underway (ClinicalTrials.gov NCT02623335) to empower patients to ask direct questions that will allow for shared decision making with their surgeons as opposed to depending on the standard informed consent process, which is often one sided and does not always incorporate individual goals and expectations.[27] Patients use prompt questions in their interactions with surgeons, with the conversations recorded, and outcomes including engagement, regret, conflict and well-being measured. Question domains include the following:

- Should I have surgery?
- What should I expect if everything goes well?
- What happens if things go wrong?

Data gathered from this work will further inform both patients and providers as to important elements of the preoperative conversation and will hopefully engage patients to become more active participants in their care decisions.

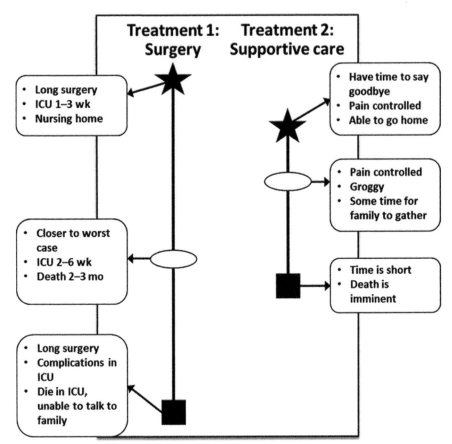

Fig. 3. The best case/worst case tool involves the drawing of a pen-and-paper diagram by the physician. A vertical bar depicts each treatment option, and the length of the bar represents the range of possible outcomes. A star represents the best case, a box the worst case, and an oval the most likely outcome. The physician describes each case using narrative derived from clinical experience and relevant evidence, and writes key points on the diagram. ICU, intensive care unit. (*From* Kruser JM, Nabozny MJ, Steffens NM, et al. "Best case/worst case": qualitative evaluation of a novel communication tool for difficult in-the-moment surgical decisions. J Am Geriatr Soc 2015;63(9):1806; with permission.)

SUMMARY

Deciding to take an older adult to surgery requires physicians to go beyond their standard process of informed consent and discussions of risks and benefits. Instead, we must begin with a model of shared decision making in which the patient can understand the impact of an operation or not having an operation on the subsequent months to years of their life. Sharing with them how their cognitive and functional status may be affected and considerations such as institutional discharge will allow them to make an informed choice that is in line with their individual goals and values.

REFERENCES

1. Robinson TN, Wu DS, Stiegmann GV, et al. Frailty predicts increased hospital and six-month healthcare cost following colorectal surgery in older adults. Am J Surg 2011. https://doi.org/10.1016/j.amjsurg.2011.06.017.

2. Kwok AC, Semel ME, Lipsitz SR, et al. The intensity and variation of surgical care at the end of life: a retrospective cohort study. Lancet 2011. https://doi.org/10.1016/S0140-6736(11)61268-3.

3. Lilley EJ, Scott JW, Goldberg JE, et al. Survival, healthcare utilization, and end-of-life care among older adults with malignancy-associated bowel obstruction: comparative study of surgery, venting gastrostomy, or medical management. Ann Surg 2017. https://doi.org/10.1097/SLA.0000000000002164.

4. Neuman MD, Silber JH, Magaziner JS, et al. Survival and functional outcomes after hip fracture among nursing home residents. JAMA Intern Med 2014. https://doi.org/10.1001/jamainternmed.2014.2362.

5. Tang VL, Sudore R, Cenzer IS, et al. Rates of recovery to pre-fracture function in older persons with hip fracture: an observational study. J Gen Intern Med 2017. https://doi.org/10.1007/s11606-016-3848-2.

6. Kazaure H, Roman S, Sosa JA. High mortality in surgical patients with do-not-resuscitate orders: analysis of 8256 patients. Arch Surg 2011. https://doi.org/10.1001/archsurg.2011.69.

7. Scarborough JE, Pappas TN, Bennett KM, et al. Failure-to-pursue rescue: explaining excess mortality in elderly emergency general surgical patients with pre-existing do-not-resuscitate orders. Ann Surg 2012. https://doi.org/10.1097/SLA.0b013e31826578fb.

8. Finlayson E, Zhao S, Boscardin WJ, et al. Functional status after colon cancer surgery in elderly nursing home residents. J Am Geriatr Soc 2012. https://doi.org/10.1111/j.1532-5415.2012.03915.x.

9. Oresanya L, Zhao S, Gan S, et al. Functional outcomes after lower extremity revascularization in nursing home residents: a national cohort study. JAMA Intern Med 2015. https://doi.org/10.1001/jamainternmed.2015.0486.

10. Hshieh TT, Saczynski J, Gou RY, et al. Trajectory of functional recovery after postoperative delirium in elective surgery. Ann Surg 2017. https://doi.org/10.1097/SLA.0000000000001952.

11. Kwon S, Symons R, Yukawa M, et al. Evaluating the association of preoperative functional status and postoperative functional decline in older patients undergoing major surgery. Am Surg 2012;78(12):1336–44.

12. Saczynski JS, Marcantonio ER, Quach L, et al. Cognitive trajectories after postoperative delirium. N Engl J Med 2012. https://doi.org/10.1056/NEJMoa1112923.

13. Vasunilashorn SM, Fong TG, Albuquerque A, et al. Delirium severity post-surgery and its relationship with long-term cognitive decline in a cohort of patients without dementia. J Alzheimers Dis 2018. https://doi.org/10.3233/JAD-170288.

14. O' Brien H, Mohan H, Hare CO, et al. Mind over matter? The hidden epidemic of cognitive dysfunction in the older surgical patient. Ann Surg 2017. https://doi.org/10.1097/SLA.0000000000001900.

15. Moskowitz EE, Overbey DM, Jones TS, et al. Post-operative delirium is associated with increased 5-year mortality. Am J Surg 2017. https://doi.org/10.1016/j.amjsurg.2017.08.034.

16. Hall DE, Arya S, Schmid KK, et al. Association of a frailty screening initiative with postoperative survival at 30, 180, and 365 days. JAMA Surg 2017. https://doi.org/10.1001/jamasurg.2016.4219.

17. Hall DE, Arya S, Schmid KK, et al. Development and initial validation of the Risk Analysis Index for measuring frailty in surgical populations. JAMA Surg 2017. https://doi.org/10.1001/jamasurg.2016.4202.

18. Legner VJ, Massarweh NN, Symons RG, et al. The significance of discharge to skilled care after abdominopelvic surgery in older adults. Ann Surg 2009. https://doi.org/10.1097/SLA.0b013e318195e12f.

19. Yeo H, Mao J, Abelson JS, et al. Development of a nonparametric predictive model for readmission risk in elderly adults after colon and rectal cancer surgery. J Am Geriatr Soc 2016. https://doi.org/10.1111/jgs.14448.

20. Cooper Z, Courtwright A, Karlage A, et al. Pitfalls in communication that lead to nonbeneficial emergency surgery in elderly patients with serious illness: description of the problem and elements of a solution. Ann Surg 2014. https://doi.org/10.1097/SLA.0000000000000721.

21. Chow WB, Rosenthal RA, Merkow RP, et al. Optimal preoperative assessment of the geriatric surgical patient: a best practices guideline from the American college of surgeons national surgical quality improvement program and the American geriatrics society. J Am Coll Surg 2012. https://doi.org/10.1016/j.jamcollsurg.2012.06.017.

22. Nabozny MJ, Kruser JM, Steffens NM, et al. Patient-reported limitations to surgical buy-in: a qualitative study of patients facing high-risk surgery. Ann Surg 2017. https://doi.org/10.1097/SLA.0000000000001645.

23. Kruser JM, Nabozny MJ, Steffens NM, et al. "best case/worst case": qualitative evaluation of a novel communication tool for difficult in-the-moment surgical decisions. J Am Geriatr Soc 2015. https://doi.org/10.1111/jgs.13615.

24. Campbell T, Schwarze M, Zelenksi A, et al. Best case/worst Case (BC/WC) communication tool - whiteboard Video - YouTube. Available at: https://www.youtube.com/watch?v=FnS3K44sbu0. Accessed December 12, 2018.

25. Taylor LJ, Nabozny MJ, Steffens NM, et al. A framework to improve surgeon communication in high-stakes surgical decisions best case/worst case. JAMA Surg 2017. https://doi.org/10.1001/jamasurg.2016.5674.

26. Kruser JM, Taylor LJ, Campbell TC, et al. "Best case/worst case": training surgeons to use a novel communication tool for high-risk acute surgical problems. J Pain Symptom Manage 2017. https://doi.org/10.1016/j.jpainsymman.2016.11.014.

27. Taylor LJ, Rathouz PJ, Berlin A, et al. Navigating high-risk surgery: protocol for a multisite, stepped wedge, cluster-randomised trial of a question prompt list intervention to empower older adults to ask questions that inform treatment decisions. BMJ Open 2017. https://doi.org/10.1136/bmjopen-2016-014002.

Preoperative Assessment of Older Adults

Sheila Ryan Barnett, MD*

KEYWORDS

- Geriatric anesthesiology • Preoperative • Preanesthesia • Risk assessment
- Frailty assessment • Cognitive dysfunction evaluation

KEY POINTS

- Geriatric syndromes such as frailty, cognitive dysfunction, polypharmacy, and malnutrition are associated with increased adverse events perioperatively and should be part of the geriatric preoperative assessment.
- A preoperative assessment of cognitive function can provide a valuable baseline and should be part of the standard assessment.
- Despite the increase in comorbidity burden, laboratory testing in older patients should be directed at the underlying disease, not driven by age alone.
- Identifying frail patients preoperatively may lead to individualized multidisciplinary consultations such as a comprehensive geriatric assessment, open discussions regarding prognosis and risk, and consideration for prehabilitation.

INTRODUCTION

In parallel with the growth observed in the aging population, the number of older adults undergoing both elective and emergent procedures is increasing steadily. This increase is accompanied by an inevitable surge in demand for preoperative testing.[1,2] Excessive and indiscriminate preoperative testing can lead to multiple unintended consequences, including delays in surgery, harm from additional work-ups, and cost to the patient and the system. In contrast, a thoughtful preoperative evaluation for an older patient provides an opportunity to review the patient's current medical condition in the context of surgical risk, potentially affecting decision making, identifying vulnerabilities, improving medication adherence, and initiating postoperative planning.[3–5] The enthusiasm for newer procedures and less invasive procedures should be balanced against the increase in risk for major complications and even mortality in older versus younger patients.[6–9]

Disclosure: The authors have nothing to disclose.
Department of Anesthesia, Critical Care and Pain Medicine, Harvard Medical School, Beth Israel Deaconess Medical Center, Boston, MA, USA
* Department of Anesthesiology, Beth Israel Deaconess Medical Center, 330 Brookline Avenue, Yamins 2, Boston, MA 02215.
E-mail address: sbarnett@bidmc.harvard.edu

Anesthesiology Clin 37 (2019) 423–436
https://doi.org/10.1016/j.anclin.2019.04.003
1932-2275/19/© 2019 Elsevier Inc. All rights reserved.

BASIC PREOPERATIVE ELEMENTS

Physiologic function is diminished with age and disease, and the preoperative evaluation of older patients is directed at the assessment of the patient's functional reserve and opportunities to minimize any potential for complications. This evaluation should be supplemented with a review of common geriatric syndromes such as frailty, cognitive impairment, dementia, polypharmacy, nutrition, and limited functional capacity[2] (**Table 1**). Depending on resources, these may be incorporated in a comprehensive geriatric assessment performed by a geriatric specialist or evaluated during the anesthesia preoperative assessment.[10,11] Ideally, an accurate risk stratification is a product of the preoperative assessment that can enable informed decision making between patients, families, and clinicians.[12,13]

SYSTEMATIC PREOPERATIVE ASSESSMENT

As with younger patients, the preoperative evaluation includes a systematic review of organ function, and documentation of comorbid conditions as well as baseline function. The American Society of Anesthesiologists (ASA) physical classification does not include age as a factor, and, although valuable as a communication tool to indicate the overall condition of cohorts of patients, it is limited as an individual risk prediction tool, especially compared with newer frailty scores (**Box 1**).[14,15]

Table 1		
Examples of factors included in the geriatric preoperative assessment		
Domain	**Assessment**	**Follow-up/Implications of Low Scores**
Cognition	Mini-Cog: clock draw and 3-item recall Montreal Cognitive Assessment	Delirium risk Decision-making potential Increased risk of nonhospital discharge Increased length of stay
Behavioral	Alcohol history Depression screening	Delirium risk Quality of life Decision making
Function	ADL Instruments ADL Timed up and go Walking speed	Increased risk of postoperative complications Increased mortality Delirium Preoperative exercise: prehabilitation opportunity
Polypharmacy	Medication list Screen for inappropriate medications	Delirium Readmission Morbidity/mortality
Nutrition	Albumin/prealbumin levels Mini–nutritional short form assessment	Preoperative nutrition supplements Increased risk of postoperative complications
Frailty	Phenotype: weight loss/grip strength/exhaustion/gait speed/low physical activity	Preoperative nutrition supplements Increased risk of postoperative complications Prehabilitation opportunity Treatment decisions

Abbreviation: ADL, activities of daily living.

Adapted from Sattar S, Alibhai SM, Wildiers H, et al. How to implement a geriatric assessment in your clinical practice. Oncologist 2014;19(10):1058–1059; and Feldman LS, Carli F. From preoperative assessment to preoperative optimization of frailty. JAMA Surg 2018;153(5):e180213; with permission.

Box 1
American Society of Anesthesiologists physical classification
ASA I: healthy patient; no organic disorder
ASA II: systemic disease that is well controlled, either by the condition that is being treated or by another pathologic process (eg, controlled hypertension, acute sinusitis, treated hypothyroidism, obesity [30<body mass index (BMI)<40])
ASA III: severe systemic disturbance from any cause or causes (eg, complicated or uncontrolled diabetes mellitus, morbid obesity (BMI>40), end-stage renal disease undergoing regular hemodialysis)
ASA IV: extreme systemic disturbance that is a constant threat to life (eg, end-stage renal disease without regular dialysis; recent myocardial infarction or cerebrovascular accident)
ASA V: condition in which the patient will not survive without surgery (eg, dissecting aortic aneurysm, massive trauma)
ASA VI: a person who is brain-dead who is presenting for organ donation
Adapted from American Society of Anesthesiologists. Standards and guidelines: ASA physical status classification system. Available at: https://www.asahq.org/standards-and-guidelines/asa-physical-status-classification-system. Accessed March 28, 2019; with permission.

Cardiac Preoperative Assessment

The incidence of cardiovascular complications is higher in older adults because of the impact of age-related changes in the cardiovascular system and the high prevalence of comorbid conditions such as coronary artery disease, hypertension, and diabetes. The decision to perform cardiac testing depends on patient-specific and surgery-specific factors as well as exercise capacity.[16,17] In general, testing should be recommended for patients who are perceived as high risk and have poor exercise capacity. Although not always appreciated, the threshold for pursuing coronary interventions should be the same during the evaluation in the perioperative period as it is when evaluated in the nonoperative setting.

The 2014 American College of Cardiology (ACC) and American Heart Association (AHA) guidelines[18] formulate a composite risk of perioperative cardiac events based on the preoperative history of cardiovascular events and risk factors. The Revised Cardiac Risk Index is the most commonly used and includes 6 independent predictors of postoperative complications after major noncardiac surgery. These predictors include high-risk surgery, a history of ischemic heart disease, congestive heart failure and cerebrovascular surgery, diabetes mellitus requiring insulin treatment, and a preoperative serum creatinine level greater than 2.0 mg/dL. The rate of major complications increases with the number of risk factors, and rates with 0, 1, 2, or greater than 3 risk factors are 0.5%, 1.3%, 4%, and 9% respectively.

Exercise tolerance

Low preoperative functional status is a reliable predictor for perioperative and long-term cardiac complications. Formal cardiopulmonary exercise testing (CPET) provides extensive information on reserve cardiovascular function, including anaerobic thresholds, peak oxygen consumption, and ventilatory equivalents for oxygen and carbon dioxide.[19–21] Alternatively, a history of activity and ability can provide a simple estimate of the patient's functional capacity; the Duke Activity Scale is one of most commonly used questionnaires[22] (**Table 2**).

Table 2	
Duke activity status index: metabolic equivalents and common activities	
Metabolic Equivalent	**Common Activities: Are You Able to…**
1.75	Walk around the house/no stairs
2.70–2.75	Light housework (dusting, dishes); self-care (eating, bathing); walk 2 blocks slowly on flat ground
3.5	Moderate housework (vacuuming, carrying groceries)
4.5	Moderate yardwork (raking leaves, weeding)
5.5	Climb a flight of stairs or a short hill
6.0	Moderate recreation activities (doubles tennis, bowling, dancing)
7.5	Strenuous sports (singles tennis, basketball, vigorous swimming)
8.0	Heavy housework (scrubbing floors, moving furniture, shoveling snow); run a short distance

Functional capacity is expressed as metabolic equivalents (METs); a MET represents the resting or basal oxygen consumption (Vo_2).

Adapted from Hlatky MA, Boineau RE, Higginbotham MB, et al. A brief self-administered questionnaire to determine functional capacity (The Duke Activity Status Index). Am J Cardiol 1989;64(10):652; with permission.

In the latest ACC/AHA guidelines, the surgery-specific risk of a major adverse cardiac event (MACE) is categorized into low, moderate, and high. Low risk carries a less than 1% risk of a postoperative event or MACE. Patients undergoing low-risk procedures can generally proceed without the need for further testing, regardless of functional status. For moderate-risk or high-risk procedures, the risk of an event is greater than 1%; in these patients, exercise capacity is required to make the decision on further testing. If the patient's reported functional ability is greater than 4 metabolic equivalents, procedures may be undertaken without further cardiac noninvasive testing. When it is not possible to establish the functional capacity of a patient who has significant clinical risk factors for coronary artery disease and is undergoing high-risk surgery, noninvasive cardiac testing may be required.[19] The rationale for further evaluation should also be determined by the impact of the test results on the plan of care for that particular surgery.

Preoperative management of β-blockers and statins
β-Blockers inhibit β-receptor activation by catecholamines, leading to slowing of heart rate and contractility, ultimately reducing myocardial oxygen consumption. Current evidence recommends continuing preoperative β-blockers in patients who are currently on this therapy. Statin therapy may reduce adverse events in patients undergoing vascular surgery,[23] and discontinuing statins is associated with increased cardiac morbidity.[24] Thus, statin therapy should be continued in patients perioperatively and initiation considered in patients with known cardiac ischemia, vascular disease, or increased low-density lipoprotein levels, as long as no contraindications exist.

Hypertension
The most recent guidelines on the treatment of hypertension change the traditional hypertension definition from a systolic blood pressure greater than or equal to 140 mm Hg or diastolic blood pressure greater than or equal to 90 mm Hg to systolic less than 130 mm Hg and diastolic 80 to 89 mm Hg.[25] The new definitions increase the

prevalence of hypertension in the older population aged 65 to 74 years to approximately 75% with a sharp increase in those more than 75 years to 80%.

Even using the older definitions, the incidence of hypertension in patients in the United States more than 60 years of age was 63%, almost double the 33% occurring in patients 40 to 59 years of age, and only 50% of older patients have their hypertension controlled, or less than the then recommended 140/90 mm Hg.[26]

The high prevalence of hypertension is relevant preoperatively because hypertension is a risk factor for stroke, renal insufficiency, congestive heart failure, and coronary artery disease, including silent myocardial infarction and ischemia.

However, despite the known health risks associated with hypertension, there is significant controversy regarding preoperative blood pressure control and the decision to treat or postpone a procedure.[16,26–28] Weksler and colleagues[29] performed a randomized prospective study in patients with poorly controlled hypertension presenting for elective surgery. Patients were randomized to a control group, in which surgery was delayed to allow blood pressure therapy, or a treatment group, who received acute treatment to bring the diastolic blood pressure to less than 110 mg Hg. There was no difference in adverse cardiac events between the groups. Similarly, a systematic review and meta-analysis of association of hypertensive disease and perioperative complications was unable to show a clear relationship between adverse events and hypertension.[28] Despite the lack of evidence linking hypertension and adverse events, the preoperative assessment provides an opportunity to evaluate patients with poorly controlled hypertension for end-organ damage, provide counseling on the importance of medication compliance, and potentially to alert the patient's primary care provider of the need for follow-up.

Pulmonary Evaluation

Age-related pulmonary changes reduce pulmonary reserve, increasing the risk of perioperative pulmonary complications.[8,30] The 5 major risk factors for postoperative respiratory failure are type of surgery (upper abdominal and thoracic carry higher risk), emergent status, poor functional status and physical dependence, preoperative sepsis, and high ASA classification. Additional risk factors predicting postoperative pulmonary complications include a history of chronic obstructive pulmonary disease; tobacco use; and signs of preoperative illness, such as an altered mental status, hypoalbuminemia, unintentional weight loss, increased serum creatinine level, and congestive heart failure. The pulmonary preoperative assessment in older patients should include a basic assessment for the risk of a pulmonary complications or failure, and, as with the cardiac assessment, functional assessment is a key component.[31,32]

Renal System

As many as 30% of older adults presenting for surgery have serious renal impairment, and age itself is associated with a decline in glomerular function, despite relatively normal creatinine levels because of a parallel decrease in muscle mass. In patients more than 85 years old, 99% have decline in glomerular filtration rate severe enough to require age-adjusted dosing. It is therefore not surprising that acute renal failure accounts for a fifth of postoperative deaths in the elderly.[33] An important aspect of the renal preoperative assessment in older adults is an acknowledgment of the underlying reduction in renal reserve and a strategy to reduce hypovolemia, hypotension, electrolyte balances, and nephrotoxic medications in the preoperative period.[34–37]

Diabetes Mellitus

The incidence of diabetes mellitus increases with age, and the duration of diabetes is also important because of increased associated complications, such as cardiac and vascular disease, delayed gastric emptying, retinopathy, and neuropathy. In addition to baseline glucose level on the day of surgery, a hemoglobin A1C can provide information on relative control of glucose levels before surgery.[38–40] Hyperglycemia has been associated with increased incidence of surgical site infections after joint surgery and cardiac surgeries and is one of the comorbidities included in the National Surgical Quality Improvement Program (NSQIP) risk calculator.[41,42]

Neurologic Assessment

The preoperative neurologic examination in older patients should include a targeted assessment for symptomatic neurologic disease.[2] For example, in patients with a prior stroke, weakness and limitations should be established preoperatively so that postoperative assessments do not lead to unnecessary alarm or testing. Cognitive impairment is discussed later.

COMMON GERIATRIC SYNDROMES

It has been recognized that aging is accompanied by an increase in occurrence of geriatric syndromes, and the anesthetic preoperative assessment for older patients should include an evaluation for these syndromes when possible (see **Table 1**).[12,43,44]

Cognitive Impairment

Postoperative neurocognitive disorders, ranging from transient delirium and delayed neurocognitive recovery to postoperative neurocognitive disorder (also collectively referred to as postoperative cognitive dysfunction), are among the most significant postoperative neurologic complications for older patients and their families. Symptoms of mild cognitive impairment, often a precursor to dementia, are frequently subtle; therefore, patients and their family members may not recognize a decline in memory as anything more than normal aging.[45] Although it is known that preoperative cognitive impairment is one of the strongest predictors of postoperative delirium, screening for cognitive impairment is not yet a routine part of the preoperative assessment.[46] There is no universally accepted cognitive screening tool, but a few exist that have acceptable sensitivity and specificity and take less than 10 minutes to administer. These tools include the Animal Fluency Test,[47] the Montreal Cognitive Assessment,[48] and the Mini-Cog[46,49]

To perform the Animal Fluency Test, patients are asked to name as many animals as possible in 60 seconds. It is generally considered a test of executive function and possibly language processing, and a low score has been associated with increased risk of delirium.[50] The Mini-Cog is easy to administer, does not require special training or equipment, and is relatively free of cultural or education bias. The instrument involves a 3-item recall test for memory and a clock drawing test that serves as a distractor. It tests visuospatial agility, basic memory through recall, and executive function. The cutoff varies; in general, scores equal to or less than 2 are consistent with some impairment and referring patients for further work-up or a geriatric or memory clinic might be considered. The Montreal Cognitive Assessment is another cognitive screening tool that can be used in the preoperative setting. It is designed as a rapid screening instrument for mild cognitive dysfunction. It assesses different cognitive domains: attention and concentration, executive functions, memory, language, visual spatial skills, conceptual thinking, calculations, and orientation.[48,51]

Although this is an evolving area, cognitive testing undertaken in preoperative testing clinics seems feasible and in one study of more than 300 patients presenting for elective surgery, with a mean age of 73 years, 22% of patients scored less than 2 on a Mini-Cog examination, consistent with previously unrecognized cognitive deficit.[49] In a separate study of orthopedic patients, 24% of 211 patients scored less than 2 on the Mini-Cog, consistent with probable cognitive impairment. These patients were almost 4 times more likely to be discharged to a place other than home, develop postoperative delirium, and have a longer length of hospital stay[46] (**Box 2**).

Regardless of the manner in which the testing is performed, the goal of preoperative cognitive testing is to identify vulnerable patients who may benefit from further testing or counseling during their preoperative evaluation. Identifying a cognitive issue preoperatively may also direct perioperative care to reduce the risk of delirium or involve geriatric consults early during the postoperative period.[1,52]

Frailty

Frailty can be defined as a decrease in physiologic capacity combined with multisystem impairments, leading to decreased ability to maintain homeostasis, and is separate from normal age-related changes. Frailty is characterized by an increased vulnerability to stressors such as surgery and anesthesia and is associated with greater postoperative mortality, increased complications, longer hospital length of stay, and increased discharge to a facility as opposed to home.[53–55] Preoperatively frail patients may benefit from individualized multidisciplinary consultations such as a comprehensive geriatric assessment, open discussions regarding prognosis and risk, and consideration for prehabilitation.

There are several approaches to frailty evaluation. Simplistically, most scales depend either on identification of a phenotype including certain physical traits (the frailty phenotype, or Fried Index), or alternatively the assessment of deficiencies

---

Box 2
Mini-Cog

Step 1: 3-item recall
    Ask patient to remember 3 of following words
    Common examples of 3 word sets:
        Banana, sunrise, chair
        Village, kitchen, baby
        Captain, garden, picture

Step 2: clock draw
    Provide sheet with or without preprinted circle
    Ask patient to place numbers and hands at specified time
    Examples of times:
        10 minutes before 2 PM
        10 minutes after 10 AM

Step 3: ask patient to repeat the 3 words provided in step 1

Scoring: add recall and clock total: 0 to 4
    Recall 3 words: score 1 to 3
        1 point for each word
    Clock draw: score 0 or 1
        0 points for abnormal clock
        1 point for normal clock

across several domains (the deficit accumulation approach, such as in the Modified Frailty Index).[56] The Fried phenotype is the best known of the clinical evaluations and consists of 5 criteria: weight loss, weak hand grip strength, exhaustion, slow gait, and low physical activity. Scores of 4 to 5 are considered frail, 2 to 3 intermediately frail, and 0 to 1 not frail. The scale is validated, and has shown good prognostic capability. One challenge to wide implementation is that the testing requires some special training and equipment, which is often beyond the ability of a standard preoperative assessment clinic. However, using just 1 or 2 of the criteria can also be useful to identify patients likely to be frail, who can then be flagged as high risk and potentially referred for further testing or a comprehensive geriatric assessment. Timed Up and Go is a popular tool used by geriatricians regularly to assess a composite of lower extremity muscle strength and gait speed and is an example of a single test that might be incorporated into a preoperative standard visit.[15,57–60] Both Timed Up and Go and slow walking speed have been correlated with an increase in complications after cardiac surgery[61] (**Box 3**, **Table 3**).

Polypharmacy

Polypharmacy is the term used to describe the use of multiple medications, and/or the administration of more medications than are clinically indicated, and/or the use of inappropriate medications. Polypharmacy is a major issue of concern because of its association with adverse health outcomes, including falls, functional impairment, adverse drug reactions, increased length of hospital stay, readmissions, and mortality.[62] Multiple factors positively associated with polypharmacy, such as drug-drug interactions, drug-disease interactions, or potentially inappropriate prescriptions, may be involved in these adverse outcomes.[63] A recent review found a positive correlation between frailty and polypharmacy, but, although an association is common, this does not establish causality, and it is difficult to know what comes first: frailty or polypharmacy. For the purpose of the preoperative evaluation, the identification of polypharmacy may lead to an opportunity to reduce numbers of medications and an active search for potential interactions.[64]

Box 3
Modified frailty index characteristics: score out of 11

1. Diabetes Mellitus

2. Dependent functional Status

3. Pulmonary disease: Chronic Obstructive Pulmonary Disease and/or pneumonia

4. Cardiac Disease:
   a. Congestive Heart Failure
   b. Myocardial Infarction
   c. Recent percutaneous intervention

5. Hypertension medication

6. Peripheral vascular disease

7. Altered sensorium

8. Transient ischemic attack

9. Neurological disease s/p CVA

Adapted from Seib CD, Rochefort H, Chomsky-Higgins K, et al. Association of patient frailty with increased morbidity after common ambulatory general surgery operations. JAMA Surg 2018;153(2):160–9.

Table 3	
Frailty phenotype description	
1	Unintentional Weight Loss
2	Weak grip strength
3	Self-reported exhaustion
4	Reduced gait speed
5	Low physical activity

Scores between 1 and 5: 4 to 5, frail; 2 to 3, intermediate frail; 0 to 1, not frail.

Adapted from Chow WB, Rosenthal RA, Merkow RP, et al. Optimal preoperative assessment of the geriatric surgical patient: a best practices guideline from the American College of Surgeons National Surgical Quality Improvement Program and the American Geriatrics Society. J Am Coll Surg 2012;215(4):458; and Fried LP, Tangen CM, Walston J, et al. Frailty in older adults: evidence for a phenotype. J Gerontol A Biol Sci Med Sci 2001;56(3):M148; with permission.

Nutrition

Malnutrition rates for older patients vary, ranging from almost 6% prevalence in community-dwelling older adults to 14% in nursing home patients, 39% of inpatients, and 50% of older patients in rehabilitation. Poor nutritional status is associated with increased length of stay and an increased risk of postoperative adverse events and mortality and morbidity. Common complications of poor nutrition are most notably related to infections: surgical site infections, pneumonia, urinary tract infections, and wound healing complications are all more common in this population.[65]

There are several ways to assess nutritional status.[66] Albumin levels less than 3.0 g/dL, although imperfect, are often used as a proxy measure for malnutrition. The Mini–Nutritional Assessment is a common tool; scores can range from 0 to 14, with 12 to 14 considered normal, 8 to 11 nutritional risk, and 7 or less suggesting malnutrition.[67] Patients with malnutrition may benefit from formal nutritional assessment and prehabilitation, designed to reverse some of the nutritional deficits.[68] Patients may also benefit in the short term from protein supplements and carbohydrate-rich drinks, as recommended by multiple enhanced recovery after surgery protocols.[69,70]

The Comprehensive Geriatric Assessment

The Comprehensive Geriatric Assessment (CGA) is a multidimensional consultation usually performed by a geriatrician and includes comorbidity, functional, psychological, and social features. The CGA is the cornerstone of the geriatric evaluation, and goes beyond what might be achieved in a standard anesthesia preoperative assessment.[9,10] A frailty assessment is frequently incorporated within the CGA. Geriatric syndromes identified through CGA can be used to provide a "roadmap" of care for older patients, including recommendations on prehabilitation, polypharmacy, nutrition, postoperative needs, and advance care planning. The value of the CGA is well described for community-dwelling older adults and also with older patients facing complex surgical procedures, such as thoracic and oncologic surgeries.[11,71] When geriatric consultations are available, creating a collaborative shared preoperative assessment with a geriatrician provides value to the patient and the clinicians involved[12] (see **Table 1**).

Preoperative Testing

Preoperative[72,73] testing protocols that include advanced age as a criterion lead to unnecessary testing, which in itself may cause harm and additional expense. For elective low-risk surgeries, preoperative laboratory testing is rarely indicated.[2,74]

Hemoglobin

Preoperative anemia is associated with increased postoperative morbidity and mortality,[8] and early identification of preoperative anemia before an elective surgery may lead to further investigation (eg, iron studies) and possible active management, such as a recommendation for iron therapy.[75] Laboratory studies for blood type and antibody screen (type and screen) should be drawn before surgeries with the potential for significant blood loss.[76]

Electrolytes and blood chemistry

Electrolyte measurements and an evaluation of renal function are useful in patients undergoing a surgery that may have significant fluid shifts or potential for ischemia. Mild hyponatremia is common in older adults, especially in patients on antihypertensive medications.[77] In older patients with low muscle mass, creatinine level may underestimate renal insufficiency.[1,36] Albumin is an imperfect measure of nutrition, but is inexpensive and lower preoperative levels have been linked to increased complications after surgery.[67,78,79]

Electrocardiograms and chest radiographs

Abnormal electrocardiograms (ECGs) are common in older patients, and preoperative ECGs should be done in patients with cardiac risk factors or a history of cardiac disease and in those undergoing intermediate-risk or high-risk surgery.[17] A prior ECG within 6 to 12 months of the surgery in the absence of new symptoms is generally acceptable.[18,27] Routine chest radiographs can lead to identification of incidental findings and additional work-ups but rarely discover findings resulting in a change in management.[12]

SUMMARY

The preoperative evaluation of older patients is complex, in part because of the increased burden of disease and the reduction in functional reserve, which can be difficult to evaluate. The high incidence of frailty, malnutrition, and cognitive impairment increase the risk of postoperative complications and even mortality, and may require additional focused testing and evaluations. Despite the challenges encountered, the anesthesia preoperative evaluation represents an opportunity to provide a realistic risk assessment so that a plan of care can be created that provides optimal and efficient patient-centered care to older adults.

REFERENCES

1. Bettelli G. Preoperative evaluation of the elderly surgical patient and anesthesia challenges in the XXI century. Aging Clin Exp Res 2018;30(3):229–35.
2. Oresanya LB, Lyons WL, Finlayson E. Preoperative assessment of the older patient. JAMA 2014;311(20):2110–1.
3. Bougeard AM, Brent A, Swart M, et al. A survey of UK peri-operative medicine: pre-operative care. Anaesthesia 2017;72(8):1010–5.
4. Mohanty S, Rosenthal RA, Russell MM, et al. Optimal perioperative management of the geriatric patient: a best practices guideline from the American college of surgeons NSQIP and the American Geriatrics Society. J Am Coll Surg 2016; 222(5):930–47.
5. Dzankic S, Pastor D, Gonzalez C, et al. The prevalence and predictive value of abnormal preoperative laboratory tests in elderly surgical patients. Anesth Analg 2001;93(2):301–8.

6. Neily J, Silla ES, Sum-Ping SJT, et al. Anesthesia adverse events voluntarily reported in the Veterans Health Administration and lessons learned. Anesth Analg 2018;126(2):471–7.

7. Cohen R-R, Lagoo-Deenadayalan SA, Heflin MT, et al. Exploring predictors of complication in older surgical patients: a deficit accumulation index and the Braden scale. J Am Geriatr Soc 2012;60(9):1609–15.

8. Earl-Royal E, Kaufman EJ, Hsu JY, et al. Age and preexisting conditions as risk factors for severe adverse events and failure to rescue after injury. J Surg Res 2016;205(2):368–77.

9. Kim S-W, Han H-S, Jung H-W, et al. Multidimensional frailty score for the prediction of postoperative mortality risk. JAMA Surg 2014;149(7):633–8.

10. Sattar S, Alibhai SMH, Wildiers H, et al. How to implement a geriatric assessment in your clinical practice. Oncologist 2014;19(10):1056–68.

11. Puts MTE, Hardt J, Monette J, et al. Use of geriatric assessment for older adults in the oncology setting: a systematic review. J Natl Cancer Inst 2012;104(15): 1134–64.

12. Chow WB, Rosenthal RA, Merkow RP, et al. Optimal preoperative assessment of the geriatric surgical patient: a best practices guideline from the American College of Surgeons National Surgical Quality Improvement Program and the American Geriatrics Society. J Am Coll Surg 2012;215(4):453–66.

13. Ajitsaria P, Eissa SZ, Kerridge RK. Risk assessment. Curr Anesthesiol Rep 2018; 8(1):1–8.

14. Hurwitz EE, Simon M, Vinta SR, et al. Adding examples to the ASA-physical status classification improves correct assignment to patients. Anesthesiology 2017;1–9. https://doi.org/10.1097/ALN.0000000000001541.

15. Makary MA, Segev DL, Pronovost PJ, et al. Frailty as a predictor of surgical outcomes in older patients. J Am Coll Surg 2010;210(6):901–8.

16. Fleisher LA. The value of preoperative assessment before noncardiac surgery in the era of value-based care. Circulation 2017;136(19):1769–71.

17. Fleisher LA. Preoperative assessment of the patient with cardiac disease undergoing noncardiac surgery. Anesthesiol Clin 2016;34(1):59–70.

18. Fleisher LA, Fleischmann KE, Auerbach AD, et al. 2014 ACC/AHA guideline on perioperative cardiovascular evaluation and management of patients undergoing noncardiac surgery: a report of the American College of Cardiology/American Heart Association Task Force on Practice Guidelines. Circulation 2014;130:e278–333.

19. Kaw R, Nagarajan V, Jaikumar L, et al. Predictive value of stress testing, revised cardiac risk index, and functional status in patients undergoing non cardiac surgery. J Cardiothorac Vasc Anesth 2019. https://doi.org/10.1053/j.jvca.2018. 07.020.

20. Kaw R, Nagarajan V, Jaikumar L, et al. 2014 ESC/ESA Guidelines on non-cardiac surgery: cardiovascular assessment and management. Eur Heart J 2014;35(35): 2383–431.

21. Moran J, Wilson F, Guinan E, et al. Role of cardiopulmonary exercise testing as a risk-assessment method in patients undergoing intra-abdominal surgery: a systematic review. Br J Anaesth 2016;116(2):177–91.

22. Hlatky MA, Robin E, Boineau MA. A brief self -administered questionnaire to determine functional capacity (the duke activity status index). Am J Cardiol 1989;64:651–4.

23. Durazzo AES, Machado FS, Ikeoka DT, et al. Reduction in cardiovascular events after vascular surgery with atorvastatin: a randomized trial. J Vasc Surg 2004; 39(5):967–75.

24. Le Manach Y, Godet G, Coriat P, et al. The impact of postoperative discontinuation or continuation of chronic statin therapy on cardiac outcome after major vascular surgery. Anesth Analg 2007;104(6):1326–33.
25. Whelton PK, Carey RM, Aronow WS, et al. 2017 ACC/AHA/AAPA/ABC/ACPM/AGS/APhA/ASH/ ASPC/NMA/PCNA guideline for the prevention, detection, evaluation, and management of high blood pressure in adults: a report of the American College of Cardiology/American Heart Association Task Force on Clinical Practice Guidelines. Hypertension 2018;71:e13–115.
26. National Center for Health Statistics, Fryar CD, Ostchega Y, Hales CM, et al. Hypertension prevalence and control among adults: United States, 2015–2016. NCHS Data Brief 2017;(289):1–8.
27. Scott IA, Shohag HA, Kam PCA, et al. Preoperative cardiac evaluation and management of patients undergoing elective non-cardiac surgery. Med J Aust 2013; 199(10):667–73.
28. Hartle A, McCormack T, Carlisle J, et al. The measurement of adult blood pressure and management of hypertension before elective surgery. Anaesthesia 2016;71(3):326–37.
29. Weksler N, Klein M, Szendro G, et al. The dilemma of immediate preoperative hypertension: to treat and operate, or to postpone surgery? J Clin Anesth 2003; 15(3):179–83.
30. Peterson B, Ghahramani M, Harris S, et al. Usefulness of the myocardial infarction and cardiac arrest calculator as a discriminator of adverse cardiac events after elective hip and knee surgery. Am J Cardiol 2016;117(12):1–4.
31. Gupta H, Gupta PK, Schuller D, et al. Development and validation of a risk calculator for predicting postoperative pneumonia. Mayo Clin Proc 2013;88(11):1241–9.
32. Miskovic A, Lumb AB. Postoperative pulmonary complications. Br J Anaesth 2017;118(3):317–34.
33. Abdelhafiz AH, Brown SHM, Bello A, et al. Chronic kidney disease in older people: physiology, pathology or both? Nephron Clin Pract 2010;116(1):c19–24.
34. Brown JR, Parikh CR, Ross CS, et al. Impact of perioperative acute kidney injury as a severity index for thirty-day readmission after cardiac surgery. Ann Thorac Surg 2014;97(1):111–7.
35. Hentschel L, Rentsch A, Lenz F, et al. A questionnaire study to assess the value of the vulnerable elders survey, g8, and predictors of toxicity as screening tools for frailty and toxicity in geriatric cancer patients. Oncol Res Treat 2016;39(4):210–6.
36. Kheterpal S, Tremper KK, Heung M, et al. Development and validation of an acute kidney injury risk index for patients undergoing general surgery: results from a national data set. Anesthesiology 2009;110(3):505–15.
37. Kheterpal S, Tremper KK, Englesbe MJ, et al. Predictors of postoperative acute renal failure after noncardiac surgery in patients with previously normal renal function. Anesthesiology 2007;107(6):892–902.
38. Harris AH, Bowe TR, Gupta S, et al. Hemoglobin A1C as a marker for surgical risk in diabetic patients undergoing total joint arthroplasty. J Arthroplasty 2013; 28(S):25–9.
39. Domek N, Dux K, Pinzur M, et al. Association between hemoglobin A1c and surgical morbidity in elective foot and ankle surgery. J Foot Ankle Surg 2016;55(5):939–43.
40. Thompson BM, Stearns JD, Apsey HA, et al. Perioperative management of patients with diabetes and hyperglycemia undergoing elective surgery. Curr Diab Rep 2015;16(1):2–9.

41. Seib CD, Rochefort H, Chomsky-Higgins K, et al. Association of patient frailty with increased morbidity after common ambulatory general surgery operations. JAMA Surg 2018;153(2):160–9.

42. McIsaac DI, Wong CA, Huang A, et al. Derivation and validation of a generalizable preoperative frailty index using population-based health administrative data. Ann Surg 2018;1–7. https://doi.org/10.1097/SLA.0000000000002769.

43. Kenis C, Bron D, Libert Y, et al. Relevance of a systematic geriatric screening and assessment in older patients with cancer: results of a prospective multicentric study. Ann Oncol 2013;24(5):1306–12.

44. Hall DE, Arya S, Schmid KK, et al. Association of a frailty screening initiative with postoperative survival at 30, 180, and 365 days. JAMA Surg 2017;152(3):233–8.

45. Bilotta F, Qeva E, Matot I. Anesthesia and cognitive disorders: a systematic review of the clinical evidence. Expert Rev Neurother 2016;16(11):1311–20.

46. Culley DJ, Flaherty D, Fahey MC, et al. Poor performance on a preoperative cognitive screening test predicts postoperative complications in older orthopedic surgical patients. Anesthesiology 2017;127(5):765–74.

47. Long LS, Wolpaw JT, Leung JM. Sensitivity and specificity of the animal fluency test for predicting postoperative delirium. [[Sensibilite et spe cificite du test de fluidite verbale sur les animaux pour la pre diction du de lirium postope ratoire]]. Can J Anaesth 2015;1–6. https://doi.org/10.1007/s12630-014-0306-7.

48. Partridge JS, Dhesi JK, Cross JD, et al. The prevalence and impact of undiagnosed cognitive impairment in older vascular surgical patients. J Vasc Surg 2014;60(4):1002–11.e3.

49. Culley DJ, Flaherty D, Reddy S, et al. Preoperative cognitive stratification of older elective surgical patients: a cross-sectional study. Anesth Analg 2016;123(1):186–92.

50. Whiteside DM, Kealey T, Semla M, et al. Verbal fluency: language or executive function measure? Appl Neuropsychol Adult 2015;23(1):29–34.

51. Smith NA, Yeow YY. Use of the Montreal Cognitive Assessment test to investigate the prevalence of mild cognitive impairment in the elderly elective surgical population. Anaesth Intensive Care 2016;44:581–7.

52. Feldman LS, Carli F. From preoperative assessment to preoperative optimization of frailty. JAMA Surg 2018. https://doi.org/10.1001/jamasurg.2018.0213.

53. Darvall JN, Gregorevic KJ, Story DA, et al. Frailty indexes in perioperative and critical care_ A systematic review. Arch Gerontol Geriatr 2018;79:88–96.

54. Griffiths R, Mehta M. Frailty and anaesthesia: what we need to know. Cont Educ Anaesth Crit Care Pain 2014;14(6):273–7.

55. Shem Tov L, Matot I. Frailty and anesthesia. Curr Opin Anaesthesiol 2017;30(3):409–17.

56. Bellamy JL, Runner RP, Vu CCL, et al. Modified frailty index is an effective risk assessment tool in primary total hip arthroplasty. J Arthroplasty 2017;32(10):2963–8.

57. Huisman MG, van Leeuwen BL, Ugolini G, et al. "Timed up & go": a screening tool for predicting 30-day morbidity in onco-geriatric surgical patients? A multicenter cohort study. PLoS One 2014;9(1). https://doi.org/10.1371/journal.pone.0086863.

58. Fried LP, Tangen CM, Walston J, et al. Frailty in older adults: evidence for a phenotype. J Gerontol A Biol Sci Med Sci 2001;56:M146–56.

59. Robinson TN, Wu DS, Sauaia A, et al. Slower walking speed forecasts increased postoperative morbidity and 1-year mortality across surgical specialties. Ann Surg 2013;1–19. https://doi.org/10.1097/SLA.0b013e3182a4e96c.

60. Furukawa H, Tanemoto K. Frailty in cardiothoracic surgery: systematic review of the literature. Gen Thorac Cardiovasc Surg 2015;63(8):1–9.
61. Townsend NT, Robinson TN. Does walking speed predict postoperative morbidity? Adv Surg 2014;48(1):53–64.
62. Barnett SR. Polypharmacy and perioperative medications in the elderly. Anesthesiol Clin 2009;27(3):377–89.
63. Nechba RB, M'barki Kadiri El M, Bennani-Ziatni M, et al. Difficulty in managing polypharmacy in the elderly: case report and review of the literature. J Clin Gerontol Geriatr 2015;6(1):30–3.
64. Gutiérrez-Valencia M, Izquierdo M, Cesari M, et al. The relationship between frailty and polypharmacy in older people: A systematic review. Br J Clin Pharmacol 2018;84(7):1432–44. https://doi.org/10.1111/bcp.13590.
65. Gupta R, Gan TJ. Preoperative nutrition and prehabilitation. Anesthesiol Clin 2016;34(1):143–53.
66. da Silva Fink J, de Mello PD, de Mello ED. Subjective global assessment of nutritional status - A systematic review of the literature. Clin Nutr 2015;34(5):785–92.
67. Bharadwaj S, Ginoya S, Tandon P, et al. Malnutrition: laboratory markers vs nutritional assessment. Gastroenterol Rep (Oxf) 2016. https://doi.org/10.1093/gastro/gow013.
68. Evans DC, Martindale RG, Kiraly LN, et al. Nutrition optimization prior to surgery. Nutr Clin Pract 2014;29(1):10–21.
69. Kehlet H. ERAS implementation—time to move forward. Ann Surg 2018;267(6):998–9.
70. Watt DG, McSorley ST, Horgan PG, et al. Enhanced recovery after surgery. Medicine 2015;94(36). https://doi.org/10.1097/MD.0000000000001286.
71. Beckert AK, Huisingh-Scheetz M, Thompson K, et al. Screening for frailty in thoracic surgical patients. Ann Thorac Surg 2017;103(3):956–61.
72. Kirkham KR, Wijeysundera DN, Pendrith C, et al. Preoperative laboratory investigations: rates and variability prior to low-risk surgical procedures. Anesthesiology 2016;1–11. https://doi.org/10.1097/ALN.0000000000001013.
73. Chen CL, Lin GA, Bardach NS, et al. Preoperative medical testing in Medicare patients undergoing cataract surgery. N Engl J Med 2015;372(16):1530–8.
74. Pasternak LR, Johns A. Ambulatory gynaecological surgery: risk and assessment. Best Pract Res Clin Obstet Gynaecol 2005;19(5):663–79.
75. Muñoz M, Gómez-Ramírez S, Kozek-Langeneker S. Pre-operative haematological assessment in patients scheduled for major surgery. Anaesthesia 2015;71:19–28.
76. Rinehart JB, Lee TC, Kaneshiro K, et al. Perioperative blood ordering optimization process using information from an anesthesia information management system. Transfusion 2016;56(4):938–45.
77. Hennrikus E, Ou G, Kinney B, et al. Prevalence, timing, causes, and outcomes of hyponatremia in hospitalized orthopaedic surgery patients. J Bone Joint Surg Am 2015;97(22):1824–32.
78. Karas PL, Goh SL, Dhital K. Is low serum albumin associated with postoperative complications in patients undergoing cardiac surgery? Interact Cardiovasc Thorac Surg 2015. https://doi.org/10.1093/icvts/ivv247.
79. Perry R, Scott LJ, Richards A, et al. Pre-admission interventions to improve outcome after elective surgery—protocol for a systematic review. Syst Rev 2016;1–9. https://doi.org/10.1186/s13643-016-0266-9.

Multimodal Prehabilitation Programs for Older Surgical Patients

Jaume Borrell-Vega, MD[a],*, Alan G. Esparza Gutierrez, BS[a],
Michelle L. Humeidan, MD, PhD[b]

KEYWORDS

- Prehabilitation • Geriatric • Surgery • Exercise • Nutrition

KEY POINTS

- Primarily through implementation of exercise protocols to improve cardiovascular fitness and muscle strength before surgery, prehabilitation programs have shown positive results, and recently have been expanded to include nutritional and cognitive/behavioral aspects.
- High-risk surgical patients seem to benefit the most from prehabilitation programs.
- Prehabilitation programs are designed to promote readiness for surgical stress and minimize functional decline postoperatively, but they have been heterogeneously studied, lacking standardized protocols and adequately powered large samples in older patients.

INTRODUCTION

At least 50 million surgeries are done annually in the United States alone, and an average American can now expect to undergo 7 operations during a lifetime.[1–3] Older adults comprise the fastest growing cohort of surgical patients.[3] Despite many advancements in perioperative care, it is indisputable that surgery is a major stressor on the body, and patients with suboptimal recovery still exist.[4] Twenty percent of patients 70 years of age or older undergoing noncardiac surgery develop 1 or more serious postoperative complications,[5] which presents a challenge to all health care providers.[6]

In the past, efforts to improve recovery have been made during the postoperative period. Because patients are healing after a surgical procedure (incisions, drains, catheters, and so forth), and often experience fatigue and anxiety awaiting return of

Disclosures: None.
[a] Department of Anesthesiology – Clinical Research, The Ohio State University Wexner Medical Center, 410 West 10th Avenue, N-411 Doan Hall, Columbus, OH 43210, USA; [b] Department of Anesthesiology, The Ohio State University Wexner Medical Center, 410 West 10th Avenue, N-411 Doan Hall, Columbus, OH 43210, USA
* Corresponding author.
E-mail addresses: Jaume.BorrellVega@osumc.edu; Jaume.borrell.93@gmail.com

function or additional treatments, this period has not proved optimal for significant changes in lifestyle that may facilitate recovery and rehabilitation.[7,8] The preoperative period seems to be a more effective time to motivate patients and actively engage them in preparation for their future recovery. In addition to physical benefits, mental health and emotional functioning can be improved by preoperative exercise.[8,9]

Introduced in 2000, prehabilitation is intended to promote successful coping with the stress of surgery by enhancing the individual's functional capacity, and therefore physiologic reserve, before an operation.[10] With prehabilitation, it is hypothesized that patients minimize postoperative functional decline compared with patients who remained inactive during the preoperative period (**Fig. 1**).[11] Several varieties of prehabilitation programs have been described, but no protocol has been universally accepted. Prehabilitation programs with exercise training before surgery are supported by the most evidence, but other programs with nutrition and cognitive as well as behavioral aspects exist and show encouraging results.[10,12]

Despite the increased risks to older patients having surgery, few prehabilitation studies have specifically targeted this population. This article presents a focused review highlighting the most current prehabilitation publications in older surgical patients (≥65 years old; randomized controlled trials, prospective studies, and retrospective studies from 2005 to July 2018). This article targets gastrointestinal, orthopedic, and urologic surgery, because most of the data have been collected in these cohorts, and the impact and mechanism for prehabilitation benefits in cardiac and pulmonary surgery patients may differ (**Table 1**). Almost all prehabilitation data are not from studies specifically targeting older patients, but include them because they are candidates for the surgical procedure being studied. Because of this, this article also discusses case series, literature reviews, integrative reviews, systematic reviews, scope reviews, and meta-analyses in surgical patients averaging 60 years of age or older (**Table 2**).

IMPORTANT CONSIDERATIONS FOR PREOPERATIVE OPTIMIZATION IN OLDER PATIENTS
Enhanced Recovery After Surgery and Prehabilitation

Enhanced Recovery After Surgery (ERAS) pathways consist of a series of preadmission, intraoperative, and postoperative evidence-based recommendations in order to achieve early, quality recovery in patients undergoing major surgery.[13] Common

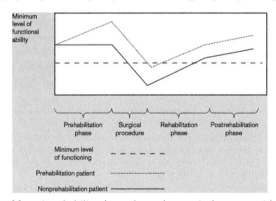

Fig. 1. Trajectory of functional ability throughout the surgical process with and without preoperative exercise training (prehabilitation). (*From* Carli F, Zavorsky GS. Optimizing functional exercise capacity in the elderly surgical population. Curr Opin Clin Nutr Metab Care 2005;8(1):23–32; with permission.)

Table 1
Description and results of prehabilitation randomized controlled trials

Author, Year	Type of Surgery	Subjects (N)	Mean Age (y)	Prehabilitation (Intervention Group)		Impact of Prehabilitation
				Program Features	Duration	
Abdominal and Colorectal Surgeries						
Jensen et al,[21] 2015	Radical cystectomy	107	69	Exercise (unsupervised aerobic, strength) Behavioral	2 wk	Improved walking capacity after surgery and ability to perform ADLs
Gillis et al,[44] 2014	Elective colorectal resection	77	65.7	Exercise (unsupervised aerobic, strength) Nutrition Behavior	4 wk	Improved walking capacity after surgery
Minnella et al,[22] 2017	Elective colorectal resection	185	68.5	Exercise (supervised or unsupervised aerobic, strength, flexibility), nutrition, behavioral	4 wk	Improved perioperative walking capacity
Barberan-Garcia et al,[36] 2018	Elective major abdominal surgery	125	71	Exercise (supervised high-intensity aerobic, unsupervised aerobic, functional) Behavioral	6 wk (±2 wk)	Increased aerobic capacity, decreased postoperative complications
Bousquet-Dion et al,[23] 2018	Colon surgery	63	71	Exercise (supervised and unsupervised aerobic and strength) Nutrition Behavioral	4 wk	No significant impact, but determined that sedentary patients more likely to benefit from prehabilitation than active patients

(continued on next page)

Table 1
(continued)

Author, Year	Type of Surgery	Subjects (N)	Mean Age (y)	Prehabilitation (Intervention Group)		Impact of Prehabilitation
				Program Features	Duration	
Orthopedic Surgeries						
Mitchell et al,[47] 2005	TKA	160	70.6	Exercise (supervised flexibility and functional)	8 wk	No improvement in patient-perceived outcomes (but home-based prehabilitation was associated with significant cost)
Siggeirsdottir et al,[56] 2005	THA	50	68	Exercise (unsupervised, unspecified) Education	4 wk	Significant decrease in LOS, better QoL
Rooks et al,[50] 2006	THA and TKA	108	65	Exercise (supervised, water-based and land-based, aerobic, strength, flexibility)	6 wk	Significant decrease in discharge to rehabilitation facility, THA patients had fewer postoperative complications
Williamson et al,[52] 2007	TKA	181	71	Arm 1: exercise (supervised aerobic, strength, functional, flexibility) Arm 2: acupuncture	6 wk	Short-term improvement in patient-reported outcomes with acupuncture only
Evgeniadis et al,[40] 2008	TKA	53	68	Exercise (supervised strength)	8 wk	Improved preoperative mental health and earlier return of basic function immediately after surgery
Topp et al,[45] 2009	TKA	54	64.1	Exercise (supervised and unsupervised strength, functional, flexibility)	V	Improved functionality before and after surgery and better postoperative surgical leg strength

Study	Surgery	N	Age	Intervention	Duration	Outcome
Bitterli et al,[49] 2011	THA	80	65.3	Exercise (unsupervised minimal intervention strategy focused on awareness of hip joint movement)	2–6 wk	Less pain and better mean balance ability before surgery, no postoperative impact of the program
Huang et al,[51] 2012	TKA	243	70.5	Exercise (unsupervised strength), education	2–4 wk	Significantly decreased LOS and medical costs
Matassi et al,[43] 2014	TKA	122	66	Exercise (supervised and unsupervised strength and flexibility)	6 wk	Significantly decreased LOS and improved knee mobility in early postoperative period
Villadsen et al,[48] 2014	THA and TKA	165	66.9	Exercise (supervised strength, functional)	8 wk	Improvement with ADLs and pain 6 wk after surgery
Biau et al,[87] 2015	THA	207	66	Education (supervised functional postoperative exercises, pain management)	1 class	Time to reach complete functional independence after surgery was not improved
Skoffer et al,[42] 2016	TKA	59	70.7	Exercise (supervised strength, flexibility)	4 wk	Improved functionality and strength 6 wk after surgery. Patient-reported outcomes (QoL, pain) unchanged

Abbreviations: ADLs, activities of daily living; LOS, length of stay; QoL, quality of life; THA, total hip arthroplasty; TKA, total knee arthroplasty; V, duration variable depending availability for surgery.

Table 2
Description and results of prehabilitation systematic reviews and meta-analysis

Author, Year	Type of Surgery	Number of Studies	Age (y)	Duration	Impact of Prehabilitation
Abdominal and Colorectal Surgeries					
Bolshinsky et al,[59] 2018	Gastrointestinal cancer surgery	20	70	21–52 d	Insufficient data for conclusions, no evidence for reduction in postoperative complications
Gillis et al,[25] 2018	Colorectal surgeries	2	68.9	29–38 d	Multimodal prehabilitation in addition to ERAS is useful for mitigating loss of body mass following surgery
Gillis et al,[24] 2018	Colorectal surgeries	9	61–71	14–38 d	Multimodal prehabilitation in addition to ERAS improved postoperative walking capacity. Nutrition prehabilitation (without or without exercise) is associated with decreased LOS
Bruns et al,[60] 2016	Colorectal surgeries	5	61–71	21–42 d	Evidence for improvement (significant) in physical function and psychological function (nonsignificant). No improvement in complication rates or LOS
Orthopedic Surgeries					
Kwok et al,[61] 2015	TKA	11	60.6–72.4	3–8 wk	Little evidence demonstrating impact of preoperative exercise on postoperative outcomes and function
Peer et al,[62] 2017	TKA	3	63.5–72.8	42 d	Preoperative strength training offered no benefit but did positively affect patient-reported WOMAC and SF-36
Wang et al,[57] 2016	Joint replacement	22	61–76	NR	Improvement in WOMAC, but no impact on pain, SF-36, LOS, or cost
Ma et al,[58] 2018	TKA	9	63.1–72.8	4–12 wk	Significant decrease in LOS, but no impact on pain, WOMAC, SF-36, or range of motion
Halloway et al,[32] 2015	Joint arthroplasty	7	65–76	2–6 wk	Evidence for improvement in multiple dimensions of physical function

Abbreviations: ERAS, enhanced recovery after surgery; NR, not reported; SF-36, short form health survey; WOMAC, Western Ontario and McMaster Universities Osteoarthritis Index.

preoperative interventions include education and counseling of the patient, elimination of smoking and alcohol consumption, and preoperative optimization of medical conditions (eg, anemia, diabetes).[14–20] Preoperative interventions in ERAS guidelines go hand in hand with the concept of prehabilitation. None of the ERAS guidelines specifically propose rigorous exercise or nutrition programs, but mention increasing exercise preoperatively may be of benefit and preoperative specialized nutritional support should be considered for malnourished patients.[16]

Although addition of a formal prehabilitation strategy to ERAS in older patients has shown improvements in walking capacity after surgery, this has not consistently translated to additional benefits in length of stay (LOS) or complication rates in individual studies.[21–23] However, a pooled analysis and meta-analysis by Gillis and colleagues[24,25] did support the utility of prehabilitation in addition to ERAS for mitigation of surgical stress, improvement in postoperative walking capacity, and reduction in LOS in older patients having colorectal surgery. In the past, ERAS protocols have been structured around the anticipated surgery, not a patient cohort such as geriatric patients. Prehabilitation therefore presents an opportunity for more individualized patient care, and a strategy for increasing the engagement of patients in their own health care and management, both important goals of ERAS and Perioperative Surgical Home models.[20,26]

High-risk Versus Low-risk Patients in Prehabilitation Studies

Frailty is a major concern when caring for older surgical patients. Defined as "multisystem impairment characterized by increased vulnerability and disabilities,"[27] frailty is associated with higher postoperative morbidity and mortality,[28] longer hospital admissions, and higher costs.[29] In general, comorbidity burden and prevalence of frailty increase with age, so older patients are considered high-risk surgical candidates.[12,30–33] Frailty can be managed, modified, and improved through structured exercise programs in nonsurgical patients[34] and surgical patients in the immediate postoperative period,[35] but evidence is less robust for a preoperative process to reduce the negative impact of frailty on recovery. The authors found only 17 randomized controlled prehabilitation trials with patients averaging greater than or equal to 65 years of age that included at least 50 patients in the study, despite a clear need for investigation of methods to mitigate perioperative risk and improve recovery in older surgical patients (see **Table 1**).

In a recent prospective study conducted by Barberan-Garcia and colleagues,[36] the investigators observed bias toward assessment of low-risk patients in prehabilitation trials, and in response conducted a randomized controlled trial on high-risk patients undergoing major abdominal surgery (American Society of Anesthesiologists class ≥III and/or ≥70 years of age). The personalized prehabilitation program included a motivational interview (to address adherence), daily activity (increasing steps per day and walking intensity), and supervised high-intensity endurance exercise training. The intervention decreased LOS and resulted in lower rates of cardiovascular complications, infections, and paralytic ileus in the prehabilitation patients. This work, along with results of a recent multimodal prehabilitation program in older colorectal surgery patients published by Bousquet-Dion and colleagues,[23] indicates that prehabilitation may be of particular utility in less heathy patients compared with healthier patients.

CORE ELEMENTS OF PREHABILITATION

Multimodal prehabilitation programs typically address 2 or more of 3 primary components: exercise, nutritional interventions, and cognitive-behavioral interventions (**Fig. 2**).[2,26]

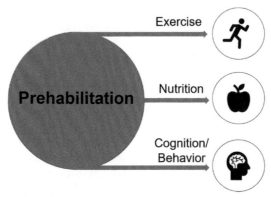

Fig. 2. Main areas of focus for prehabilitation programs.

Exercise

First published in 1993 by Older and colleagues,[37] the association of low preoperative fitness levels with higher morbidity and mortality after major surgery has been validated by several publications.[12,30,38,39] This consideration is important for older adults because more than 60% of individuals more than 65 years of age do not meet recommended daily activity guidelines.[32]

Exercise program features

Exercise programs are highly variable in the literature. A common trend is to individualize the training programs and adapt to each individual's needs. These training protocols must exceed normal activities of daily living (ADL) and be more than what the patient is used to performing, without being excessive and irrational, in order to maintain good adherence rates.[2,7,12] Typically, exercise is categorized into 1 of 4 categories. Strength exercises, including resistance training and weight lifting, build muscle mass[38,40–44] and are popular in prehabilitation for orthopedic surgeries.[43,45] Aerobic exercise for cardiopulmonary enhancement can be achieved with devices such as a stationary bicycle[7,36] or with unassisted exercises such as walking, jogging, or swimming.[22,44,46] Stretching/flexibility and breathing exercises are also used.[43,45–47] Training for postural control, orientation, and positioning control has been described as well.[47–49] Of note, land-based exercises are significantly more used than water-based exercise, despite what could be perceived as benefits of water activities in aging populations, such as decreased joint stress.[50] The mode of delivery for prehabilitation exercise sessions varies, and can include one-on-one exercise sessions with a therapist or other health professional,[23,36,40,47,50–52] group sessions,[42,48] and/or unsupervised home sessions.[21,43,44,47,53]

Assessment of exertion and functional reserve during exercise requires objective and subjective tools. The 6-minute walk test (6MWT) measuring the distance traveled on a treadmill in the stated time period is a popular primary outcome measure for objective progression of functional capacity, and has no ceiling effect.[7,22,23,44] Maximal oxygen uptake (Vo_{2max}), is considered the current gold standard for objective aerobic fitness tests, but it requires specialized personnel and expensive equipment, therefore it is not as regularly reported as the 6MWT.[9,54,55] A common subjective tool to assess the perceived level of exertion is the Borg Scale or the shorter Modified Borg Scale. A visual, color-coded, 12-point scale ranging from "no intensity" to "very, very hard intensity," the Borg Scale is often accompanied by cartoons representing effort for easy use.[2] Measurements of other variables, such as muscle capacity, muscle strength, and joint mobility, are not reported as often.[38]

Impact of preoperative exercise in older patients

Several studies in older patients have reported improved postoperative physical function, including improved mobility,[43] increased aerobic capacity,[36] walking capacity,[21,22,44] and strength[42,45] with prehabilitation that included exercise. Faster postoperative return of basic function[40,42,45] and ability to perform ADLs[21,48] has been shown as well. In addition, fewer postoperative complications have been reported.[36,50] Older orthopedic patients have benefitted from decreased postoperative LOS[50,56] and need for discharge to rehabilitation facilities after exercise prehabilitation.[50] For example, Hung and colleagues[51] conducted a randomized controlled trial with a supervised prehabilitation exercise program (quadriceps muscle strength training) in older patients (mean age, 70.4 years) undergoing total knee arthroplasty (TKA). These investigators showed a shorter LOS in the intervention group and, therefore, lower medical costs. However, not all studies have shown postoperative benefits. Mitchell and colleagues[47] reported increased costs associated with supervised exercise, and no postoperative benefits. Likewise, although less pain and better balance ability were described preoperatively, no postoperative impact was reported in older orthopedic patients following total hip arthroplasty (THA), possibly because the exercise intervention was an unsupervised minimal intervention strategy solely focused on awareness of hip joint movement.[49]

Results from exercise-based prehabilitation studies should be carefully examined because of the variety of activity and measurement strategies used. Also, it is common to find that a significant number of patients do not respond to an exercise intervention, despite completing it. This finding may be explained by several factors, such as age, gender, disease state, compliance, type of exercise, and dietary intake.[26] The small number of randomized prehabilitation studies specifically targeting older adults, and lack of common exercise type, duration, intensity, and measurement strategies, has limited meta-analysis of the data. However, because older patients make up an ever-growing proportion of surgical candidates, several reviews exist in which the average age of patients included is 60 years or older. For gastrointestinal, colorectal, and orthopedic surgeries, no clear conclusions can be drawn regarding the impact of preoperative exercise on recovery. With regard to physical status, LOS, and complications, both benefit[57,58] and lack of benefit[59–62] have been reported in pooled data studies (see **Table 2**).

Understanding the mechanisms behind exercise-induced improvement in postoperative recovery will facilitate design of future trials and guide achievement of maximum benefit from prehabilitation. Both preclinical and clinical studies support the value of exercise. In a rodent model of metabolic syndrome showing several risk factors for poor postoperative recovery, including low functional capacity and insulin resistance, Feng and colleagues[63] showed attenuation of neuroinflammation and cognitive decline after surgical repair of a tibial fracture in animals completing 10 weeks of treadmill exercise preoperatively. In healthy older humans, 1 year of aerobic exercise was associated with an increase in brain-derived neurotrophic factor, insulinlike growth factor type 1, and vascular endothelial growth factor in certain areas of the brain, promoting functional connectivity and neuroplasticity.[64] Pain relief resulting from regular exercise in nonsurgical patients may be secondary to central nervous system changes in N-methyl-D-aspartate receptor phosphorylation, serotonin receptor expression, and neurotransmitter levels and endogenous opiate levels.[65] Less pain following exercise in older orthopedic surgical patients has been reported before surgery, although the mechanism is unclear and the pain relief effect was lost after surgery.[49] Following resistance training, improvements in muscle function are thought to be caused by changes at many levels in the neuromuscular system, including increased protein synthesis, changes in type II muscle fibers, and a shift toward anabolic pathways (and away from catabolism).[66] Aerobic exercise increases cardiac output and changes vasculature number, structure, and compliance to promote oxygen delivery, and also promotes more efficient oxygen extraction,[67] which can prepare surgical patients for the "stress test" of an operation.

Nutrition

In the last decade, large amounts of data have been published linking malnutrition to poor postoperative outcomes,[68] including increased rates of morbidity and mortality.[68,69] A crucial element of malnutrition is protein-energy deficit, especially when requirements are high with surgery-induced inflammatory and catabolic states.[24,70,71] One in 5 outpatients with colorectal cancer are reported to be malnourished, with more than half experiencing weight loss before surgery.[24] Furthermore, advanced age is an independent risk factor for malnourishment and sarcopenia (reduced muscle mass and protein body composition).[72]

In combination with exercise programs, multimodal prehabilitation interventions include preprocedure nutritional supplementation (1.2–1.5 g of protein per kilogram per day)[73] in order to reverse the basal impoverished state and improve muscle strength and mass.[22,23,44] Other than protein supplementation, interventions can include counseling sessions with a nutritionist to assess overall diet, glycemic control and body composition, among other parameters.[23,44,74] Bruns and colleagues[60] conducted a meta-analysis on the effect of preoperative nutritional support in patients undergoing colorectal surgery ranging from 60 to 72 years old. Malnourishment rates varied from 6% to 68% preoperatively, and the intervention consisted of oral protein supplementation, along with other supplements in certain studies, such as carbohydrates. No significant reduction in the overall complication rate was found in the intervention groups, although this was attributed to the heterogeneity of studies included. Older patients given multimodal prehabilitation before colorectal surgery had improved walking capacity postoperatively in 2 reports,[22,44] but a subsequent study showed no benefit.[23] Although results are still controversial, combined exercise and protein-replacement prehabilitation in older patients seems to be beneficial for reducing loss of lean body and fat masses after a surgical procedure,[25] and seems to reduce the number of days spent in the hospital.[24]

Cognitive and Behavioral Interventions

Complications like postoperative delirium (POD), postoperative cognitive dysfunction (POCD), anxiety, and depression can be detrimental to recovery and are associated with longer LOS, impaired ADL, distress, reduced autonomy, and increased morbidity and mortality.[75–79] These complications are associated with significant cost, so prevention is beneficial not only to patient wellbeing but also to the health care system.[80,81] In additional to evidence supporting postoperative cognitive benefits from preoperative exercise,[63] multimodal prehabilitation can include cognitive and psychological (behavioral) components to improve recovery. Acupuncture as a complementary intervention may also be considered, because one study showed that TKA patients with an average age in the 70s had no postoperative benefit from weekly exercise but did report better postoperative function and pain with the Oxford Knee Score[52] after weekly acupuncture.[52] Evidence for other complementary and alternative medicine interventions, such as reiki or chiropractic care, is limited.

Cognitive prehabilitation
Cognitive reserve is a concept that is theorized to be linked to complications after surgery, such as POD and POCD.[82] The cause of these complications is not yet clear, but advanced age and preexisting cognitive dysfunction before surgery are significant risk factors.[75,83] Cognitive exercise has been shown to exert protective effects on longitudinal neuropsychological performance and prevent neurologic decline, and therefore could be a potential form of prophylaxis for POD and POCD.[81,84,85] Saleh and colleagues[86] showed that simple preoperative mnemonic skill training sessions in elderly patients scheduled for gastrointestinal surgery can reduce POCD rates 1 week after surgery. In an ongoing study, Humeidan and colleagues[81] theorize that a minimum of 10 hours of preoperative cognitive exercise focused on memory, speed, attention, flexibility, and problem solving can increase cognitive reserve and reduce the incidence of postoperative delirium by 50% in older patients having noncardiac, nonneurologic surgeries.

Patient education
Inclusion of education in prehabilitation protocols can have positive impact in older surgical patients. LOS was reduced, and overall better quality of life was reported by Siggeirdottir and colleagues[56] in their study of THA patients with an average age of 68 years when detailed education about the surgery and postoperative activity was provided preoperatively. However, addition of hands-on education about postoperative activities such as use of crutches conferred no additional benefit in time to reach postoperative functional independence compared with standard education without hands-on instruction in older THA patients.[87] To date, the number of studies in older patients incorporating use of education in prehabilitation protocols does not allow meta-analysis[57]

Psychological and psychosocial prehabilitation
Tsimopoulou and colleagues[76] conducted a systematic review of psychological interventions before cancer surgery with most included patients being older than 50 years. In general, preoperative psychological interventions were shown to decrease postoperative LOS, anxiety, depression, and cortisol levels, with improvements in wound healing reported too. Despite this, studies in older patients incorporating psychological consultation and techniques for anxiety reduction and relaxation into prehabilitation have shown no impact on anxiety or quality of life.[22,23,44] Regarding postoperative functionality, multimodal prehabilitation with psychological components has had mixed results, with 2 studies reporting improved postoperative walking capacity[22,44] and 1 study showing no improvement.[23]

SUMMARY

Primarily through implementation of exercise programs for better cardiovascular fitness and muscle strength, prehabilitation programs have shown positive impact on postoperative recovery and have been expanded to include nutritional and cognitive/behavioral aspects. A major limitation of the prehabilitation literature is heterogeneity across studies, making it difficult to generalize. Despite growing evidence for efficacy, thus far there are few prehabilitation studies that have focused specifically on aging patients. Older adults will be the largest cohort of surgical patients in the future, and frailty and postoperative complications occur with increased frequency in this group, highlighting the opportunity to use prehabilitation for physical, physiologic, and mental optimization before surgical stress. In general, providing each patient with a supervised, multimodal prehabilitation program focused on the individual needs for the upcoming surgical procedure will be crucial to ensure adherence and achieve significantly improved outcomes.[26]

REFERENCES

1. Gawande A. Two hundred years of surgery. N Engl J Med 2012;366(18):1716–23.
2. Carli F, Scheede-Bergdahl C. Prehabilitation to enhance perioperative care. Anesthesiol Clin 2015;33(1):17–33.
3. Lee PHU, Gawande AA. The number of surgical procedures in an American lifetime in 3 states. J Am Coll Surg 2008;207(3):S75.
4. Schilling PL, Dimick JB, Birkmeyer JD. Prioritizing quality improvement in general surgery. J Am Coll Surg 2008;207(5):698–704.
5. Harari D, Hopper A, Dhesi J, et al. Proactive care of older people undergoing surgery ('POPS'): designing, embedding, evaluating and funding a comprehensive geriatric assessment service for older elective surgical patients. Age Ageing 2007;36(2):190–6.
6. Kazaure HS, Roman SA, Sosa JA. Association of postdischarge complications with reoperation and mortality in general surgery. Arch Surg 2012;147(11):1000–7.
7. Carli F, Charlebois P, Stein B, et al. Randomized clinical trial of prehabilitation in colorectal surgery. Br J Surg 2010;97(8):1187–97.
8. van Rooijen S, Carli F, Dalton SO, et al. Preoperative modifiable risk factors in colorectal surgery: an observational cohort study identifying the possible value of prehabilitation. Acta Oncol 2017;56(2):329–34.
9. Dunne DF, Jack S, Jones RP, et al. Randomized clinical trial of prehabilitation before planned liver resection. Br J Surg 2016;103(5):504–12.
10. Gillis C, Loiselle SE, Fiore JF Jr, et al. Prehabilitation with whey protein supplementation on perioperative functional exercise capacity in patients undergoing colorectal resection for cancer: a pilot double-blinded randomized placebo-controlled trial. J Acad Nutr Diet 2016;116(5):802–12.
11. Carli F, Zavorsky GS. Optimizing functional exercise capacity in the elderly surgical population. Curr Opin Clin Nutr Metab Care 2005;8(1):23–32.
12. Pouwels S, Hageman D, Gommans LN, et al. Preoperative exercise therapy in surgical care: a scoping review. J Clin Anesth 2016;33:476–90.
13. Society ERAS. Enhanced recovery after surgery (ERAS) 2016. Available at: http://erassociety.org/. Accessed June 21, 2018.
14. Gustafsson U, Scott M, Schwenk W, et al. Guidelines for perioperative care in elective colonic surgery: enhanced Recovery After Surgery (ERAS®) Society recommendations. World J Surg 2013;37(2):259–84.
15. Nygren J, Thacker J, Carli F, et al. Guidelines for perioperative care in elective rectal/pelvic surgery: Enhanced Recovery After Surgery (ERAS®) Society recommendations. Clin Nutr 2012;31(6):801–16.
16. Thorell A, MacCormick A, Awad S, et al. Guidelines for perioperative care in bariatric surgery: enhanced recovery after surgery (ERAS) society recommendations. World J Surg 2016;40(9):2065–83.
17. Feldheiser A, Aziz O, Baldini G, et al. Enhanced Recovery After Surgery (ERAS) for gastrointestinal surgery, part 2: consensus statement for anaesthesia practice. Acta Anaesthesiol Scand 2016;60(3):289–334.
18. Melloul E, Hübner M, Scott M, et al. Guidelines for perioperative care for liver surgery: enhanced Recovery After Surgery (ERAS) society recommendations. World J Surg 2016;40(10):2425–40.

19. Temple-Oberle C, Shea-Budgell MA, Tan M, et al. Consensus review of optimal perioperative care in breast reconstruction: enhanced recovery after surgery (ERAS) society recommendations. Plast Reconstr Surg 2017;139(5):1056e–71e.

20. Shanahan JL, Leissner KB. Prehabilitation for the enhanced recovery after surgery patient. J Laparoendosc Adv Surg Tech A 2017;27(9):880–2.

21. Jensen BT, Petersen AK, Jensen JB, et al. Efficacy of a multiprofessional rehabilitation programme in radical cystectomy pathways: a prospective randomized controlled trial. Scand J Urol 2015;49(2):133–41.

22. Minnella EM, Bousquet-Dion G, Awasthi R, et al. Multimodal prehabilitation improves functional capacity before and after colorectal surgery for cancer: a five-year research experience. Acta Oncol 2017;56(2):295–300.

23. Bousquet-Dion G, Awasthi R, Loiselle SE, et al. Evaluation of supervised multimodal prehabilitation programme in cancer patients undergoing colorectal resection: a randomized control trial. Acta Oncol 2018;57(6):849–59.

24. Gillis C, Buhler K, Bresee L, et al. Effects of nutritional prehabilitation, with and without exercise, on outcomes of patients who undergo colorectal surgery: a systematic review and meta-analysis. Gastroenterology 2018;155(2):391–410.e4.

25. Gillis C, Fenton TR, Sajobi TT, et al. Trimodal prehabilitation for colorectal surgery attenuates post-surgical losses in lean body mass: A pooled analysis of randomized controlled trials. Clinical Nutrition 2019;38(3):1053–60.

26. Minnella EM, Carli F. Prehabilitation and functional recovery for colorectal cancer patients. Eur J Surg Oncol 2018;44(7):919–26.

27. Clegg A, Young J, Iliffe S, et al. Frailty in elderly people. Lancet 2013;381(9868): 752–62.

28. Afilalo J, Eisenberg MJ, Morin J-F, et al. Gait Speed as an incremental predictor of mortality and major morbidity in elderly patients undergoing cardiac surgery. J Am Coll Cardiol 2010;56(20):1668–76.

29. Abreu A. Prehabilitation: expanding the concept of cardiac rehabilitation. Eur J Prev Cardiol 2018;25(9):970–3.

30. Jack S, West M, Grocott MP. Perioperative exercise training in elderly subjects. Best Pract Res Clin Anaesthesiol 2011;25(3):461–72.

31. Turrentine FE, Wang H, Simpson VB, et al. Surgical risk factors, morbidity, and mortality in elderly patients. J Am Coll Surg 2006;203(6):865–77.

32. Halloway S, Buchholz SW, Wilbur J, et al. Prehabilitation interventions for older adults: an integrative review. West J Nurs Res 2015;37(1):103–23.

33. Shen Y, Hao Q, Zhou J, et al. The impact of frailty and sarcopenia on postoperative outcomes in older patients undergoing gastrectomy surgery: a systematic review and meta-analysis. BMC Geriatr 2017;17(1):188.

34. Theou O, Stathokostas L, Roland KP, et al. The effectiveness of exercise interventions for the management of frailty: a systematic review. J Aging Res 2011; 2011:19.

35. Nordstrom P, Thorngren KG, Hommel A, et al. Effects of geriatric team rehabilitation after hip fracture: meta-analysis of randomized controlled trials. J Am Med Dir Assoc 2018;19(10):840–5.

36. Barberan-Garcia A, Ubre M, Roca J, et al. Personalised prehabilitation in high-risk patients undergoing elective major abdominal surgery: a randomized blinded controlled trial. Ann Surg 2018;267(1):50–6.

37. Older R, Smith R, Courtney B, et al. Preoperative evaluation of cardiac failure and ischemia in elderly patients by cardiopulmonary exercise testing. Chest 1993; 104(3):701–4.

38. Cabilan CJ, Hines S, Munday J. The effectiveness of prehabilitation or preoperative exercise for surgical patients: a systematic review. JBI Database System Rev Implement Rep 2015;13(1):146–87.
39. Wilson RJ, Davies S, Yates D, et al. Impaired functional capacity is associated with all-cause mortality after major elective intra-abdominal surgery. Br J Anaesth 2010;105(3):297–303.
40. Evgeniadis G, Beneka A, Malliou P, et al. Effects of pre-or postoperative therapeutic exercise on the quality of life, before and after total knee arthroplasty for osteoarthritis. J Back Musculoskelet Rehabil 2008;21(3):161–9.
41. Clode NJ, Perry MA, Wulff L. Does physiotherapy prehabilitation improve pre-surgical outcomes and influence patient expectations prior to knee and hip joint arthroplasty? Int J Orthop Trauma Nurs 2018;30:14–9.
42. Skoffer B, Maribo T, Mechlenburg I, et al. Efficacy of preoperative progressive resistance training on postoperative outcomes in patients undergoing total knee arthroplasty. Arthritis Care Res (Hoboken) 2016;68(9):1239–51.
43. Matassi F, Duerinckx J, Vandenneucker H, et al. Range of motion after total knee arthroplasty: the effect of a preoperative home exercise program. Knee Surg Sports Traumatol Arthrosc 2014;22(3):703–9.
44. Gillis C, Li C, Lee L, et al. Prehabilitation versus rehabilitation: a randomized control trial in patients undergoing colorectal resection for cancer. Anesthesiology 2014;121(5):937–47.
45. Topp R, Swank AM, Quesada PM, et al. The effect of prehabilitation exercise on strength and functioning after total knee arthroplasty. PM R 2009;1(8):729–35.
46. Mazzola M, Bertoglio C, Boniardi M, et al. Frailty in major oncologic surgery of upper gastrointestinal tract: How to improve postoperative outcomes. Eur J Surg Oncol 2017;43(8):1566–71.
47. Mitchell C, Walker J, Walters S, et al. Costs and effectiveness of pre- and postoperative home physiotherapy for total knee replacement: randomized controlled trial. J Eval Clin Pract 2005;11(3):283–92.
48. Villadsen A, Overgaard S, Holsgaard-Larsen A, et al. Postoperative effects of neuromuscular exercise prior to hip or knee arthroplasty: a randomised controlled trial. Ann Rheum Dis 2014;73(6):1130–7.
49. Bitterli R, Sieben JM, Hartmann M, et al. Pre-surgical sensorimotor training for patients undergoing total hip replacement: a randomised controlled trial. Int J Sports Med 2011;32(9):725–32.
50. Rooks DS, Huang J, Bierbaum BE, et al. Effect of preoperative exercise on measures of functional status in men and women undergoing total hip and knee arthroplasty. Arthritis Rheum 2006;55(5):700–8.
51. Huang SW, Chen PH, Chou YH. Effects of a preoperative simplified home rehabilitation education program on length of stay of total knee arthroplasty patients. Orthop Traumatol Surg Res 2012;98(3):259–64.
52. Williamson L, Wyatt MR, Yein K, et al. Severe knee osteoarthritis: a randomized controlled trial of acupuncture, physiotherapy (supervised exercise) and standard management for patients awaiting knee replacement. Rheumatology (Oxford) 2007;46(9):1445–9.
53. Nagarajan K, Bennett A, Agostini P, et al. Is preoperative physiotherapy/pulmonary rehabilitation beneficial in lung resection patients? Interact Cardiovasc Thorac Surg 2011;13(3):300–2.
54. Kim DJ, Mayo NE, Carli F, et al. Responsive measures to prehabilitation in patients undergoing bowel resection surgery. Tohoku J Exp Med 2009;217(2):109–15.

55. West MA, Loughney L, Lythgoe D, et al. Effect of prehabilitation on objectively measured physical fitness after neoadjuvant treatment in preoperative rectal cancer patients: a blinded interventional pilot study. Br J Anaesth 2015;114(2): 244–51.

56. Siggeirsdottir K, Olafsson O, Jonsson H, et al. Short hospital stay augmented with education and home-based rehabilitation improves function and quality of life after hip replacement: randomized study of 50 patients with 6 months of follow-up. Acta Orthop 2005;76(4):555–62.

57. Wang L, Lee M, Zhang Z, et al. Does preoperative rehabilitation for patients planning to undergo joint replacement surgery improve outcomes? A systematic review and meta-analysis of randomised controlled trials. BMJ Open 2016;6(2): e009857.

58. Ma JX, Zhang LK, Kuang MJ, et al. The effect of preoperative training on functional recovery in patients undergoing total knee arthroplasty: a systematic review and meta-analysis. Int J Surg 2018;51:205–12.

59. Bolshinsky V, Li MH, Ismail H, et al. Multimodal prehabilitation programs as a bundle of care in gastrointestinal cancer surgery: a systematic review. Dis Colon Rectum 2018;61(1):124–38.

60. Bruns ER, van den Heuvel B, Buskens CJ, et al. The effects of physical prehabilitation in elderly patients undergoing colorectal surgery: a systematic review. Colorectal Dis 2016;18(8):O267–77.

61. Kwok IH, Paton B, Haddad FS. Does pre-operative physiotherapy improve outcomes in primary total knee arthroplasty? - A systematic review. J Arthroplasty 2015;30(9):1657–63.

62. Peer MA, Rush R, Gallacher PD, et al. Pre-surgery exercise and post-operative physical function of people undergoing knee replacement surgery: a systematic review and meta-analysis of randomized controlled trials. J Rehabil Med 2017; 49(4):304–15.

63. Feng X, Uchida Y, Koch L, et al. Exercise prevents enhanced postoperative neuroinflammation and cognitive decline and rectifies the gut Microbiome in a rat Model of Metabolic syndrome. Front Immunol 2017;8:1768.

64. Voss MW, Erickson KI, Prakash RS, et al. Neurobiological markers of exercise-related brain plasticity in older adults. Brain Behav Immun 2013;28:90–9.

65. Lima LV, Abner TS, Sluka KA. Does exercise increase or decrease pain? Central mechanisms underlying these two phenomena. J Physiol 2017;595(13):4141–50.

66. McCormick R, Vasilaki A. Age-related changes in skeletal muscle: changes to life-style as a therapy. Biogerontology 2018;19(6):519–36.

67. Hellsten Y, Nyberg M. Cardiovascular adaptations to exercise training. Compr Physiol 2015;6(1):1–32.

68. Martindale RG, McClave SA, Taylor B, et al. Perioperative nutrition: what is the current landscape? JPEN J Parenter Enteral Nutr 2013;37(5 Suppl):5s–20s.

69. Torgersen Z, Balters M. Perioperative nutrition. Surg Clin North Am 2015;95(2): 255–67.

70. Arora RC, Brown CH, Sanjanwala RM, et al. "NEW" prehabilitation: a 3-way approach to improve postoperative survival and health-related quality of life in cardiac surgery patients. Can J Cardiol 2018;34(7):839–49.

71. Tang JE, Manolakos JJ, Kujbida GW, et al. Minimal whey protein with carbohydrate stimulates muscle protein synthesis following resistance exercise in trained young men. Appl Physiol Nutr Metab 2007;32(6):1132–8.

72. van Stijn MF, Korkic-Halilovic I, Bakker MS, et al. Preoperative nutrition status and postoperative outcome in elderly general surgery patients: a systematic review. JPEN J Parenter Enteral Nutr 2013;37(1):37–43.
73. Braga M, Ljungqvist O, Soeters P, et al. ESPEN Guidelines on Parenteral Nutrition: Surgery. Clin Nutr 2009;28(4):378–86.
74. Chia CL, Mantoo SK, Tan KY. 'Start to finish trans-institutional transdisciplinary care': a novel approach improves colorectal surgical results in frail elderly patients. Colorectal Dis 2016;18(1):O43–50.
75. Neuner B, Hadzidiakos D, Bettelli G. Pre-and postoperative management of risk factors for postoperative delirium: who is in charge and what is its essence? Aging Clin Exp Res 2018;30(3):245–8.
76. Tsimopoulou I, Pasquali S, Howard R, et al. Psychological prehabilitation before cancer surgery: a systematic review. Ann Surg Oncol 2015;22(13):4117–23.
77. Pignay-Demaria V, Lespérance F, Demaria RG, et al. Depression and anxiety and outcomes of coronary artery bypass surgery. Ann Thorac Surg 2003;75(1):314–21.
78. Mayo NE, Feldman L, Scott S, et al. Impact of preoperative change in physical function on postoperative recovery: argument supporting prehabilitation for colorectal surgery. Surgery 2011;150(3):505–14.
79. Rosenberger PH, Jokl P, Ickovics J. Psychosocial factors and surgical outcomes: an evidence-based literature review. J Am Acad Orthop Surg 2006;14(7):397–405.
80. Rubin FH, Williams JT, Lescisin DA, et al. Replicating the Hospital Elder Life Program in a community hospital and demonstrating effectiveness using quality improvement methodology. J Am Geriatr Soc 2006;54(6):969–74.
81. Humeidan ML, Otey A, Zuleta-Alarcon A, et al. Perioperative cognitive protection—cognitive exercise and cognitive reserve (the neurobics trial): a single-blind randomized trial. Clin Ther 2015;37(12):2641–50.
82. Satz P. Brain reserve capacity on symptom onset after brain injury: a formulation and review of evidence for threshold theory. Neuropsychology 1993;7(3):273.
83. Culley DJ, Crosby G. Prehabilitation for prevention of postoperative cognitive dysfunction? Anesthesiology 2015;123(1):7–9.
84. Valenzuela M, Sachdev P. Can cognitive exercise prevent the onset of dementia? Systematic review of randomized clinical trials with longitudinal follow-up. Am J Geriatr Psychiatry 2009;17(3):179–87.
85. Wilson RS, De Leon CFM, Barnes LL, et al. Participation in cognitively stimulating activities and risk of incident Alzheimer disease. JAMA 2002;287(6):742–8.
86. Saleh AJ, Tang G-X, Hadi SM, et al. Preoperative cognitive intervention reduces cognitive dysfunction in elderly patients after gastrointestinal surgery: a randomized controlled trial. Med Sci Monit 2015;21:798.
87. Biau DJ, Porcher R, Roren A, et al. Neither pre-operative education or a minimally invasive procedure have any influence on the recovery time after total hip replacement. Int Orthop 2015;39(8):1475–81.

Geriatric Physiology and the Frailty Syndrome

Kashif T. Khan, MD, SM[a], Kaveh Hemati, MD[b], Anne L. Donovan, MD[c],*

KEYWORDS

- Frailty • Perioperative • Surgery • Elderly • Older adult • Geriatric • Aging
- Physiology

KEY POINTS

- As the population ages, older adults will comprise a greater proportion of perioperative patients.
- Changes to the physiology of organ systems with aging present a unique set of challenges to the provision of safe and effective perioperative care.
- Frailty is an emerging concept that predicts perioperative morbidity and mortality better than age or American Society of Anesthesiologists classification alone.
- There is a diverse array of instruments to facilitate diagnosis of frailty in the medical and surgical settings, but lack of consensus criteria for frailty precludes identification of a single best diagnostic tool.
- Frailty plays an increasing role in perioperative decision-making, guiding perioperative optimization, prognosis, informed consent, and advanced directives.

INTRODUCTION

The prevalence of older adults undergoing surgery is expected to increase as the population ages.[1] Because of physiologic decline and loss of functional reserve, older patients are at a higher risk of developing perioperative complications.[2] A paradigm shift is occurring in the perioperative care of older adults to focus on prevention of complications that have a substantial impact on quality of life, including functional decline, cognitive decline, and loss of independence.[3–6] Perioperative healthcare providers therefore seek to better characterize, understand, evaluate, and intervene on the contributors of increased morbidity and mortality among older adults.[7–11]

Disclosure Statement: Dr A.L. Donovan has received pilot grant funding from NIDUS. Other authors have nothing to disclose.
[a] Department of Anesthesia and Perioperative Care, Division of Critical Care Medicine, University of California, San Francisco, 505 Parnassus Avenue, Room M-917, San Francisco, CA 94143, USA; [b] Department of Anesthesia and Perioperative Care, University of California, San Francisco, 513 Parnassus Avenue, San Francisco, CA 94143, USA; [c] Department of Anesthesia and Perioperative Care, Division of Critical Care Medicine, University of California, San Francisco, 513 Parnassus Avenue, Box 0648, San Francisco, CA 94143, USA
* Corresponding author.
E-mail address: anne.donovan@ucsf.edu

1932-2275/19/© 2019 Elsevier Inc. All rights reserved.

Although predictable changes to physiologic function occur with aging, age alone is not a sufficient predictor of a patient's risk for perioperative morbidity and mortality.[12] Frailty is increasingly recognized as a critical predictor of poor perioperative outcomes; however, challenges remain regarding the definition, measurement, and effective clinical intervention of frailty. Recent effort to translate this complex and multidimensional term into clinical use suggests possibilities to identify, prevent, and treat frailty in surgical patients. This article first reviews physiologic changes occurring with age, and then integrates the importance of these changes into a more comprehensive discussion of the frailty syndrome.

AGE-RELATED PHYSIOLOGIC CHANGES

Aging is associated with a decline in organ function in all body systems, resulting from a complex interplay of many processes occurring throughout one's lifetime.[13] Genetic, environmental, molecular, and evolutionary processes have all been proposed as contributors to aging. Organ system decline leads to a reduction in overall functional reserve and limits an individual's capacity to respond to acute stressors.[14–16] Physiologic changes occurring with aging have important implications for providing safe anesthesia care to elderly surgical patients. Age-related organ systems changes, and implications for anesthetic management, are described in **Table 1**.[13,14,16–19]

Although it is critical for the anesthesia provider to have an understanding of the physiologic changes associated with aging, it is also important to know that these changes are necessary, but not sufficient, to predict perioperative risk for elderly surgical patients.

THE FRAILTY SYNDROME

Frailty is a state of reduced physiologic reserve beyond that which would be expected with normal aging, and is thought to result from the cumulative effect of multiple physiologic changes over time.[14,15,20] The prevalence of frailty in community-dwelling elders increases with age: 4% in 65 to 69 year olds, 7% in 70 to 74 year olds, 9% in 75 to 79 year olds, 16% in 80 to 84 year olds, and 26% in 85 year olds and older.[21] Three systematic reviews have recently reported the prevalence of frailty in surgical and critical care populations: 10.4% to 37% in general surgery patients[22]; 19% to 62% among general, vascular, cardiac, thoracic, and orthopedic surgery patients[23]; and 30% in critically ill patients.[24] Another transnational prospective cohort study reported the prevalence of frailty in the intensive care unit population as 43.1%.[25] Frailty, which accounts for factors beyond age-related physiologic changes alone, is increasingly appreciated as a predictor of adverse postoperative outcomes (**Box 1**).[14,15,20]

Definition

Although frailty is widely recognized, there is lack of consensus on clinical and operational definitions of the term.[28–31] The evolving geriatric "syndrome" of frailty is described as a state of vulnerability to ongoing physiologic decline after a stressor event (eg, disease, illness, injury, surgery, changes in medication) as a consequence of cumulative decline in many physiologic systems over the course of a lifetime. Frail patients have reduced capacity to recover to their baseline health state after being exposed to a stressor (**Fig. 1**).

Table 1
Age-related organ system changes and anesthetic considerations

Organ System	Structural Changes	Functional Changes	Considerations for Anesthetic Management
Central nervous	↓ Brain volume ↓ DA, 5-HT, ACh, NE receptors ↓ Epidural space area ↓ CSF volume ↓ Number/diameter of dorsal and ventral nerve root fibers ↑ Monoamine oxidase levels ↑ Distance between Schwann cells in peripheral nerves	↓ Cerebral metabolic rate ↑ BBB permeability	↓ Ability to perform IADLs ↑ Memory decline ↑ Risk of postoperative delirium ↑ Risk of POCD ↑ Sensitivity to anesthetic agents ↑ Sensitivity to neuraxial and regional anesthesia
Cardiovascular	↓ Elastin and collagen ↓ Cardiomyocyte number ↓ Conduction fiber density ↓ SA node cell number ↑ LV hypertrophy ↑ Vascular rigidity	↓ β-adrenergic receptor response ↓ Baroreceptor sensitivity ↓ Vascular compliance ↓ Contractility ↑ Pulse pressure ↑ Endothelial dysfunction ↑ Diastolic LV dysfunction ↑ LV filling pressures ↑ MAP	↓ SV and CO ↓ Maximal HR ↑ SVR and SBP ↑ Hemodynamic instability Risk of CAD, CHF, arrhythmias, valvular disease Autonomic dysfunction: postural hypotension or cardiogenic syncope

(continued on next page)

Table 1
(continued)

Organ System	Structural Changes	Functional Changes	Considerations for Anesthetic Management
Pulmonary	↓ Respiratory muscle strength ↓ Elastic tissue ↓ Small airway diameter ↓ Surfactant production ↓ Cross-sectional surface area of pulmonary vascular bed ↑ Chest wall rigidity ↑ Central airway size ↑ Collagen	↓ Chest wall compliance ↓ Central responses to hypoxia, hypercarbia, mechanical stress, and exercise ↓ Functional alveolar surface area ↓ Vital capacity ↓ FEV$_1$ ↓ Hypoxic pulmonary vasoconstriction ↓ Protective cough/swallow ↑ Closing capacity ↑ Lung compliance ↑ Expiratory flow limitation ↑ Anatomic dead space ↑ Residual volume ↑ V/Q mismatch ↑ A-a gradient ↑ Pulmonary arterial pressure	↓ Time to desaturation ↑ Atelectasis ↑ Hypoxia, hypercarbia ↑ Sensitivity to respiratory depressants ↑ Risk of airway obstruction, bronchospasm ↑ Aspiration risk ↑ Infection risk
Gastrointestinal and hepatic	↓ Small intestine surface area ↓ Liver volume ↓ Hepatic and splanchnic blood flow	↓ Esophageal motility ↓ Gastric acid secretion ↓ Hepatic drug metabolism ↓ Synthesis of coagulation factors ↑ Gastric emptying time	↓ Speed of drug metabolism ↑ Aspiration risk ↑ Constipation ↑ Bleeding risk ↑ Drug toxicity risk
Renal	↓ Renal tissue mass ↓ Nephrons ↓ Renal blood flow	↓ GFR, creatinine clearance ↓ Ability to conserve sodium ↓ Ability to concentrate urine ↓ Thirst response ↑ Sodium retention	↓ Clearance of renally excreted medications ↑ Risk of dehydration ↑ Electrolyte (sodium) abnormalities ↑ Risk of AKI

Body composition and clinical pharmacology	↓ Skeletal muscle mass	↓ O$_2$ consumption and heat production	↑ Hypothermia
	↓ Total body water	↓ Size of central compartment	↑ Serum concentration after bolus
	↓ Lean body mass	↓ Renal and hepatic drug clearance	↑ t$_{1/2}$ of fat-soluble drugs
	↓ Albumin	↑ Volume of distribution for water soluble drugs	↑ Drug toxicity risk
	↑ Percentage of body fat	↑ Volume of distribution for lipid soluble drugs	Prolonged drug effect
	↑ α$_1$-acid glycoprotein	↑ Target organ drug sensitivity	Increased sensitivity to anesthetics
			Changes to unbound drug fraction

Abbreviations: 5-HT, serotonin; A-a, alveolar-arterial; ACh, acetylcholine; AKI, acute kidney injury; BBB, blood-brain barrier; CAD, coronary artery disease; CHF, congestive heart failure; CO, cardiac output; CSF, cerebrospinal fluid; DA, dopamine; FEV$_1$, forced expiratory volume in 1 s; GFR, glomerular filtration rate; HR, heart rate; IADLs, instrumental activities of daily living; LV, left ventricle; MAP, mean arterial pressure; NE, norepinephrine; POCD, postoperative cognitive dysfunction; SA, sinoatrial; SBP, systolic blood pressure; SV, stroke volume; SVR, systemic vascular resistance; t1/2, half-life; V/Q, ventilation/perfusion.

> **Box 1**
> **The significance of frailty**
>
> *Why does frailty matter?*
>
> Frailty increases the risk of adverse outcomes in community, inpatient, and perioperative patient populations including loss of function, falls, delirium, disability, hospitalization, and death.
>
> Therefore, diagnosis, prevention, and treatment of frailty is critical for health promotion.
>
> *Data from Refs.*[7,8,26,27]

Frail Organ Systems

The pathophysiologic basis of frailty involves several interrelated organ systems (brain, cardiovascular, respiratory, renal, endocrine, immune, skeletal), independent of age and comorbidity (**Fig. 2**):[27,32–36]

- The aging brain experiences various structural and physiologic changes. Frailty is associated with delirium,[37] cognitive impairment,[38] and dementia.[39,40]
- The neuroendocrine system is involved with metabolism through hormone mediators. Persistently high levels of cortisol are associated with increased catabolism, loss of muscle mass, anorexia, weight loss, and reduced energy

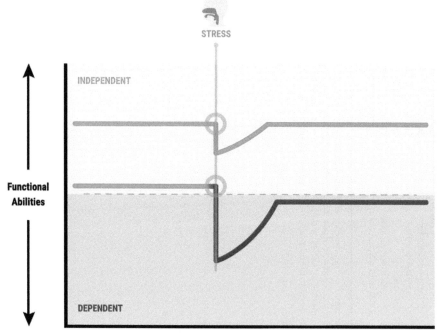

Fig. 1. Vulnerability of older adults following acute stress. The *upper green line* represents a fit older adult who is functionally independent at baseline. Following an acute stressor, such as a low-risk surgery, the fit elder decreases in his functional abilities but quickly returns to baseline independence. The *lower green* and *red line* represents a near-frail older individual who deteriorates more markedly and does not return to his prior baseline functional status after experiencing a similar stressor. (*Reprinted with permission from* Elsevier [Clegg A, Young J, Iliffe S, et al. Frailty in elderly people. Lancet 2013;381(9868):752–62.])

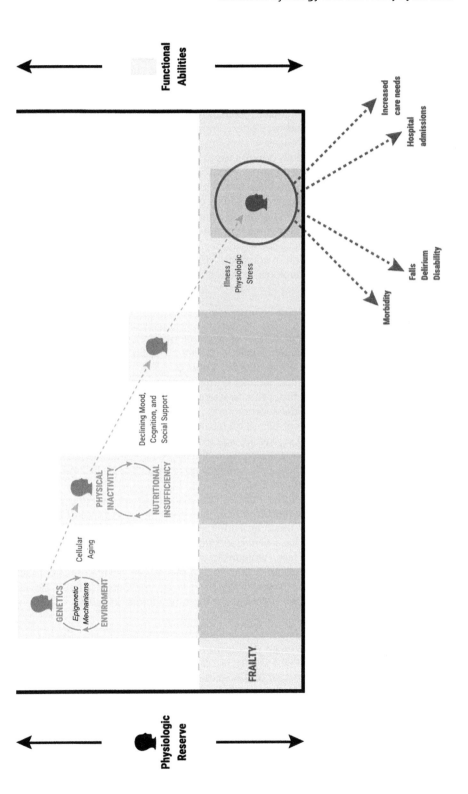

expenditure.[41,42] Frailty is independently associated with higher levels of cortisol[43] and blunted variation of diurnal cortisol concentrations.[43,44]

- The cardiovascular system undergoes structural and functional changes over time. Frailty is associated with cardiovascular morbidity and mortality[45,46] and may be a risk factor for cardiovascular disease.[47]
- The respiratory system is subject to pathology including airflow limitation and lung restriction. Frailty and respiratory impairment are associated, and risk of death is substantially increased when both are present.[36]
- The renal system significantly contributes to fluid and electrolyte balance and the excretion of waste. A systematic review noted that the incidence of frailty increased with reduced glomerular filtration rate.[48]
- Changes to the immune system caused by aging[49,50] may contribute to an inadequate response to the stress of acute inflammation.[50] An abnormal, low-grade inflammatory response contributes to the development of frailty.[51]
- The skeletal system experiences loss of muscle mass, muscle strength, and muscle power as a function of aging.[52–54] The skeletal system is linked to effective functioning of the neurologic, endocrine, and immune systems.

Models

A wide variety of frailty instruments have been developed for use in different settings (ie, research, clinical, community dwelling, facility dwelling, primary care, acute care).[23,55–64] Selected models are featured in **Table 2**.[12,36,65–77]

Comprehensive geriatric assessment is the frailty detection model most widely supported by evidence; however, the resource-intensive nature of this process prevents its widespread use in busy clinical environments.[27] Formal identification of frailty helps the clinician risk stratify a patient based on biologic age (ie, presence or absence of frailty) rather than on chronologic age (ie, age alone). Proposed instruments to measure and operationalize frailty have a basis in differing conceptual views. Two main frailty models, which have been validated against adverse outcomes in large community cohorts, have emerged (**Boxes 2 and 3**).

Box 2 describes the physical frailty phenotype, also known as the Fried Index.[7] In this model, a person is considered frail if he or she meets three or more of the listed criteria, prefrail with a score of 1 to 2, and not frail (ie, robust) with a score of 0. Frailty as measured by this definition has been associated with numerous long-term adverse outcomes including incident falls, worsening mobility or activities of daily living, disability, hospitalization, and death.[7] Criticisms of this model include: development from a secondary analysis of a prospective cohort study, the Cardiovascular Health Study,[27] and absence of other potentially important factors including cognition, mood, and social support.[56]

◄————————————————————————————

Fig. 2. Pathophysiology of frailty. Image depicts the process leading to frailty in one individual. Physiologic reserve and functional abilities are at their peak initially, but slowly begin to decline with normal aging. Additional factors, such as physical inactivity, nutritional insufficiency, and declining mood, cognition, and social support combine to hasten the decline of reserve and functional abilities. An acute physiologic stressor, such as illness or surgery, ultimately causes the patient to cross the threshold into frailty (*dashed horizontal line*). Frail individuals experience a variety of poor outcomes, including falls, delirium, and disability; increased care needs; hospital admissions; and morbidity. These sequelae, in addition to ongoing interplay among the conditions leading to frailty, may reduce physiologic reserve and functional abilities further.

Table 2
Selected frailty detection instruments for the general population

Type of Instrument	Name	Description	Reference	Population
Questionnaire, scale, screen	Clinical Frailty Scale	Clinical judgment used to determine fitness and function by domains: very fit; well; well, with treated comorbid disease; apparently vulnerable; mildly frail; moderately frail; severely frail.	Rockwood et al,[71] 2005 PMID: 16129869	Prospective cohort clinical examination of 2305 patients ≥65 y
	Edmonton Frail Scale	0–2 points assigned to multiple domains: cognition, general health status, functional independence, social support, medication use, nutrition, mood, continence, functional performance. Maximum 17 total points. Reliable and valid compared with a geriatrician's clinical assessment of frailty.	Rolfson et al,[72] 2006 PMID: 16757522	Community-based referral sample of 158 patients age ≥65 y in acute care wards, rehabilitation units, day hospitals, and outpatient clinics
	Frailty Index–Comprehensive Geriatric Assessment	Rating of 10 frailty dimensions based on clinical judgment and comorbidity: cognition, mood and motivation, communication, mobility, balance, bowel function, bladder function, IADL and ADL, nutrition, and social resources.	Jones et al,[69] 2004 PMID: 15507074	Secondary analysis of an RCT of specialized mobile geriatric assessment team evaluating participants in their homes
			Jones et al,[70] 2005 PMID: 16485864	Secondary analysis of a prospective cohort study involving clinical examinations of 2305 people
	Groningen Frailty Indicator	15-item questionnaire on 8 frailty factors: mobility, physical fitness, vision, hearing, nourishment, morbidity, cognition, psychosocial.	Schuurmans et al,[12] 2004 PMID: 15472162	Community sample of people aged ≥65 y randomly drawn from 6 municipalities

(continued on next page)

Table 2
(continued)

Type of Instrument	Name	Description	Reference	Population
	Tilburg Frailty Indicator	Self-report questionnaire in two parts: part one contains 10 questions on determinants of frailty and diseases; part two contains 3 domains (physical, psychological, social) of frailty with a total of 15 questions on components of frailty.	Gobbens et al,[75] 2010 PMID: 20511102	479 community-dwelling persons aged ≥75 y comprising 2 representative samples
	Balducci Frailty Criteria from Comprehensive Geriatric Assessment	Based on: age >85, dependence for ≥1 ADL, presence of ≥3 comorbid conditions, presence of ≥1 geriatric syndrome (dementia, delirium, depression, incontinence, falls, osteoporosis, neglect/abuse, failure to thrive).	Balducci and Beghe,[66] 2000 PMID: 10960797	Expert consensus for elderly patients with cancer categorized as fit, vulnerable, or frail; no formal validation of prognostic performance
	FRAIL Scale/ Questionnaire	Includes 5 domains: fatigue, resistance (1 flight of stairs), ambulation (1 block), illnesses (>5), loss of weight (>5%).	Morley et al,[77] 2012 PMID: 22836700	Longitudinal study of 582 African Americans aged 49–65
	Study of Osteoporotic Fractures Scale	Presence of 2 or more out of 3 frailty factors: weight loss, inability to rise from chair, reduced energy level.	Ensrud 2008[73] PMID: 18299493	Prospective cohort study of 6701 women aged ≥69 y
			Ensrud et al,[74] 2009 PMID: 19245414	Prospective cohort study of 3132 men ≥67 y
	Vulnerable Elders Survey-13	Self-report 13-item questionnaire on physical functioning.	Saliba et al,[67] 2001 PMID: 11844005	Nationally representative, longitudinal, community-based survey data of 6205 Medicare beneficiaries aged ≥65 y

Single factor assessment	Timed-up-and-go test	Patient is observed and timed while patient rises from an armchair, walks 3 m, turns, walks back, and sits down again.	Podsiadlo and Richardson,[65] 1991 PMID: 1991946	60 patients referred to a geriatric day hospital, mean age 79.5 y
	Hand grip strength test	Grip strength evaluation with dynamometer.	Syddall et al,[68] 2003 PMID: 14600007	Cross-sectional study of 717 men and women aged 64–74 y
	Pulmonary function test	Spirometry evaluating respiratory impairment (airflow limitation or restrictive pattern).	Vaz Fragoso et al,[36] 2012 PMID: 22195532	Cross-sectional study of 3578 white participants aged 65–80 y
	Gait speed	Walk distance between 8 ft and 6 m, timed.	Studenski et al,[76] 2011 PMID: 21205966	Pooled analysis of 9 cohort studies including 34,485 community-dwelling adults aged ≥65 y

Abbreviations: ADL, activities of daily living; IADL, instrumental activities of daily living; RCT, randomized controlled trial.

> **Box 2**
> **Physical phenotype model of frailty**
>
> Physical frailty phenotype (Cardiovascular Health Study Frailty Phenotype): a list of components designed to assess an individual patient, consisting of five criteria based on hypothesized signs and symptoms of frailty:
> - Weight loss: self-reported weight loss of >4.5 kg or recorded weight loss of ≥5% per year
> - Exhaustion: self-reported exhaustion on US Center for Epidemiologic Studies depression scale (3–4 days per week or most of the time)
> - Low energy expenditure: energy expenditure <383 kcal/wk (men) or <270 kcal/wk (women)
> - Slow gait speed: standardized cutoff times to walk 4.57 m, stratified by sex and height
> - Weak grip strength: grip strength, stratified by sex and body mass index
>
> *Data from* Fried LP, Tangen CM, Walston J, et al. Frailty in older adults: evidence for a phenotype. J Gerontol A Biol Sci Med Sci 2001;56(3):M146–156.

Box 3 describes the deficit accumulation model of frailty.[8,71,78,79] The original model as described by Mitnitski and coworkers[8] defined frailty based on 92 baseline variables including symptoms, signs, abnormal laboratory values, disease states, and disabilities. Subsequent models reduced the number of variables to 30 without loss of predictive validity.[80,81] Level of frailty is constructed by counting the number of deficits; with more deficits, likelihood of frailty increases. This model, therefore, allows frailty to be gradable on a scale, rather than simply present or absent. Critics of this model suggest that time pressures of a clinical setting may preclude its use given the larger number of variables[82]; however, there is potential for integration of automatically collected data, particularly with electronic records permitting a robust, valid, and comparable frailty measure, using no additional clinician time.[23,83] Another criticism is that all variables are weighted equally with the assumption that each variable contributes equally to the condition of frailty.

Frailty in the Perioperative Setting

In the geriatric population at large, assessment of risk based on frailty status has yielded important insights linking physiologic age with risk of morbidity and mortality. The potential for modifiability of frailty has generated a great amount of interest for targeting interventions and optimization of care in the perioperative setting based on frailty status. Frailty has been recently associated with a variety of postoperative complications, such as mortality,[84–89] nonroutine recovery,[90,91] delirium,[92] major adverse cardiac and cerebral events,[84] increased length of stay,[89] discharge to institution,[86] functional decline,[93,94] readmission,[89] and decline in quality of life.[88] A variety of frailty

> **Box 3**
> **Deficit accumulation model of frailty**
>
> Deficit accumulation index (Canadian Study of Health and Aging Frailty Index): frailty is the accumulation of biophysical deficits over time resulting in reduced resistance to external insults. There are no set deficits that need to be measured in a frailty index, and scales may be constructed as long as they adhere to the following criteria:
> - Variables must be deficits associated with health status
> - Deficits must generally increase with age
> - Chosen deficits must not saturate too early with age
> - The deficits that make up the frailty index must cover a range of systems
> - On serial use on the same people, the items in the frailty index must be the same
>
> *Data from* Refs.[8,71,78,79]

Table 3
Selected frailty detection instruments in the surgical population

Name	Description	Reference	Surgical Population
Comprehensive Geriatric Assessment	Multidimensional interdisciplinary diagnostic process focused on determining a frail elderly person's medical, psychological, and functional capability to develop a coordinated and integrated plan for treatment and long-term follow-up	Kristjansson et al,[90] 2010 PMID: 20005123 Lasithiotakis et al,[105] 2013 PMID: 23052539	Elective colorectal cancer Elective laparoscopic cholecystectomy
Deficit Accumulation Index/Modified Frailty Index	Compilation of individual deficits/impairments into an index incorporating variables evaluating symptoms, signs, abnormal laboratory values, disease states, disabilities; Searle 2008 criteria include: • Variables must be deficits associated with health status • Deficits must generally increase with age • Chosen deficits must not saturate too early with age • The deficits that make up the frailty index must cover a range of systems • On serial use on the same people, the items in the frailty index must be the same	Saxton and Velanovich,[102] 2011 PMID: 21412145 Farhat et al,[103] 2012 PMID: 22695416 Joseph et al,[110] 2016 PMID: 27113515 Lin et al,[112] 2017 PMID: 29137576 Sridharan et al,[118] 2018 PMID: 28689950 Wahl et al,[113] 2017 PMID: 28467535	Elective general Emergency general Emergency general surgery Intermediate to high risk Carotid endarterectomy Orthopedic, general, vascular
Physical Frailty Phenotype/ Hopkins Frailty Score	Decline in 5 domains: shrinking/weight loss, decreased grip strength/weakness, exhaustion, low physical activity, slowed walking speed	Makary et al,[9] 2010 PMID: 20510798 Revenig et al,[106] 2013 PMID: 24054409 Andreou et al,[115] 2018 PMID: 30014293	Elective surgery General, oncologic, urologic Elective general
Comprehensive Assessment of Frailty	Assessment of weakness, self-reported exhaustion, slowness of gait speed, low activity, balance assessment, albumin,	Sundermann et al,[108] 2014 PMID: 24497604	Elective cardiac

(continued on next page)

Table 3
(continued)

Name	Description	Reference	Surgical Population
	creatinine, brain natriuretic peptide, FEV₁, and Clinical Frailty Scale		
Clinical Frailty Scale	Use of clinical judgment to interpret the results of history-taking and clinical examination to determine fitness and function separated into domains of: very fit; well; well, with treated comorbid disease; apparently vulnerable; mildly frail; moderately frail; severely frail	Hewitt et al,[89] 2015 PMID: 25173599 McIsaac et al,[117] 2018 PMID: 30048320 Li et al,[116] 2018 PMID: 29565018	Emergency general surgery Elective noncardiac surgery Emergency abdominal surgery
Edmonton Frail Scale	Multifactorial scale that is quick and easy to administer	Dasgupta et al,[99] 2009 PMID: 18068828 Amabili et al,[114] 2018 PMID: 30049520	Elective noncardiac Elective cardiac
FRAIL Scale	Includes 5 domains: fatigue, resistance (1 flight of stairs), ambulation (1 block), illnesses (>5), loss of weight (>5%)	Gleason et al,[111] 2017 PMID: 28866353	Trauma
Balducci Frailty Criteria	Comprised of Cumulative Illness Rating Scale–Geriatrics, activities of daily living, polypharmacy, mini nutritional assessment, mini-mental state examination, Geriatric Depression Scale	Ommundsen et al,[87] 2014 PMID: 25355846	Elective colorectal cancer
Groningen Frailty Indicator	15-item questionnaire on 8 frailty factors: mobility, physical fitness, vision, hearing, nourishment, morbidity, cognition, psychosocial	Tegels et al,[109] 2014 PMID: 24420730	Elective gastric cancer
Gait speed	Slow gait speed defined as a time taken to walk 5 m of ≥6 s	Afilalo et al,[100] 2010 PMID: 21050978	Cardiac
Timed-up-and-go test	Stand from chair, walk 10 ft, return to chair, sit down; fast ≤10 s, intermediate 11–14 s, slow ≥15 s	Robinson et al,[107] 2013 PMID: 23979272	Elective colorectal and cardiac
Skeletal muscle mass	Muscle mass assessed by computed tomography or total psoas area	Lee et al,[101] 2011 PMID: 21215580 Peng et al,[104] 2012 PMID: 22692586	Elective open AAA Pancreatic

Abbreviations: AAA, abdominal aortic aneurysm; FEV₁, forced expiratory volume in 1 s.

instruments have been identified for use in surgical populations to evaluate postoperative adverse outcomes and surgical risk.[22,23,95–98] Selected instruments are described in **Table 3**.[3,9,87,89,90,99–118]

Unfortunately, an ideal tool, which would provide a highly specific comprehensive patient assessment, but would also be feasible to use in the time-, space-, and resource-pressured perioperative environment, has not yet been identified. These constraints have prevented consensus around a particular frailty instrument for use in surgical patients. An effective frailty tool may assist patients and clinicians with perioperative informed consent, decision-making, and management whether used in a surgical clinic, anesthesia preoperative clinic, preoperative holding area, inpatient setting, or emergency department. Additional research may help identify the best frailty tool, or different frailty tools for different type of surgeries and patients, for the perioperative environment.

Interventions

Prevention or reduction of frailty may improve health outcomes; however, there are sparse data on proven interventions for modification of outcomes in frail patients.[119,120] In a Cochrane Review, inpatient comprehensive geriatric assessment for frail patients has increased the likelihood of returning home, decreased the likelihood of cognitive or functional decline, and decreased in-hospital mortality rates.[119] Exercise may prove beneficial for frail elderly in terms of muscle strength and functional ability.[121–123] There remains insufficient evidence for exercise intensity, sustained improvement, and cost-effectiveness. The effect of "prehabilitation" before elective surgery in frail patients has been studied. Although more study is needed, some preliminary results have been encouraging.[124,125]

SUMMARY

Surgical patients are getting older, and more often present with increasing quantity and severity of comorbid illness. Understanding geriatric physiology is critical for successful perioperative management of older surgical patients. Furthermore, the frailty syndrome is evolving as an important, potentially modifiable process capturing a patient's biologic age, which accounts for additive physiologic insults occurring over the course of a patient's lifetime, and is more predictive of adverse perioperative outcomes than simply chronologic age. Use of frailty in risk stratification and perioperative decision-making allows providers to effectively diagnose, risk stratify, prevent, and treat patients in the perioperative setting. Frailty will likely play an increasing role in discussions with patients, families, and health care providers around issues of perioperative optimization, prognosis, informed consent, and advanced directives. Further study is needed to develop a universal definition of frailty, to identify comprehensive yet feasible screening tools that allow for the accurate detection of frailty in the perioperative setting, and to refine treatment programs for frail surgical patients.

REFERENCES

1. Dall TM, Gallo PD, Chakrabarti R, et al. An aging population and growing disease burden will require a large and specialized health care workforce by 2025. Health Aff (Millwood) 2013;32(11):2013–20.
2. Turrentine FE, Wang H, Simpson VB, et al. Surgical risk factors, morbidity, and mortality in elderly patients. J Am Coll Surg 2006;203(6):865–77.
3. Finlayson E, Zhao S, Boscardin WJ, et al. Functional status after colon cancer surgery in elderly nursing home residents. J Am Geriatr Soc 2012;60(5):967–73.

4. Mohanty S, Liu Y, Paruch JL, et al. Risk of discharge to postacute care: a patient-centered outcome for the American College of Surgeons national surgical quality improvement program surgical risk calculator. JAMA Surg 2015; 150(5):480–4.

5. Berian JR, Mohanty S, Ko CY, et al. Association of loss of independence with readmission and death after discharge in older patients after surgical procedures. JAMA Surg 2016;151(9):e161689.

6. Robinson TN, Berian JR. Incorporating patient-centered outcomes into surgical care. Ann Surg 2017;265(4):654–5.

7. Fried LP, Tangen CM, Walston J, et al. Frailty in older adults: evidence for a phenotype. J Gerontol A Biol Sci Med Sci 2001;56(3):M146–56.

8. Mitnitski AB, Mogilner AJ, Rockwood K. Accumulation of deficits as a proxy measure of aging. ScientificWorldJournal 2001;1:323–36.

9. Makary MA, Segev DL, Pronovost PJ, et al. Frailty as a predictor of surgical outcomes in older patients. J Am Coll Surg 2010;210(6):901–8.

10. Beggs T, Sepehri A, Szwajcer A, et al. Frailty and perioperative outcomes: a narrative review. Can J Anaesth 2015;62(2):143–57.

11. Hall DE, Arya S, Schmid KK, et al. Development and initial validation of the risk analysis index for measuring frailty in surgical populations. JAMA Surg 2017; 152(2):175–82.

12. Schuurmans H, Steverink N, Lindenberg S, et al. Old or frail: what tells us more? J Gerontol A Biol Sci Med Sci 2004;59(9):M962–5.

13. Alvis BD, Hughes CG. Physiology considerations in geriatric patients. Anesthesiol Clin 2015;33(3):447–56.

14. Miller RD, Pardo M, Stoelting RK. Basics of anesthesia. 6th edition. Philadelphia: Elsevier/Saunders; 2011.

15. Partridge JS, Harari D, Dhesi JK. Frailty in the older surgical patient: a review. Age Ageing 2012;41(2):142–7.

16. Oresanya LB, Lyons WL, Finlayson E. Preoperative assessment of the older patient: a narrative review. JAMA 2014;311(20):2110–20.

17. Tonner PH, Kampen J, Scholz J. Pathophysiological changes in the elderly. Best Pract Res Clin Anaesthesiol 2003;17(2):163–77.

18. Colloca G, Santoro M, Gambassi G. Age-related physiologic changes and perioperative management of elderly patients. Surg Oncol 2010;19(3):124–30.

19. Miller RD. Miller's anesthesia. 8th edition. Philadelphia: Elsevier/Saunders; 2015.

20. Joseph B, Pandit V, Sadoun M, et al. Frailty in surgery. J Trauma Acute Care Surg 2014;76(4):1151–6.

21. Collard RM, Boter H, Schoevers RA, et al. Prevalence of frailty in community-dwelling older persons: a systematic review. J Am Geriatr Soc 2012;60(8): 1487–92.

22. Hewitt J, Long S, Carter B, Bach S, McCarthy K, Clegg A. The prevalence of frailty and its association with clinical outcomes in general surgery: a systematic review and meta-analysis. Age Ageing 2018;47(6):793–800.

23. Darvall JN, Gregorevic KJ, Story DA, et al. Frailty indexes in perioperative and critical care: a systematic review. Arch Gerontol Geriatr 2018;79:88–96.

24. Muscedere J, Waters B, Varambally A, et al. The impact of frailty on intensive care unit outcomes: a systematic review and meta-analysis. Intensive Care Med 2017;43(8):1105–22.

25. Flaatten H, De Lange DW, Morandi A, et al. The impact of frailty on ICU and 30-day mortality and the level of care in very elderly patients (/= 80 years). Intensive Care Med 2017;43(12):1820–8.

26. Xue QL. The frailty syndrome: definition and natural history. Clin Geriatr Med 2011;27(1):1–15.
27. Clegg A, Young J, Iliffe S, et al. Frailty in elderly people. Lancet 2013;381(9868): 752–62.
28. Gobbens RJ, Luijkx KG, Wijnen-Sponselee MT, et al. In search of an integral conceptual definition of frailty: opinions of experts. J Am Med Dir Assoc 2010; 11(5):338–43.
29. Morley JE, Vellas B, van Kan GA, et al. Frailty consensus: a call to action. J Am Med Dir Assoc 2013;14(6):392–7.
30. Rodriguez-Manas L, Feart C, Mann G, et al. Searching for an operational definition of frailty: a Delphi method based consensus statement: the frailty operative definition-consensus conference project. J Gerontol A Biol Sci Med Sci 2013; 68(1):62–7.
31. Soong JT, Poots AJ, Bell D. Finding consensus on frailty assessment in acute care through Delphi method. BMJ Open 2016;6(10):e012904.
32. Walston J, Hadley EC, Ferrucci L, et al. Research agenda for frailty in older adults: toward a better understanding of physiology and etiology: summary from the American Geriatrics Society/National Institute on Aging Research Conference on Frailty in Older Adults. J Am Geriatr Soc 2006;54(6):991–1001.
33. Afilalo J, Karunananthan S, Eisenberg MJ, et al. Role of frailty in patients with cardiovascular disease. Am J Cardiol 2009;103(11):1616–21.
34. Fried LP, Xue QL, Cappola AR, et al. Nonlinear multisystem physiological dysregulation associated with frailty in older women: implications for etiology and treatment. J Gerontol A Biol Sci Med Sci 2009;64(10):1049–57.
35. Abadir PM. The frail renin-angiotensin system. Clin Geriatr Med 2011;27(1): 53–65.
36. Vaz Fragoso CA, Enright PL, McAvay G, et al. Frailty and respiratory impairment in older persons. Am J Med 2012;125(1):79–86.
37. Eeles EM, White SV, O'Mahony SM, et al. The impact of frailty and delirium on mortality in older inpatients. Age Ageing 2012;41(3):412–6.
38. Boyle PA, Buchman AS, Wilson RS, et al. Physical frailty is associated with incident mild cognitive impairment in community-based older persons. J Am Geriatr Soc 2010;58(2):248–55.
39. Buchman AS, Boyle PA, Wilson RS, et al. Frailty is associated with incident Alzheimer's disease and cognitive decline in the elderly. Psychosom Med 2007; 69(5):483–9.
40. Song X, Mitnitski A, Rockwood K. Nontraditional risk factors combine to predict Alzheimer disease and dementia. Neurology 2011;77(3):227–34.
41. Attaix D, Mosoni L, Dardevet D, et al. Altered responses in skeletal muscle protein turnover during aging in anabolic and catabolic periods. Int J Biochem Cell Biol 2005;37(10):1962–73.
42. Menconi M, Fareed M, O'Neal P, et al. Role of glucocorticoids in the molecular regulation of muscle wasting. Crit Care Med 2007;35(9 Suppl):S602–8.
43. Varadhan R, Walston J, Cappola AR, et al. Higher levels and blunted diurnal variation of cortisol in frail older women. J Gerontol A Biol Sci Med Sci 2008; 63(2):190–5.
44. Johar H, Emeny RT, Bidlingmaier M, et al. Blunted diurnal cortisol pattern is associated with frailty: a cross-sectional study of 745 participants aged 65 to 90 years. J Clin Endocrinol Metab 2014;99(3):E464–8.
45. Afilalo J. Frailty in patients with cardiovascular disease: why, when, and how to measure. Curr Cardiovasc Risk Rep 2011;5(5):467–72.

46. Afilalo J, Alexander KP, Mack MJ, et al. Frailty assessment in the cardiovascular care of older adults. J Am Coll Cardiol 2014;63(8):747–62.

47. Veronese N, Cereda E, Stubbs B, et al. Risk of cardiovascular disease morbidity and mortality in frail and pre-frail older adults: results from a meta-analysis and exploratory meta-regression analysis. Ageing Res Rev 2017;35:63–73.

48. Chowdhury R, Peel NM, Krosch M, et al. Frailty and chronic kidney disease: a systematic review. Arch Gerontol Geriatr 2017;68:135–42.

49. Miller RA. The aging immune system: primer and prospectus. Science 1996; 273(5271):70–4.

50. Sahin E, Depinho RA. Linking functional decline of telomeres, mitochondria and stem cells during ageing. Nature 2010;464(7288):520–8.

51. Soysal P, Stubbs B, Lucato P, et al. Inflammation and frailty in the elderly: a systematic review and meta-analysis. Ageing Res Rev 2016;31:1–8.

52. Howard C, Ferrucci L, Sun K, et al. Oxidative protein damage is associated with poor grip strength among older women living in the community. J Appl Physiol (1985) 2007;103(1):17–20.

53. Cruz-Jentoft AJ, Baeyens JP, Bauer JM, et al. Sarcopenia: European consensus on definition and diagnosis: report of the European Working Group on Sarcopenia in Older People. Age Ageing 2010;39(4):412–23.

54. Manini TM, Clark BC. Dynapenia and aging: an update. J Gerontol A Biol Sci Med Sci 2012;67(1):28–40.

55. Sternberg SA, Wershof Schwartz A, Karunananthan S, et al. The identification of frailty: a systematic literature review. J Am Geriatr Soc 2011;59(11):2129–38.

56. de Vries NM, Staal JB, van Ravensberg CD, et al. Outcome instruments to measure frailty: a systematic review. Ageing Res Rev 2011;10(1):104–14.

57. Hoogendijk EO, van der Horst HE, Deeg DJ, et al. The identification of frail older adults in primary care: comparing the accuracy of five simple instruments. Age Ageing 2013;42(2):262–5.

58. Clegg A, Rogers L, Young J. Diagnostic test accuracy of simple instruments for identifying frailty in community-dwelling older people: a systematic review. Age Ageing 2015;44(1):148–52.

59. Buta BJ, Walston JD, Godino JG, et al. Frailty assessment instruments: systematic characterization of the uses and contexts of highly-cited instruments. Ageing Res Rev 2016;26:53–61.

60. McIsaac DI, Taljaard M, Bryson GL, et al. Comparative assessment of two frailty instruments for risk-stratification in elderly surgical patients: study protocol for a prospective cohort study. BMC Anesthesiol 2016;16(1):111.

61. O'Neill BR, Batterham AM, Hollingsworth AC, et al. Do first impressions count? Frailty judged by initial clinical impression predicts medium-term mortality in vascular surgical patients. Anaesthesia 2016;71(6):684–91.

62. Ambagtsheer R, Visvanathan R, Cesari M, et al. Feasibility, acceptability and diagnostic test accuracy of frailty screening instruments in community-dwelling older people within the Australian general practice setting: a study protocol for a cross-sectional study. BMJ Open 2017;7(8):e016663.

63. Apostolo J, Cooke R, Bobrowicz-Campos E, et al. Predicting risk and outcomes for frail older adults: an umbrella review of frailty screening tools. JBI Database Syst Rev Implement Rep 2017;15(4):1154–208.

64. Sadiq F, Kronzer VL, Wildes TS, et al. Frailty phenotypes and relations with surgical outcomes: a latent class analysis. Anesth Analg 2018;127(4):1017–27.

65. Podsiadlo D, Richardson S. The timed "Up & Go": a test of basic functional mobility for frail elderly persons. J Am Geriatr Soc 1991;39(2):142–8.

66. Balducci L, Beghe C. The application of the principles of geriatrics to the management of the older person with cancer. Crit Rev Oncol Hematol 2000;35(3): 147–54.

67. Saliba D, Elliott M, Rubenstein LZ, et al. The Vulnerable Elders Survey: a tool for identifying vulnerable older people in the community. J Am Geriatr Soc 2001; 49(12):1691–9.

68. Syddall H, Cooper C, Martin F, et al. Is grip strength a useful single marker of frailty? Age Ageing 2003;32(6):650–6.

69. Jones DM, Song X, Rockwood K. Operationalizing a frailty index from a standardized comprehensive geriatric assessment. J Am Geriatr Soc 2004;52(11): 1929–33.

70. Jones D, Song X, Mitnitski A, et al. Evaluation of a frailty index based on a comprehensive geriatric assessment in a population based study of elderly Canadians. Aging Clin Exp Res 2005;17(6):465–71.

71. Rockwood K, Song X, MacKnight C, et al. A global clinical measure of fitness and frailty in elderly people. CMAJ 2005;173(5):489–95.

72. Rolfson DB, Majumdar SR, Tsuyuki RT, et al. Validity and reliability of the Edmonton Frail Scale. Age Ageing 2006;35(5):526–9.

73. Ensrud KE, Ewing SK, Taylor BC, et al. Comparison of 2 frailty indexes for prediction of falls, disability, fractures, and death in older women. Arch Intern Med 2008;168(4):382–9.

74. Ensrud KE, Ewing SK, Cawthon PM, et al. A comparison of frailty indexes for the prediction of falls, disability, fractures, and mortality in older men. J Am Geriatr Soc 2009;57(3):492–8.

75. Gobbens RJ, van Assen MA, Luijkx KG, et al. The Tilburg Frailty Indicator: psychometric properties. J Am Med Dir Assoc 2010;11(5):344–55.

76. Studenski S, Perera S, Patel K, et al. Gait speed and survival in older adults. JAMA 2011;305(1):50–8.

77. Morley JE, Malmstrom TK, Miller DK. A simple frailty questionnaire (FRAIL) predicts outcomes in middle aged African Americans. J Nutr Health Aging 2012; 16(7):601–8.

78. Mitnitski AB, Song X, Rockwood K. The estimation of relative fitness and frailty in community-dwelling older adults using self-report data. J Gerontol A Biol Sci Med Sci 2004;59(6):M627–32.

79. Searle SD, Mitnitski A, Gahbauer EA, et al. A standard procedure for creating a frailty index. BMC Geriatr 2008;8:24.

80. Mitnitski A, Song X, Skoog I, et al. Relative fitness and frailty of elderly men and women in developed countries and their relationship with mortality. J Am Geriatr Soc 2005;53(12):2184–9.

81. Song X, Mitnitski A, Rockwood K. Prevalence and 10-year outcomes of frailty in older adults in relation to deficit accumulation. J Am Geriatr Soc 2010;58(4): 681–7.

82. Cesari M, Gambassi G, van Kan GA, et al. The frailty phenotype and the frailty index: different instruments for different purposes. Age Ageing 2014;43(1):10–2.

83. Hubbard RE, Peel NM, Samanta M, et al. Derivation of a frailty index from the interRAI acute care instrument. BMC Geriatr 2015;15:27.

84. Stortecky S, Schoenenberger AW, Moser A, et al. Evaluation of multidimensional geriatric assessment as a predictor of mortality and cardiovascular events after transcatheter aortic valve implantation. JACC Cardiovasc Interv 2012;5(5): 489–96.

85. Neuman HB, Weiss JM, Leverson G, et al. Predictors of short-term postoperative survival after elective colectomy in colon cancer patients >/= 80 years of age. Ann Surg Oncol 2013;20(5):1427–35.
86. Kim SW, Han HS, Jung HW, et al. Multidimensional frailty score for the prediction of postoperative mortality risk. JAMA Surg 2014;149(7):633–40.
87. Ommundsen N, Wyller TB, Nesbakken A, et al. Frailty is an independent predictor of survival in older patients with colorectal cancer. Oncologist 2014;19(12):1268–75.
88. Green P, Arnold SV, Cohen DJ, et al. Relation of frailty to outcomes after transcatheter aortic valve replacement (from the PARTNER trial). Am J Cardiol 2015;116(2):264–9.
89. Hewitt J, Moug SJ, Middleton M, et al. Prevalence of frailty and its association with mortality in general surgery. Am J Surg 2015;209(2):254–9.
90. Kristjansson SR, Nesbakken A, Jordhoy MS, et al. Comprehensive geriatric assessment can predict complications in elderly patients after elective surgery for colorectal cancer: a prospective observational cohort study. Crit Rev Oncol Hematol 2010;76(3):208–17.
91. Kenig J, Zychiewicz B, Olszewska U, et al. Six screening instruments for frailty in older patients qualified for emergency abdominal surgery. Arch Gerontol Geriatr 2015;61(3):437–42.
92. Persico I, Cesari M, Morandi A, et al. Frailty and delirium in older adults: a systematic review and meta-analysis of the literature. J Am Geriatr Soc 2018;66(10):2022–30.
93. Schoenenberger AW, Stortecky S, Neumann S, et al. Predictors of functional decline in elderly patients undergoing transcatheter aortic valve implantation (TAVI). Eur Heart J 2013;34(9):684–92.
94. Partridge JS, Fuller M, Harari D, et al. Frailty and poor functional status are common in arterial vascular surgical patients and affect postoperative outcomes. Int J Surg 2015;18:57–63.
95. Sepehri A, Beggs T, Hassan A, et al. The impact of frailty on outcomes after cardiac surgery: a systematic review. J Thorac Cardiovasc Surg 2014;148(6):3110–7.
96. Lin HS, Watts JN, Peel NM, et al. Frailty and post-operative outcomes in older surgical patients: a systematic review. BMC Geriatr 2016;16(1):157.
97. Oakland K, Nadler R, Cresswell L, et al. Systematic review and meta-analysis of the association between frailty and outcome in surgical patients. Ann R Coll Surg Engl 2016;98(2):80–5.
98. Watt J, Tricco AC, Talbot-Hamon C, et al. Identifying older adults at risk of harm following elective surgery: a systematic review and meta-analysis. BMC Med 2018;16(1):2.
99. Dasgupta M, Rolfson DB, Stolee P, et al. Frailty is associated with postoperative complications in older adults with medical problems. Arch Gerontol Geriatr 2009;48(1):78–83.
100. Afilalo J, Eisenberg MJ, Morin JF, et al. Gait speed as an incremental predictor of mortality and major morbidity in elderly patients undergoing cardiac surgery. J Am Coll Cardiol 2010;56(20):1668–76.
101. Lee JS, He K, Harbaugh CM, et al. Frailty, core muscle size, and mortality in patients undergoing open abdominal aortic aneurysm repair. J Vasc Surg 2011;53(4):912–7.
102. Saxton A, Velanovich V. Preoperative frailty and quality of life as predictors of postoperative complications. Ann Surg 2011;253(6):1223–9.

103. Farhat JS, Velanovich V, Falvo AJ, et al. Are the frail destined to fail? Frailty index as predictor of surgical morbidity and mortality in the elderly. J Trauma Acute Care Surg 2012;72(6):1526–30 [discussion: 1530–1].

104. Peng P, Hyder O, Firoozmand A, et al. Impact of sarcopenia on outcomes following resection of pancreatic adenocarcinoma. J Gastrointest Surg 2012; 16(8):1478–86.

105. Lasithiotakis K, Petrakis J, Venianaki M, et al. Frailty predicts outcome of elective laparoscopic cholecystectomy in geriatric patients. Surg Endosc 2013;27(4): 1144–50.

106. Revenig LM, Canter DJ, Taylor MD, et al. Too frail for surgery? Initial results of a large multidisciplinary prospective study examining preoperative variables predictive of poor surgical outcomes. J Am Coll Surg 2013;217(4):665–70.e1.

107. Robinson TN, Wu DS, Sauaia A, et al. Slower walking speed forecasts increased postoperative morbidity and 1-year mortality across surgical specialties. Ann Surg 2013;258(4):582–8 [discussion: 588–90].

108. Sundermann SH, Dademasch A, Seifert B, et al. Frailty is a predictor of short- and mid-term mortality after elective cardiac surgery independently of age. Interact Cardiovasc Thorac Surg 2014;18(5):580–5.

109. Tegels JJ, de Maat MF, Hulsewe KW, Hoofwijk AG, Stoot JH. Value of geriatric frailty and nutritional status assessment in predicting postoperative mortality in gastric cancer surgery. J Gastrointest Surg 2014;18(3):439–45 [discussion: 445–6].

110. Joseph B, Zangbar B, Pandit V, et al. Emergency general surgery in the elderly: too old or too frail? J Am Coll Surg 2016;222(5):805–13.

111. Gleason LJ, Benton EA, Alvarez-Nebreda ML, et al. FRAIL questionnaire screening tool and short-term outcomes in geriatric fracture patients. J Am Med Dir Assoc 2017;18(12):1082–6.

112. Lin H, Peel NM, Scott IA, et al. Perioperative assessment of older surgical patients using a frailty index-feasibility and association with adverse postoperative outcomes. Anaesth Intensive Care 2017;45(6):676–82.

113. Wahl TS, Graham LA, Hawn MT, et al. Association of the modified frailty index with 30-day surgical readmission. JAMA Surg 2017;152(8):749–57.

114. Amabili P, Wozolek A, Noirot I, et al. The Edmonton frail scale improves the prediction of 30-day mortality in elderly patients undergoing cardiac surgery: a prospective observational study. J Cardiothorac Vasc Anesth 2019;33(4):945–52.

115. Andreou A, Lasithiotakis K, Venianaki M, et al. A comparison of two preoperative frailty models in predicting postoperative outcomes in geriatric general surgical patients. World J Surg 2018;42(12):3897–902.

116. Li Y, Pederson JL, Churchill TA, et al. Impact of frailty on outcomes after discharge in older surgical patients: a prospective cohort study. CMAJ 2018; 190(7):E184–90.

117. McIsaac DI, Taljaard M, Bryson GL, et al. Frailty as a predictor of death or new disability after surgery: a prospective cohort study. Ann Surg 2018. [Epub ahead of print].

118. Sridharan ND, Chaer RA, Wu BB, et al. An accumulated deficits model predicts perioperative and long-term adverse events after carotid endarterectomy. Ann Vasc Surg 2018;46:97–103.

119. Ellis G, Whitehead MA, O'Neill D, Langhorne P, Robinson D. Comprehensive geriatric assessment for older adults admitted to hospital. Cochrane Database Syst Rev 2011;(7):CD006211.

120. Fairhall N, Langron C, Sherrington C, et al. Treating frailty: a practical guide. BMC Med 2011;9:83.
121. Fiatarone MA, O'Neill EF, Ryan ND, et al. Exercise training and nutritional supplementation for physical frailty in very elderly people. N Engl J Med 1994; 330(25):1769–75.
122. Forster A, Lambley R, Hardy J, et al. Rehabilitation for older people in long-term care. Cochrane Database Syst Rev 2009;(1):CD004294.
123. de Vries NM, van Ravensberg CD, Hobbelen JS, et al. Effects of physical exercise therapy on mobility, physical functioning, physical activity and quality of life in community-dwelling older adults with impaired mobility, physical disability and/or multi-morbidity: a meta-analysis. Ageing Res Rev 2012;11(1):136–49.
124. Swank AM, Kachelman JB, Bibeau W, et al. Prehabilitation before total knee arthroplasty increases strength and function in older adults with severe osteoarthritis. J Strength Cond Res 2011;25(2):318–25.
125. Gillis C, Li C, Lee L, et al. Prehabilitation versus rehabilitation: a randomized control trial in patients undergoing colorectal resection for cancer. Anesthesiology 2014;121(5):937–47.

Geriatric Pharmacology
An Update

Tate M. Andres, MD[a],*, Tracy McGrane, MD, MPH[b],
Matthew D. McEvoy, MD[c], Brian F.S. Allen, MD[d]

KEYWORDS

- Geriatric • Elderly • Aging • Pharmacology • Physiology • Anesthesiology
- Pharmacokinetic • Pharmacodynamic

KEY POINTS

- An aging worldwide population demands that anesthesiologists consider geriatrics a unique subset of patients requiring customization of practice.
- The physiology of elderly patients causes pharmacokinetic and pharmacodynamic changes that must be taken into consideration when planning and providing anesthetic care.
- The dosing of most commonly used anesthetic and analgesic agents must be adjusted for the safe practice and care of elderly patients.
- Because many rigorous studies often exclude geriatric patients from research populations, the establishment of best practices for the elderly deserves ongoing special attention and investigation.

INTRODUCTION

The geriatric population (>65 years) is growing much faster than the population as a whole, with projections of more than 100 million people greater than 65 years old in the United States population by the year 2060.[1] The number of adults aged 65 or older

Disclosure Statement: M.D. McEvoy: GE Foundation—funding for education research unrelated to this article; Cheetah Medical—funding for research unrelated to this article; and Edwards Lifesciences—funding for research unrelated to this article. All other authors have nothing to disclose.
[a] Department of Anesthesiology, Vanderbilt University Medical Center, 1301 Medical Center Drive, 4648 TVC, Nashville, TN, USA; [b] Division of Anesthesiology Critical Care Medicine, Department of Anesthesiology, Vanderbilt University Medical Center, 1301 Medical Center Drive, 4648 TVC, Nashville, TN 37232, USA; [c] Perioperative Consult Service, Division of Multi-specialty Anesthesiology, Department of Anesthesiology, Vanderbilt University Medical Center, 1301 Medical Center Drive, 4648 TVC, Nashville, TN 37232, USA; [d] Regional and Acute Pain Medicine Fellowship, Regional and Acute Pain Medicine Service, Division of Multispecialty Anesthesiology, Department of Anesthesiology, Vanderbilt University Medical Center, 1301 Medical Center Drive, 4648 TVC, Nashville, TN 37232, USA
* Corresponding author.
E-mail address: tate.m.andres.1@vumc.org

Anesthesiology Clin 37 (2019) 475–492
https://doi.org/10.1016/j.anclin.2019.04.007
1932-2275/19/© 2019 Elsevier Inc. All rights reserved.
anesthesiology.theclinics.com

is expected to exceed half of the US population by the year 2020,[2] and likewise these patients are expected to represent a greater fraction of surgical patients with each coming year. Older adults already represent a majority of the surgical patient population for such specialties as cardiac surgery and ophthalmology.[2] Simultaneously, the elderly population is at greatest risk of morbidity and mortality with any given complication after surgery.[3,4] This magnifies the importance of tailored care for these patients by all providers involved in the surgical process, including anesthesiologists. It is well known that older adults require less anesthetic than their younger counterparts, a phenomenon largely attributable to declining organ function and reserve, including alterations in medication response due to pharmacokinetic (PK) and pharmacodynamic (PD) changes. The mechanisms underlying these changes should be well understood by all anesthesiologists in order to provide the safest care for older adults undergoing surgery.

PKs describes the manner in which the body affects a drug, whereas PDs describes the manner in which the drug affects the body. The specific PK and PD changes associated with aging include changes related to reduced end-organ function, receptor sensitivity, homeostasis patterns, concurrent medication use, and complexity of concomitant disease states. Changes in organ system function, body composition, nutritional state, and a lifetime of metabolic insults, including changes to DNA processing, can occur with wide variation between older patients. Such variety serves to complicate the effort to understand how drug activity changes with age.[5,6] Furthermore, older adults often are excluded from clinical trials due to comorbidity, despite their increased use of medication relative to other populations.[6,7]

Inadequate understanding of pharmacologic changes in geriatric patients undergoing anesthesia unfortunately is common and can have disastrous consequences. Since the advent of modern anesthesiology, however, great strides have been made in understanding how drug absorption, distribution, activity, and elimination change with age. This article discusses the major PK and PD changes associated with aging; the PD changes that occur in the neurologic, respiratory, and cardiovascular systems with aging for the most common anesthetics in use today also are covered. The final section discusses the PK and PD changes associated with aging and gives practical recommendations regarding the clinical applications of these principles with commonly used anesthetic medications.

PHARMACOKINETIC CHANGES IN THE ELDERLY
Drug Absorption

There are substantial changes in the aging gastrointestinal (GI) tract that have an impact on uptake and absorption of orally administered medications. Transmucosal absorption of medications seems preserved, as demonstrated in a study of transmucosal fentanyl administration in young and old patients without apparent difference in the incidence of negative side effects.[8] More substantial research has been directed toward changes in the stomach and distal GI tract. Commonly observed decreases in gastric acid secretion with resultant elevated gastric pH in the elderly can reduce absorption of medications that rely on ionization within the stomach for proper absorption distally. Furthermore, use of proton-pump inhibitors and antacids can interfere with drug ionization.[6,9–11] The stomach's role in absorption can be altered further by changes in gastric motility and transit time; slower gastric emptying time, decreased peristalsis, and slower colonic transit overall can be attributed to a loss of neuronal activity in the GI tract.[6,12,13] Conversely, gastric emptying time may be increased in elderly patients due to a history of partial gastrectomy or use of laxatives or cholinergic agents, such as physostigmine. Increased or decreased gastric emptying can have variable impacts on drug absorption depending on a given drug's site of absorption.[10,14] Additionally, decreases in gastric blood flow, whether from chronic vascular disease or another cause, may play a role in preventing effective drug ionization and uptake.[9–11]

More distally, decreased peristalsis and slower colonic transit time due to neuron loss or other concomitant disease can have a further impact on drug absorption. Prolonged exposure of the digestive tract to medications or failure to efficiently deliver compounds to the site of absorption may be of greatest consequence when considering medications with low solubility or permeability.[6,12,13] In conjunction with these changes to the proximal GI tract, the peak concentration of a medication as well as the time it takes to reach it may be widely variable in older patients with multiple comorbidities. The ultimate bioavailability of orally administered drugs is influenced by the amount of drug absorbed by the GI mucosa, the amount of drug that flows unchanged to the liver, and the amount of first-pass metabolism that occurs. Hepatic mass may decrease as much as 25% to 35% with age, and flow may decrease as much as 35% to 40%[15,16]; however, in the absence of concomitant disease, the structure of the liver and its synthetic function seem preserved with age and the extent to which liver mass and blood flow have an impact on first-pass metabolism remains unclear.[7] Understanding the liver's role in drug bioavailability is complicated further by the variability in cytochrome p pathways and the large number of drugs that interact with them. Further research into how each of these pathways is affected with age is required for a better understanding of medication-specific changes in the elderly.

Drug absorption through other administration methods also seems impacted by age. Older adults were found more vulnerable to the side effects of transdermal fentanyl than younger subjects.[17] Although the enhanced vulnerability of the elderly to narcotics likely is attributable to multiple physiologic changes, older adults experience thinning of the epidermis and structural weakening of the dermis that may alter and likely augment transdermal drug absorption.[18–20]

Older adults are also known to be more vulnerable to the effects of inhaled anesthetics, and the decreased minimum alveolar concentration (MAC) of inhaled anesthetics in the elderly has been widely accepted.[21] Lung physiology has been researched extensively and changes dramatically with age. Older patients demonstrate reduced airway elasticity, which can be enhanced by chronic smoking, as well as decreased chest wall compliance due to intervertebral disk height loss, ossification of costal cartilage, and weakening of respiratory muscles. These changes contribute to an overall profile of decreased tidal volume, loss of functional residual capacity, increased closing capacity, and ventilation/perfusion mismatch.[22,23] These changes reduce the efficiency of gas exchange across the alveolar membrane, likely translating to altered translocation of inhaled anesthetics impacting both induction and emergence. The uptake and offloading of inhaled anesthetics also are particularly vulnerable to acute changes in cardiac function. This has been observed in cases of significant and sudden drops in cardiac output correlated with dramatic increases in end-tidal volatile anesthetic, likely due to enhanced uptake of the anesthetic due to slower transit times through the pulmonary vasculature.[24] Although a full review of the cardiac changes with age is outside of the scope of this section, significant changes to cardiac output and flow through the pulmonary vasculature are common in elderly patients and affect uptake and offloading of volatile anesthetics.

Drug Distribution

Older adults experience clinically significant change in their volume of distribution due to a few key physiologic changes. Total body water decreases by 10% to 15% in elderly compared with younger persons.[25] This effectively decreases the volume of distribution for hydrophilic agents in elderly persons and, therefore, water-soluble drugs have higher peak plasma concentrations at a given dose compared with younger patients. Decreases in parenteral loading doses of 10% to 20% are recommended in older adults.[6,15] Although total body water decreases with age, there is an increased volume of distribution of lipophilic drugs due a combination of muscle wasting and increase in body fat, in particular central adiposity and visceral body fat with aging.[26,27] Body fat in older adults has been shown to increase up to 20% to 40%. Dosing for the parenteral loading of highly lipophilic drugs may be increased by approximately 10% to 20%.[6,15] Lipophilic drugs, however, have an increased elimination half-life and thus lead to drug accumulation.

Age-related changes in protein binding have been studied extensively. The pH of the drug and the protein binding should be taken into consideration when determining dosing adjustments in elderly patients. One notable change includes a linear decrease in serum albumin levels with increasing age. This decrease in serum albumin predominately affects highly protein-bound, acidic drugs because they more commonly bind albumin.[11] Even when there is a small reduction in the protein binding of extensively bound drugs, this may result in a clinically significant increase in free drug concentration.[11] There also is a slight increase in α_1-acid glycoprotein in elderly patients, however, which is probably due to age-associated inflammatory changes.[28] This increase in α_1-acid acid glycoprotein theoretically can affect the circulating free drug concentrations, particularly of lipophilic basic drugs[11] Notable anesthetic drugs that may be affected by age-related protein-binding changes are those highly extracted by the liver, extensively protein bound, and administered intravenously (IV).

In addition to a reduced central circulating volume in elderly patients, central organ perfusion undergoes change with aging. The aging brain is accompanied by a decrease in neuronal volume, which starts earlier in men but progresses more rapidly in women once it begins.[29] The aging brain also sustains a change in vascular distribution. Capillaries that normally are packed densely in areas of the brain that have higher processing demands decrease in number and show increased microvessel deformities starting in approximately the fifth decade of life.[30] Increasing age is associated with increasing blood-brain barrier permeability,[31] which can allow inappropriate passage of mediators from the plasma into the central nervous system (CNS).

Older adults have increased sensitivity to IV anesthetic agents due to fundamental changes in drug binding and distribution, described previously. Unfortunately, the changes in drug effect vary between patients of different ages in a nonlinear, exponential fashion.[32] Likewise, changes in drug effect with age depend heavily on PK and PD parameters for a given drug, with wide variation between different medications, even within a given class. Thus, easy-to-remember recommendations for medication dose adjustments applicable to multiple drugs over a range of patient ages, comorbidities, weights, nutritional statuses, and so forth, are impossible. Even so, most experts believe it prudent to significantly reduce medication doses in older patients.[33,34] Examples include fentanyl, haloperidol, lidocaine, midazolam, and propofol,[34] for which dose reductions should be considered.

Drug Metabolism and Excretion

Metabolism of drugs is another area of PK change in older adults. Hepatic metabolism of drugs is affected by aging due to a decrease in hepatic blood flow of approximately 40% in elderly patients,[6] thereby decreasing rate of drug delivery. Additionally, there is an age-related decrease in liver mass, reducing hepatic microsomal enzymes and extending the half-life of many drugs, including anesthetics. Because many older adults have multiple chronic comorbidities that require use of medicines, anesthetic drug metabolism is effectively further decreased due to saturation of the reduced number of hepatic microsomal enzymes. When controlling for volume of distribution, terminal elimination half-life of fentanyl was markedly prolonged in the elderly (patients more than 60 years old) compared with patients less than 50 years old (945 min vs 265 min).[33] The exact influence a reduction of hepatic microsomal enzymes has on anesthetic dosing, however, in the aging population is less clear, because other studies evaluating the effect of age on anesthetic drug clearance have been inconclusive.[35,36]

It is currently unknown whether extrahepatic metabolism of drugs is impacted by aging. Pulmonary metabolism of drugs is well described but the implications of lung metabolism in older adults, particularly for anesthetic drugs, have not been well studied. The extent to which ester metabolism changes in the elderly also is unclear, with conflicting studies regarding different commonly used agents. Ornstein and colleagues[37] studied changes in ester metabolism in older (65–82 years old) compared with younger (30–49 years old) individuals and found that although the onset of action of cisatracurium was delayed, the elimination half-life was unchanged, suggesting there is no difference in ester metabolism in the elderly. APK model of remifentanil, however, showed a decrease in metabolism with age.[38]

Renal function decreases in older adults, with a progressive reduction in renal mass, creatinine clearance, and glomerular filtration rate. Some studies have shown the decrease in glomerular filtration rate to be approximately 1 mL/min/1.73 m^2 per year after approximately 40 years of age, which is due to a reduced number of functioning glomeruli.[39] Serum creatinine is commonly used as a marker of renal function and, therefore, drug elimination, but it should be recognized that this is affected by muscle mass, physical activity, protein intake, and active secretion of creatinine by the renal proximal tubules.[39] Because of this reduction in renal clearance, the plasma half-life of a renally excreted drug is prolonged and the steady-state concentration increases.[11] There is a reduction in renal blood flow with age after the fourth decade of life, resulting in a 10% decrease with each decade of life.[40] Accompanying this decrease in renal blood flow is a decrease in autoregulation of volume status and autoregulation of blood flow in hypertensive and hypotensive states, called renal vascular dysautonomy.[41,42] Drugs that are renally cleared by the kidney and eliminated unchanged also warrant a reduction in dosing in the elderly.

There seems to be heterogeneity in geriatric PKs, which likely is due to a difference in fit versus frail older adults. Physiologic changes that affect PKs in older adults are certainly affected by the increased prevalence of chronic comorbidities. More research is needed, however, to further categorize pharmacokinetics in relation to chronologic versus functional aging.[43]

PHARMACODYNAMIC CHANGES IN THE ELDERLY
Central Nervous System

It is well known that older adults are more sensitive to inhaled anesthetics and opioids than younger adults. MAC correlates with the degree to which an anesthetic enhances the function of γ-aminobutyric acid (GABA)-A receptors in the brain, and PET scans have shown this interaction dependent on the blood concentration of the anesthetic.[22,44,45] The MAC value for volatile anesthetics decreases by 6% per decade and that for nitrous oxide decreases by approximately 8% per decade over the age of 40 years.[46] Similarly, the best research suggests that older adults are more sensitive to sedative and possibly deliriogenic effects of opioids, and thus dosing should be reduced.[47] At least 1 prospective trial currently is ongoing that may give more insight into whether opioid-free anesthesia is of benefit.[48]

Overall, the CNS of older adults is approximately 30% more sensitive to propofol than younger patients, which has been reported for both induction doses and infusions (**Fig. 1**).[49] During induction, patients greater than 70 years old reach significantly deeper electroencephalographic (EEG) stages and need more time until a normal EEG returns compared with younger patients.[50] Propofol has favorable effects on CNS parameters, because it lowers cerebral metabolic rate ($CMRO_2$), cerebral blood flow (CBF), and intracranial pressure (ICP).[51] When given as a bolus, propofol can lower the mean arterial pressure (MAP) considerably, possibly lowering cerebral perfusion pressure (CPP) below a critical level. This latter consideration is of prime importance in older adults because they are more apt to have critical carotid or aortic valvular stenosis. The range of cerebral autoregulation may be altered significantly if the patient has chronic hypertension; these patients are more apt to have blood pressure lability with induction. Thus, it seems that increasing age causes changes in the brain that increase the effective potency of propofol for the geriatric patient.

The mechanism of action of benzodiazepines on the GABA receptor (and its various subtypes) is reasonably well understood.[52–54] The onset and duration of action of a bolus IV administration of midazolam depend largely on the dose given and time at which the dose is administered; the higher the dose given over a shorter time (bolus), the faster the onset. The time to establish equilibrium between plasma concentration and EEG effect of midazolam is approximately 2 minutes to 3 minutes and is not affected by age.[55] Although there may not be a PK change, however, there seems to be a clear PD effect of increased risk of delirium with benzodiazepines, especially in older adults, when used as an infusion in the intensive care unit (ICU).[56,57] Whether

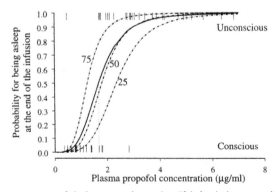

Fig. 1. Effect of age on propofol pharmacodynamics. This logistic regression shows the age-related probability of being asleep after a 1-hour infusion of propofol. A 75-year-old patient is 30% to 50% more sensitive to propofol than is a 25-year-old patient. (*From* Schnider TW, Minto CF, Shafer SL, et al. The influence of age on propofol pharmacodynamics. Anesthesiology 1999;90(6):1510; with permission.)

this is true for small doses in the perioperative period has not been definitively shown.[58] Recommendations by the American Geriatrics Society (with representation from both surgery and anesthesiology) recommend avoidance of benzodiazepines, limiting their use to special circumstances.[59]

Etomidate induces changes in CBF, $CMRO_2$, and ICP similar to propofol, but it does not result in the same changes in MAP.[60] This is of particular importance in the older patient at risk for ischemic stroke secondary to carotid occlusion. Overall, there are no PD changes with age with respect to etomidate as measured by EEG,[60] but etomidate is associated with a higher rate of postoperative nausea and vomiting than other induction drugs, and this seems unchanged in the elderly.[61,62]

Ketamine has received particular attention in older adults over the past few years because there was a concern that its use may be associated with increased delirium after surgery. Several studies in the past decade have shown a decreased incidence of postoperative delirium after cardiopulmonary bypass in anesthetized elderly patients treated with ketamine (0.5 mg/kg–1 mg/kg) compared with placebo.[63,64] More recently, a large international, multicenter, randomized controlled trial demonstrated that ketamine neither increased nor decreased postoperative delirium.[65] A planned substudy showed that intraoperative ketamine infusions were not associated with any reduction in new depressive symptoms after surgery, which is interesting given the interest of prolonged outpatient ketamine infusions for reducing depression.[66] Overall, there are no reports of PD changes in the elderly compared with in young adults.

Finally, dexmedetomidine has emerged as a medication frequently used for sedation in the perioperative period and the ICU setting, as discussed previously. Few studies have addressed whether there are PD changes with aging that would affect dexmedetomidine dosing. One small study comparing elderly and young patients showed no difference in PD parameters, although the elderly did require more interventions from a hemodynamic perspective.[67]

Respiratory System

In addition to age-related PD changes in the CNS, there are important age-related changes in the respiratory system that should be understood in order to provide optimal care related to anesthesia pharmacology. Propofol causes dose-related depression of ventilation.[68,69] In standard induction doses, propofol causes apnea whereas infusions for sedation cause increasing levels of respiratory depression.[70] Additionally, airway reflexes are depressed and both the hypoxic and hypercapnic ventilatory responses are blunted with propofol administration, all of which are greatly enhanced by the addition of opioids.[70–74] Due to changes in pulmonary anatomy and mechanics in older adults (increased closing capacity, decreased functional residual capacity, and decreased strength of cough to clear secretions), all these effects of propofol can have profound consequences.[75] Similar to propofol, older age and debilitating disease increase the incidence and severity of respiratory depression with midazolam.[76] Conversely, etomidate, dexmedetomidine, and ketamine all cause less respiratory depression in older patients than benzodiazepines or propofol, even in induction doses.[77–80] This advantage can make these medications useful choices in the setting of an elderly patient with diminished respiratory reserve, although care would need to be taken related to cardiovascular effects of dexmedetomidine.

Cardiovascular System

Another major consideration in older adults involves the interaction of PD changes in the cardiovascular system related to anesthetic agents. Propofol can cause profound changes in MAP through reduced vascular resistance when given in induction bolus doses.[81] In the young adult patient, this is well tolerated and easily reversed by airway manipulation. In elderly patients, many of whom are hypertensive at baseline, the degree of hypotension is increased due to reduced baroreceptor reflex responses, a higher likelihood of ventricular dysfunction, and greater likelihood of hypovolemia due to chronic diuretic therapy.[82] As such, propofol may be avoided for patients with severe cardiovascular disease (eg, severe/critical aortic stenosis or ventricular dysfunction). Many of these deleterious effects can be greatly reduced if a slower induction is performed rather than a rapid bolus.[83]

Unlike propofol, etomidate has minimal effects on the cardiovascular system during induction. Reduction in vascular resistance is minimal, and myocardial contractility, heart rate, and cardiac output usually are unchanged.[84] These aspects of the PD profile of etomidate make it useful for older adults who may have reduced preload, coronary artery disease, valvular disease, or reduced ventricular function. Like etomidate, midazolam alone has modest hemodynamic effects. But, the addition of opioids, especially fentanyl and sufentanil, to benzodiazepines result in greater reductions in blood pressure than either alone.[85–87] Ketamine also has a favorable hemodynamic profile, even in the elderly. It can cause transient increases in heart rate, blood pressure, and cardiac output but these parameters return to baseline within minutes and can be controlled with a short-acting β-blocker, such as esmolol.[88] Overall, titrated doses are well tolerated in older adults, including the critically ill, but ketamine should be used with great caution in patients with severe stenotic valvular lesions, active myocardial ischemia, or decompensated heart failure.

Finally, dexmedetomidine has been shown to be of benefit in reducing delirium in the ICU setting (likely by avoiding benzodiazepines). It can, however, have significant hemodynamic effects through bradycardia and peripheral vasodilation. Accordingly, for the reasons discussed previously, the hemodynamic effects of dexmedetomidine tend to be more pronounced in elderly patients and this means dosing should be reduced or boluses administered more slowly than in young adults.[89]

IMPLICATIONS FOR PRACTICE: ANESTHETIC DOSING RECOMMENDATIONS IN THE ELDERLY
Opioids

A large variety of opioids with heterogeneous pharmacokinetics are available for perioperative use, with properties ranging from lipophilic to hydrophilic and clearance by the liver or in plasma, with and without active or toxic metabolites. Coverage of the breadth of opioids is beyond the scope of this article, but in general, older adults experience prolonged clearance of morphine, fentanyl, remifentanil, and meperidine but not sufentanil.[33,90–92] Reduced renal clearance of active or toxic metabolites make meperidine and morphine particularly risky in older or renally impaired individuals. In contrast, the PD changes with aging are more uniform across medications. Older individuals are markedly more sensitive to the analgesic effects as well as the sedative and respiratory depressant side effects of opioids.[93,94] Considering the PD and PK changes and their interindividual variability, opioid titration in the elderly should proceed carefully, with significantly reduced doses (25%–50%), longer redosing intervals, and avoidance of drugs with toxic metabolites.

Benzodiazepines

Although PK changes in midazolam do not affect drug onset, clearance of the drug is reduced by up to 30% with increased age, resulting in prolonged drug effect.[95] PD changes result in increased sensitivity to benzodiazepine effect with age or comorbid conditions. Early work advised a dose reduction of 20% to 50% in older patients and those with ASA physical status of 3 or 4.[96] Dose reduction of 75% in 90-year-old patients compared with 20-year-old patients produces similar sedative effects (**Fig. 2**).[97] The deliriogenic effects of benzodiazepine infusions in elderly and critically ill patients are well documented and warrant some hesitation when administering even low-dose midazolam in the elderly. This is especially true when opioid coadministration is planned, due to synergistic respiratory depression.[98,99] In summation, benzodiazepines should be used cautiously at significantly decreased doses in the elderly (if they are used at all) (**Table 1**).

Propofol

The overall effects of propofol are pronounced in elderly patients, resulting in higher plasma drug levels, increased sensitivity, and reduced clearance.[49,82,83,100] Suggested alterations in propofol administration with age include a 20% reduction in induction dose, a decrease in speed of induction dose administration, and a 30% to 50% reduction in infusion rates for anesthetic maintenance.[97] For example, a 75 year old requires only half the maintenance infusion rate that a 25 year old would receive (**Fig. 3**). The context-sensitive half-time of propofol is approximately 20 minutes to 30 minutes after a 1-hour to 2-hour infusion in the elderly compared with only 10 minutes to 15 minutes in younger patients. The practical effect of this is that propofol infusions should be stopped significantly earlier in the elderly to allow for timely awakening and recovery[101] (see **Table 1**).

Etomidate

Etomidate PD parameters have not been shown to vary based on age, although PK factors do change. Aging decreases etomidate clearance, lengthens elimination

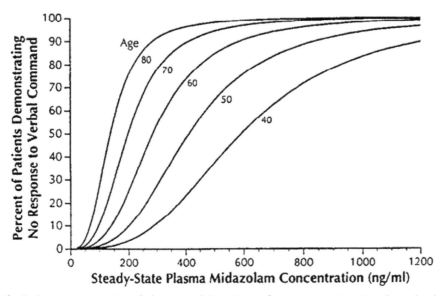

Fig. 2. Response curves to verbal commands in patients of various ages at varying plasma levels of midazolam. This demonstrates a pharmacodynamic change associated with aging in response to midazolam. (*From* Jacobs JR, Reves JG, Marty J, et al. Aging increases pharmacodynamic sensitivity to the hypnotic effects of midazolam. Anesth Analg 1995;80(1):143–148; with permission.)

Table 1
Uses and doses of commonly used nonopiate drugs

Drug	Sedation Dose (Intravenous)	Induction/Bolus Dose	Maintenance/ Infusion Dose	Dose Reduction (%) for Older Adults
Dexmedetomidine	0.5–1 µg/kg[a]	0.5–3 µg/kg[a]	0.1–2.5 µg/kg/h	30–50
Etomidate	N/A	0.2–0.4 mg/kg	N/A	20–50
Ketamine	0.2–0.5 mg/kg	1–2 mg/kg	10–20 µg/kg/min	0/unknown
Midazolam	0.02 mg/kg	0.025–0.1 mg/kg	0.3–1.5 µg/kg/min	20
Propofol	25–50 µg/kg/min	1.0–1.5 mg/kg	75–150 µg/kg/min	20
Thiopental	N/A	2–5 mg/kg	N/A	20

[a] Over 10 minutes to 20 minutes.
Data from Refs.[109,112,118–121]

half-life, and, most significantly, decreases the initial volume of distribution, raising drug plasma levels relative to younger controls. These PK changes are significant, with a 50% to 66% reduction required for anesthetic induction in 80 year olds compared with 20 year olds.[102] (see **Table 1**). Although it is prized for its hemodynamic stability during induction of anesthesia compared with other IV anesthetic agents, etomidate does produce significant, clinically relevant suppression of the adrenocortical system lasting 6 hours to 8 hours with single doses.[62] In patients experiencing sepsis or trauma, etomidate can suppress cortisol levels for 24 hours to 72 hours. This potent suppression of cortisol synthesis occurs even at low doses. A recent meta-analysis did not find any effects, however, on mortality in critically ill patients.[103] Additionally, repeated use of etomidate for electroconvulsive therapy in patients who are not critically ill does not seem to have any harmful effects and likely promotes better seizure duration.[104]

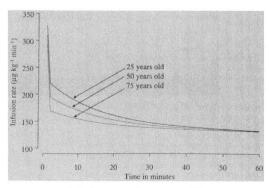

Fig. 3. Effect of age on propofol pharmacodynamics with a computer-controlled target-controlled infusion. In younger people, higher infusion rates must be maintained during the first 20 minutes to 30 minutes. In elderly people, after the first minute, a constant infusion rate is adequate for maintaining a constant plasma concentration. A 75-year-old patient is 30% to 50% more sensitive to propofol than is a 25-year-old patient. (*From* Schnider TW, Minto CF, Gambus PL, et al. The influence of method of administration and covariates on the pharmacokinetics of propofol in adult volunteers. Anesthesiology 1998;88(5):1180; with permission.)

Ketamine

Studies evaluating ketamine anesthesia do not provide guidance on dosing adjustments with age.[88,105] Studies of age-related dose adjustments for its modern usage as an analgesic given in subanesthetic doses are lacking. The impact of subanesthetic doses of ketamine on outcome varies by study, but there is no strong evidence of benefit or harm on postoperative cognitive outcomes or rates of delirium.[63,65,106,107] Because recommended doses for subanesthetic ketamine vary by an order of magnitude depending on the source, providing a dose recommendation is outside the scope of this discussion[108] (see **Table 1**).

Dexmedetomidine

Although the PKs of dexmedetomidine were not previously believed to vary with age, more recent work suggests a prolonged clearance and increased context-sensitive half-time in older adults.[109] In patients with hypoalbuminemia, these changes are more pronounced. Changes in dexmedetomidine PDs have not been elucidated, so the increased effects of the drug in the elderly may reflect either the PK changes or a combination of PD and PK changes. Regardless, a dose reduction of 33% is recommended for dexmedetomidine in the elderly, with titration to the appropriate level of sedation.[110] Adjustments should be made to the doses used in younger individuals for both bolus (0.5–1.0 μg/kg over 10 minutes) and infusion (0.2–1.0 μg/kg/h) dosing.[109] Although dexmedetomidine side effects, such as hypotension and bradycardia, are more common in the elderly (especially with bolus dosing), the drug offers several advantages, such as decreases in anesthetic requirements, opioid doses, agitation scores, and delirium incidence.[110–112] (see **Table 1**).

Nondepolarizing Neuromuscular Blockers

The PD parameters for neuromuscular blocking (NMB) drugs from the tetrahydroisoquinoline class (cisatracurium) and aminosteroid class (rocuronium and vecuronium) do not change with age. This means that age-related differences in clinical effect are entirely explained by PK changes, with no difference in receptor sensitivity related to aging.[113] Clearance of rocuronium, primarily by the liver, decreases with age, resulting in longer elimination half-life and prolonged drug effect in older adults. To demonstrate the magnitude of this difference, 1 study showed the half-life of a single 0.6 mg/kg-dose rocuronium in septuagenarians to be 98 minutes, which is 16 minutes longer than in younger controls.[113] Thus, the redosing interval for rocuronium should be longer in the elderly.

Cisatracurium is degraded largely by Hofmann elimination, with clearance independent of age and an only slightly increased volume of distribution and elimination half-life in the elderly. Onset in older patients is 1 minute slower (3.4 minutes vs 2.5 minutes), possibly related to slower circulation time.[113] For cisatracurium, duration of effect and redosing interval are only trivially lengthened whereas time to optimal intubating conditions may be delayed.

Sugammadex

Sugammadex, a selective relaxant binding agent, was approved in the United States in 2015 for reversal of NMB caused by rocuronium or vecuronium. Its γ-cyclodextrin structure selectively encapsulates aminosteroid NMB and is cleared primarily by the kidneys. Hypersensitivity (anaphylactic) reactions are the most severe complication related to sugammadex use, with a reported incidence of 0.039% in 1 study.[114] This is comparable in frequency to anaphylaxis with succinylcholine or rocuronium.

Other issues with sugammadex include an up to 5% risk of residual NMB when train-of-four (TOF) monitoring is not used to monitor relaxation and guide therapy.

Older adults differ in response to sugammadex therapy in several ways. They experience a slower spontaneous recovery of TOF, a slower onset of sugammadex effect, and a higher incidence of recurarization (worsening of TOF ratio) after sugammadex therapy compared with younger patients.[115] Patients with severe renal impairment also experience prolonged time to spontaneous recovery of TOF and slower onset of sugammadex.[116] This may be related to renal clearance of sugammadex and the sugammadex/NMB complex. In all groups, it is important to recognize that recovery to a TOF ratio greater than 0.9 is still significantly faster than with neostigmine reversal of NMB activity. All patients, but especially older adults and those with renal insufficiency, should receive TOF monitoring to appropriately guide sugammadex therapy.[117]

Volatile Anesthetics

As discussed previously, MAC requirements for all volatile anesthetics decrease with age.[21] Targeting a lower end-tidal anesthetic concentration in the elderly is advisable and iso-MAC charts or electronic resources can provide guidance.

SUMMARY

Providing the highest level of anesthetic care for elderly patients requires a thoughtful approach that accounts for the many physiologic PK and PD changes that occur with aging. Because older adults often are excluded from large trials due to age or comorbidity, developing a thorough understanding of their needs can be challenging but not impossible. Ongoing research, particularly with respect to the pharmacologic changes of aging, continues to expand understanding and improve care of older patients throughout the perioperative period.

REFERENCES

1. Bureau, U.S.C. From Pyramid to PIllar: a Century of change, population of the U.S. 2018. Available at: https://www.census.gov/library/visualizations/2018/comm/century-of-change.html. Accessed October 9, 2018.
2. Etzioni DA, Liu JH, Maggard MA, et al. The aging population and its impact on the surgery workforce. Ann Surg 2003;238(2):170–7.
3. Sankar A, Beattie WS, Wijeysundera DN. How can we identify the high-risk patient? Curr Opin Crit Care 2015;21(4):328–35.
4. Hamidi M, Joseph B. Changing epidemiology of the American population. Clin Geriatr Med 2019;35(1):1–12.
5. Crooks J. Aging and drug disposition–pharmacodynamics. J Chronic Dis 1983;36(1):85–90.
6. McLean AJ, Le Couteur DG. Aging biology and geriatric clinical pharmacology. Pharmacol Rev 2004;56(2):163–84.
7. Klotz U. Pharmacokinetics and drug metabolism in the elderly. Drug Metab Rev 2009;41(2):67–76.
8. Kharasch ED, Hoffer C, Whittington D. Influence of age on the pharmacokinetics and pharmacodynamics of oral transmucosal fentanyl citrate. Anesthesiology 2004;101(3):738–43.
9. Bender AD. Effect of age on intestinal absorption: implications for drug absorption in the elderly. J Am Geriatr Soc 1968;16(12):1331–9.

10. Evans MA, Triggs EJ, Cheung M, et al. Gastric emptying rate in the elderly: implications for drug therapy. J Am Geriatr Soc 1981;29(5):201–5.
11. Tumer N, Scarpace PJ, Lowenthal DT. Geriatric pharmacology: basic and clinical considerations. Annu Rev Pharmacol Toxicol 1992;32:271–302.
12. Orr WC, Chen CL. Aging and neural control of the GI tract: IV. Clinical and physiological aspects of gastrointestinal motility and aging. Am J Physiol Gastrointest Liver Physiol 2002;283(6):G1226–31.
13. Wiley JW. Aging and neural control of the GI tract: III. Senescent enteric nervous system: lessons from extraintestinal sites and nonmammalian species. Am J Physiol Gastrointest Liver Physiol 2002;283(5):G1020–6.
14. Nimmo WS. Drugs, diseases and altered gastric emptying. Clin Pharmacokinet 1976;1(3):189–203.
15. Le Couteur DG, McLean AJ. The aging liver. Drug clearance and an oxygen diffusion barrier hypothesis. Clin Pharmacokinet 1998;34(5):359–73.
16. Zeeh J, Platt D. The aging liver: structural and functional changes and their consequences for drug treatment in old age. Gerontology 2002;48(3):121–7.
17. Holdsworth MT, Forman WB, Killilea TA, et al. Transdermal fentanyl disposition in elderly subjects. Gerontology 1994;40(1):32–7.
18. Daly CH, Odland GF. Age-related changes in the mechanical properties of human skin. J Invest Dermatol 1979;73(1):84–7.
19. Montagna W, Carlisle K. Structural changes in aging human skin. J Invest Dermatol 1979;73(1):47–53.
20. Roskos KV, Maibach HI. Percutaneous absorption and age. Implications for therapy. Drugs Aging 1992;2(5):432–49.
21. Nickalls RW, Mapleson WW. Age-related iso-MAC charts for isoflurane, sevoflurane and desflurane in man. Br J Anaesth 2003;91(2):170–4.
22. Campagna JA, Miller KW, Forman SA. Mechanisms of actions of inhaled anesthetics. N Engl J Med 2003;348(21):2110–24.
23. Corcoran TB, Hillyard S. Cardiopulmonary aspects of anaesthesia for the elderly. Best Pract Res Clin Anaesthesiol 2011;25(3):329–54.
24. Kennedy RR, Baker AB. The effect of cardiac output changes on end-tidal volatile anaesthetic concentrations. Anaesth Intensive Care 2001;29(5):535–8.
25. Beaufrere B, Morio B. Fat and protein redistribution with aging: metabolic considerations. Eur J Clin Nutr 2000;54(Suppl 3):S48–53.
26. Lei SF, Liu MY, Chen XD, et al. Relationship of total body fatness and five anthropometric indices in Chinese aged 20-40 years: different effects of age and gender. Eur J Clin Nutr 2006;60(4):511–8.
27. Chang SH, Beason TS, Hunleth JM, et al. A systematic review of body fat distribution and mortality in older people. Maturitas 2012;72(3):175–91.
28. Grandison MK, Boudinot FD. Age-related changes in protein binding of drugs: implications for therapy. Clin Pharmacokinet 2000;38(3):271–90.
29. Small SA. Age-related memory decline: current concepts and future directions. Arch Neurol 2001;58(3):360–4.
30. Trollor JN, Valenzuela MJ. Brain ageing in the new millennium. Aust N Z J Psychiatry 2001;35(6):788–805.
31. Farrall AJ, Wardlaw JM. Blood-brain barrier: ageing and microvascular disease–systematic review and meta-analysis. Neurobiol Aging 2009;30(3):337–52.
32. Homer TD, Stanski DR. The effect of increasing age on thiopental disposition and anesthetic requirement. Anesthesiology 1985;62(6):714–24.
33. Bentley JB, Borel JD, Nenad RE Jr, et al. Age and fentanyl pharmacokinetics. Anesth Analg 1982;61(12):968–71.

34. Benet LZ, Hoener BA. Changes in plasma protein binding have little clinical relevance. Clin Pharmacol Ther 2002;71(3):115–21.
35. Lemmens HJ, Bovill JG, Hennis PJ, et al. Age has no effect on the pharmacodynamics of alfentanil. Anesth Analg 1988;67(10):956–60.
36. Lemmens HJ, Burm AG, Hennis PJ, et al. Influence of age on the pharmacokinetics of alfentanil. Gender dependence. Clin Pharmacokinet 1990;19(5):416–22.
37. Ornstein E, Lien CA, Matteo RS, et al. Pharmacodynamics and pharmacokinetics of cisatracurium in geriatric surgical patients. Anesthesiology 1996;84(3):520–5.
38. Minto CF, Howe C, Wishart S, et al. Pharmacokinetics and pharmacodynamics of nandrolone esters in oil vehicle: effects of ester, injection site and injection volume. J Pharmacol Exp Ther 1997;281(1):93–102.
39. McLachlan AJ, Pont LG. Drug metabolism in older people–a key consideration in achieving optimal outcomes with medicines. J Gerontol A Biol Sci Med Sci 2012;67(2):175–80.
40. Silva FG. The aging kidney: a review–part II. Int Urol Nephrol 2005;37(2):419–32.
41. Perico N, Remuzzi G, Benigni A. Aging and the kidney. Curr Opin Nephrol Hypertens 2011;20(3):312–7.
42. Karsch-Volk M, Schmid E, Wagenpfeil S, et al. Kidney function and clinical recommendations of drug dose adjustment in geriatric patients. BMC Geriatr 2013;13:92.
43. Kinirons MT, O'Mahony MS. Drug metabolism and ageing. Br J Clin Pharmacol 2004;57(5):540–4.
44. Zimmerman SA, Jones MV, Harrison NL. Potentiation of gamma-aminobutyric acidA receptor Cl- current correlates with in vivo anesthetic potency. J Pharmacol Exp Ther 1994;270(3):987–91.
45. Gyulai FE, Mintun MA, Firestone LL. Dose-dependent enhancement of in vivo GABA(A)-benzodiazepine receptor binding by isoflurane. Anesthesiology 2001;95(3):585–93.
46. Stevens WC, Dolan WM, Gibbons RT, et al. Minimum alveolar concentrations (MAC) of isoflurande with and without nitrous oxide in patients of various ages. Anesthesiology 1975;42(2):197–200.
47. Prostran M, Vujović KS, Vučković S, et al. Pharmacotherapy of pain in the older population: the place of opioids. Front Aging Neurosci 2016;8:144.
48. Beloeil H, Laviolle B, Menard C, et al. POFA trial study protocol: a multicentre, double-blind, randomised, controlled clinical trial comparing opioid-free versus opioid anaesthesia on postoperative opioid-related adverse events after major or intermediate non-cardiac surgery. BMJ Open 2018;8(6):e020873.
49. Schnider TW, Minto CF, Shafer SL, et al. The influence of age on propofol pharmacodynamics. Anesthesiology 1999;90(6):1502–16.
50. Schultz A, Grouven U, Zander I, et al. Age-related effects in the EEG during propofol anaesthesia. Acta Anaesthesiol Scand 2004;48(1):27–34.
51. Ludbrook GL, Visco E, Lam AM. Propofol: relation between brain concentrations, electroencephalogram, middle cerebral artery blood flow velocity, and cerebral oxygen extraction during induction of anesthesia. Anesthesiology 2002;97(6):1363–70.
52. Amrein R, Hetzel W, Bonetti EP, et al. Clinical pharmacology of dormicum (midazolam) and anexate (flumazenil). Resuscitation 1988;16(Suppl):S5–27.

53. Mohler H, Richards JG. The benzodiazepine receptor: a pharmacological control element of brain function. Eur J Anaesthesiol Suppl 1988;2:15–24.
54. Mould DR, DeFeo TM, Reele S, et al. Simultaneous modeling of the pharmacokinetics and pharmacodynamics of midazolam and diazepam. Clin Pharmacol Ther 1995;58(1):35–43.
55. Haefely W. The preclinical pharmacology of flumazenil. Eur J Anaesthesiol Suppl 1988;2:25–36.
56. Pandharipande PP, Pun BT, Herr DL, et al. Effect of sedation with dexmedetomidine vs lorazepam on acute brain dysfunction in mechanically ventilated patients: the MENDS randomized controlled trial. JAMA 2007;298(22):2644–53.
57. Barr J, Fraser GL, Puntillo K, et al. Clinical practice guidelines for the management of pain, agitation, and delirium in adult patients in the intensive care unit. Crit Care Med 2013;41(1):263–306.
58. Christe C, Janssens JP, Armenian B, et al. Midazolam sedation for upper gastrointestinal endoscopy in older persons: a randomized, double-blind, placebo-controlled study. J Am Geriatr Soc 2000;48(11):1398–403.
59. Mohanty S, Rosenthal RA, Russell MM, et al. Optimal perioperative management of the geriatric patient: a best practices guideline from the American College of Surgeons NSQIP and the American Geriatrics Society. J Am Coll Surg 2016;222(5):930–47.
60. Doenicke AW, Roizen MF, Kugler J, et al. Reducing myoclonus after etomidate. Anesthesiology 1999;90(1):113–9.
61. Watcha MF, White PF. Postoperative nausea and vomiting. Its etiology, treatment, and prevention. Anesthesiology 1992;77(1):162–84.
62. Forman SA. Clinical and molecular pharmacology of etomidate. Anesthesiology 2011;114(3):695–707.
63. Hudetz JA, Patterson KM, Iqbal Z, et al. Ketamine attenuates delirium after cardiac surgery with cardiopulmonary bypass. J Cardiothorac Vasc Anesth 2009; 23(5):651–7.
64. Hudetz JA, Pagel PS. Neuroprotection by ketamine: a review of the experimental and clinical evidence. J Cardiothorac Vasc Anesth 2010;24(1):131–42.
65. Avidan MS, Maybrier HR, Abdallah AB, et al. Intraoperative ketamine for prevention of postoperative delirium or pain after major surgery in older adults: an international, multicentre, double-blind, randomised clinical trial. Lancet 2017; 390(10091):267–75.
66. Mashour GA, Ben Abdallah A, Pryor KO, et al. Intraoperative ketamine for prevention of depressive symptoms after major surgery in older adults: an international, multicentre, double-blind, randomised clinical trial. Br J Anaesth 2018; 121(5):1075–83.
67. Kuang Y, Zhang RR, Pei Q, et al. Pharmacokinetic and pharmacodynamic study of dexmedetomidine in elderly patients during spinal anesthesia. Int J Clin Pharmacol Ther 2015;53(12):1005–14.
68. Conti G, Dell'Utri D, Vilardi V, et al. Propofol induces bronchodilation in mechanically ventilated chronic obstructive pulmonary disease (COPD) patients. Acta Anaesthesiol Scand 1993;37(1):105–9.
69. Brown RH, Greenberg RS, Wagner EM. Efficacy of propofol to prevent bronchoconstriction: effects of preservative. Anesthesiology 2001;94(5):851–5 [discussion: 6A].
70. Blouin RT, Conard PF, Gross JB. Time course of ventilatory depression following induction doses of propofol and thiopental. Anesthesiology 1991;75(6):940–4.

71. Van Keer L, Van Aken H, Vandermeersch E, et al. Propofol does not inhibit hypoxic pulmonary vasoconstriction in humans. J Clin Anesth 1989;1(4):284–8.

72. Blouin RT, Seifert HA, Babenco HD, et al. Propofol depresses the hypoxic ventilatory response during conscious sedation and isohypercapnia. Anesthesiology 1993;79(6):1177–82.

73. Abe K, Shimizu T, Takashina M, et al. The effects of propofol, isoflurane, and sevoflurane on oxygenation and shunt fraction during one-lung ventilation. Anesth Analg 1998;87(5):1164–9.

74. Tagaito Y, Isono S, Nishino T. Upper airway reflexes during a combination of propofol and fentanyl anesthesia. Anesthesiology 1998;88(6):1459–66.

75. Zaugg M, Lucchinetti E. Respiratory function in the elderly. Anesthesiol Clin North America 2000;18(1):47–58, vi.

76. Parlak M, Parlak I, Erdur B, et al. Age effect on efficacy and side effects of two sedation and analgesia protocols on patients going through cardioversion: a randomized clinical trial. Acad Emerg Med 2006;13(5):493–9.

77. Choi SD, Spaulding BC, Gross JB, et al. Comparison of the ventilatory effects of etomidate and methohexital. Anesthesiology 1985;62(4):442–7.

78. Kolenda H, Gremmelt A, Rading S, et al. Ketamine for analgosedative therapy in intensive care treatment of head-injured patients. Acta Neurochir (Wien) 1996; 138(10):1193–9.

79. Green SM, Krauss B. The semantics of ketamine. Ann Emerg Med 2000;36(5): 480–2.

80. Erstad BL, Patanwala AE. Ketamine for analgosedation in critically ill patients. J Crit Care 2016;35:145–9.

81. Kirkbride DA, Parker JL, Williams GD, et al. Induction of anesthesia in the elderly ambulatory patient: a double-blinded comparison of propofol and sevoflurane. Anesth Analg 2001;93(5):1185–7.

82. John AD, Sieber FE. Age associated issues: geriatrics. Anesthesiol Clin North America 2004;22(1):45–58.

83. Kazama T, Ikeda K, Morita K, et al. Comparison of the effect-site k(eO)s of propofol for blood pressure and EEG bispectral index in elderly and younger patients. Anesthesiology 1999;90(6):1517–27.

84. Kettler D, Sonntag H, Donath U, et al. Haemodynamics, myocardial mechanics, oxygen requirement and oxygenation of the human heart during induction of anaesthesia with etomidate (author's transl). Anaesthesist 1974;23(3):116–21 [in German].

85. Heikkila H, Jalonen J, Arola M, et al. Midazolam as adjunct to high-dose fentanyl anaesthesia for coronary artery bypass grafting operation. Acta Anaesthesiol Scand 1984;28(6):683–9.

86. Reves JG. Valium-fentanyl interaction, in common problems in cardiac anaesthesia. Chicago: Mosby, Incorporated; 1987. p. 356.

87. Windsor JP, Sherry K, Feneck RO, et al. Sufentanil and nitrous oxide anaesthesia for cardiac surgery. Br J Anaesth 1988;61(6):662–8.

88. Idvall J, Ahlgren I, Aronsen KR, et al. Ketamine infusions: pharmacokinetics and clinical effects. Br J Anaesth 1979;51(12):1167–73.

89. Chrysostomou C, Schmitt CG. Dexmedetomidine: sedation, analgesia and beyond. Expert Opin Drug Metab Toxicol 2008;4(5):619–27.

90. Odar-Cederlof I, Boréus LO, Bondesson U, et al. Comparison of renal excretion of pethidine (meperidine) and its metabolites in old and young patients. Eur J Clin Pharmacol 1985;28(2):171–5.

91. Matteo RS, Schwartz AE, Ornstein E, et al. Pharmacokinetics of sufentanil in the elderly surgical patient. Can J Anaesth 1990;37(8):852–6.
92. Minto CF, Schnider TW, Egan TD, et al. Influence of age and gender on the pharmacokinetics and pharmacodynamics of remifentanil. I. Model development. Anesthesiology 1997;86(1):10–23.
93. Scott JC, Ponganis KV, Stanski DR. EEG quantitation of narcotic effect: the comparative pharmacodynamics of fentanyl and alfentanil. Anesthesiology 1985;62(3):234–41.
94. Macintyre PE, Jarvis DA. Age is the best predictor of postoperative morphine requirements. Pain 1996;64(2):357–64.
95. Polasek TM, Patel F, Jensen BP, et al. Predicted metabolic drug clearance with increasing adult age. Br J Clin Pharmacol 2013;75(4):1019–28.
96. Reves JG, Fragen RJ, Vinik HR, et al. Midazolam: pharmacology and uses. Anesthesiology 1985;62(3):310–24.
97. Shafer SL. The pharmacology of anesthetic drugs in elderly patients. Anesthesiol Clin North America 2000;18(1):1–29, v.
98. Gross JB, Zebrowski ME, Carel WD, et al. Time course of ventilatory depression after thiopental and midazolam in normal subjects and in patients with chronic obstructive pulmonary disease. Anesthesiology 1983;58(6):540–4.
99. Brogden RN, Goa KL. Flumazenil. A reappraisal of its pharmacological properties and therapeutic efficacy as a benzodiazepine antagonist. Drugs 1991; 42(6):1061–89.
100. Schnider TW, Minto CF, Gambus PL, et al. The influence of method of administration and covariates on the pharmacokinetics of propofol in adult volunteers. Anesthesiology 1998;88(5):1170–82.
101. Schuttler J, Ihmsen H. Population pharmacokinetics of propofol: a multicenter study. Anesthesiology 2000;92(3):727–38.
102. Arden JR, Holley FO, Stanski DR. Increased sensitivity to etomidate in the elderly: initial distribution versus altered brain response. Anesthesiology 1986; 65(1):19–27.
103. Bruder EA, Ball IM, Ridi S, et al. Single induction dose of etomidate versus other induction agents for endotracheal intubation in critically ill patients. Cochrane Database Syst Rev 2015;(1):CD010225.
104. Wang N, Wang XH, Lu J, et al. The effect of repeated etomidate anesthesia on adrenocortical function during a course of electroconvulsive therapy. J ECT 2011;27(4):281–5.
105. Stefansson T, Wickstrom I, Haljamae H. Hemodynamic and metabolic effects of ketamine anesthesia in the geriatric patient. Acta Anaesthesiol Scand 1982; 26(4):371–7.
106. Lee KH, Kim JY, Kim JW, et al. Influence of ketamine on early postoperative cognitive function after orthopedic surgery in elderly patients. Anesth Pain Med 2015;5(5):e28844.
107. Rascon-Martinez DM, Fresán-Orellana A, Ocharán-Hernández ME, et al. The effects of ketamine on cognitive function in elderly patients undergoing ophthalmic surgery: a pilot study. Anesth Analg 2016;122(4):969–75.
108. Schwenk ES, Viscusi ER, Buvanendran A, et al. Consensus guidelines on the use of intravenous ketamine infusions for acute pain management from the American Society of regional anesthesia and pain medicine, the American Academy of Pain Medicine, and the American Society of Anesthesiologists. Reg Anesth Pain Med 2018;43(5):456–66.

109. Iirola T, Ihmsen H, Laitio R, et al. Population pharmacokinetics of dexmedetomidine during long-term sedation in intensive care patients. Br J Anaesth 2012; 108(3):460–8.

110. Kim DJ, Kim SH, So KY, et al. Effects of dexmedetomidine on smooth emergence from anaesthesia in elderly patients undergoing orthopaedic surgery. BMC Anesthesiol 2015;15:139.

111. Ergenoglu P, Akin S, Bali C, et al. Effect of low dose dexmedetomidine premedication on propofol consumption in geriatric end stage renal disease patients. Braz J Anesthesiol 2015;65(5):326–32.

112. Kim J, Kim WO, Kim HB, et al. Adequate sedation with single-dose dexmedetomidine in patients undergoing transurethral resection of the prostate with spinal anaesthesia: a dose-response study by age group. BMC Anesthesiol 2015; 15:17.

113. Matteo RS, Ornstein E, Schwartz AE, et al. Pharmacokinetics and pharmacodynamics of rocuronium (Org 9426) in elderly surgical patients. Anesth Analg 1993;77(6):1193–7.

114. Miyazaki Y, Sunaga H, Kida K, et al. Incidence of anaphylaxis associated with sugammadex. Anesth Analg 2018;126(5):1505–8.

115. Muramatsu T, Isono S, Ishikawa T, et al. Differences of recovery from rocuronium-induced deep paralysis in response to small doses of sugammadex between elderly and nonelderly patients. Anesthesiology 2018;129(5):901–11.

116. Panhuizen IF, Gold SJ, Buerkle C, et al. Efficacy, safety and pharmacokinetics of sugammadex 4 mg kg-1 for reversal of deep neuromuscular blockade in patients with severe renal impairment. Br J Anaesth 2015;114(5):777–84.

117. Naguib M, Brull SJ, Kopman AF, et al. Consensus statement on perioperative use of neuromuscular monitoring. Anesth Analg 2018;127(1):71–80.

118. Sun GC, Hsu MC, Chia YY, et al. Effects of age and gender on intravenous midazolam premedication: a randomized double-blind study. Br J Anaesth 2008; 101(5):632–9.

119. Center for Drug Evaluation and Research: Dexmedetomidine Hydrochloride (Precedex). 2010. Available at: https://www.accessdata.fda.gov/drugsatfda_docs/nda/2010/021038Orig1s017.pdf. Accessed October 9, 2018.

120. Giovannitti JA Jr, Thoms SM, Crawford JJ. Alpha-2 adrenergic receptor agonists: a review of current clinical applications. Anesth Prog 2015;62(1):31–9.

121. Hansen TG. Sedative medications outside the operating room and the pharmacology of sedatives. Curr Opin Anaesthesiol 2015;28(4):446–52.

Emergency General Surgery in Older Adults: A Review

Sylvie Aucoin, MD, FRCPC[a], Daniel I. McIsaac, MD, MPH, FRCPC[a,b],*

KEYWORDS

- Surgery • Anesthesia • Geriatrics • Acute care • Frailty • Outcomes • Epidemiology

KEY POINTS

- Older age is a strong risk factor for adverse events after emergency general surgery.
- The presence of frailty and sarcopenia substantially increases risk.
- Anesthesiologists play a key role in preoperative risk stratification, communication, and establishing goals of care.
- Preoperative optimization should be goal directed and time limited.
- Anesthesiologists play a key role in applying acute postoperative monitoring strategies and facilitating multidisciplinary care.

OVERVIEW AND RATIONALE

More than 500,000 emergency general surgery (EGS) procedures are performed annually in the United States, with an estimated cost in excess of $6 billion.[1] Compared with major elective surgery, where 30-day morbidity and mortality rates are 10% to 20% and 1% to 2%, respectively, major complications occur in more than 40% of EGS patients and mortality rates exceed 10%.[2–4] Costs also are substantially increased when surgery is performed on an emergent basis.[5]

Older people (ie, aged ≥65 years) are the fastest growing segment of the population.[6] This rapid population aging has a substantial impact on provision of emergency perioperative care. Older people have surgery at a higher rate than other age groups[7]; despite making up only 15% of the population, more than 30% of EGS cases are performed for older people.[8] Recent data demonstrate a steady increase in the age of people, in particular men, admitted to EGS services over time.[8] As the population continues to age, this demographic shift is predicted to have an impact on patient outcomes and increase health system costs.

Disclosure Statement: The authors have nothing to disclose.
a Department of Anesthesiology & Pain Medicine, The Ottawa Hospital, University of Ottawa, Room B311, 1053 Carling Avenue, Ottawa, Ontario K1S 2Z3, Canada; b Ottawa Hospital Research Institute, School of Epidemiology & Public Health, University of Ottawa, Room B311, 1053 Carling Avenue, Ottawa, Ontario K1S 2Z3, Canada
* Corresponding author. Department of Anesthesiology & Pain Medicine, The Ottawa Hospital, University of Ottawa, Room B311, 1053 Carling Avenue, Ottawa, Ontario K1S 2Z3 Canada.
E-mail address: dmcisaac@toh.ca

Anesthesiology Clin 37 (2019) 493–505
https://doi.org/10.1016/j.anclin.2019.04.008   anesthesiology.theclinics.com
1932-2275/19/Crown Copyright © 2019 Published by Elsevier Inc. All rights reserved.

Given the growing number of older people presenting for EGS, it is important that anesthesiologists understand (1) the outcome burden associated with advanced age in EGS patients, (2) strategies for risk stratification, (3) current evidence-based interventions that may improve outcomes, and (4) key knowledge gaps that must be addressed to support improved care and outcomes. Therefore, this article's objective is to provide a narrative review of key perioperative issues facing older surgical patients having EGS procedures.

APPROACH

Articles informing this review were limited to those describing care and/or outcomes for EGS procedures as outlined by the core set of surgeries recommended by Scott and colleagues[1] (laparotomies, lysis of adhesions, large and small bowel resection, peptic ulcer repairs, cholecystectomies, and appendectomies performed on a nonelective basis[3] [**Box 1**]). These 7 procedures represent 80% of all procedures, deaths, complications, and costs related to EGS in the United States.[1]

This review is structured as follows. First, the association of older age with perioperative outcomes for older people having EGS procedures is discussed. Next, approaches to risk stratification using multivariable risk models as well as the geriatric syndromes of frailty and sarcopenia are discussed. Then, key themes related to each phase of the perioperative period identified through a systematic search are discussed. Finally, key knowledge gaps to be addressed in future research are described.

EPIDEMIOLOGY AND OUTCOMES OF OLDER PEOPLE HAVING EMERGENCY GENERAL SURGERY
Advanced Age and Mortality

Mortality is a tier 1 priority outcome for older people.[9] Across EGS procedures in older people, 30-day mortality rates exceed 15%[2,10] and, in the year after surgery, 1 in 4 older people die.[3] Mortality rates differ, however, between EGS procedures and tend to increase with advancing age.[10] For example, after lower-risk EGS procedures (such as cholecystectomy or appendectomy), 30-day mortality rates are approximately 3% to 4%,[4,11] whereas after laparotomy, 30-day mortality rates exceed 10% in people 60 years to 69 years of age, and death occurs in more than 20% of people

---

Box 1
Core procedures in emergency general surgery

Appendectomy

Cholecystectomy

Excision of large intestine

Lysis of adhesions

Excision of small intestine

Control and suture of stomach or duodenal ulcer

Laparotomy

Procedures are listed by prevalence in derivation study.

Data from Scott JW, Olufajo OA, Brat GA, et al. Use of national burden to define operative emergency general surgery. JAMA Surg 2016;151(6):e160480.

greater than 90 years of age.[12] Overall, existing data suggest that compared with younger individuals, older age is associated with a 2-fold to 5-fold increase in the odds of postoperative mortality after adjustment for patient, clinical, and procedural variables.

Advanced Age and Complications

Older people also frequently experience complications after EGS procedures. Using health administrative data, Kuy and colleagues[4] reported a 27% complication rate after emergency cholecystectomy in people 65 years to 79 years old and a 38% rate in people more than 80 years of age. Ingraham and colleagues[2] reported a 27% complication rate across EGS procedures in people more than 65 years of age. After adjustment for patient, clinical, and procedural factors, advanced age is consistently associated with postoperative complications, with studies reporting a 1.2-fold to 2.4-fold increase in risk.

Advanced Age and Loss of Independence

Despite the increasing focus on patient-reported outcomes[13] and preference expressed by older people to have access to data reflecting functional recovery,[14] few studies describe the typical functional recovery trajectory of older people after EGS.[10,15] Berian and colleagues[16] reported that almost 80% of older people suffer a loss of independence (defined as a decrease in ability to perform activities of daily living, need for a new mobility aid, or increase in care needs) after emergency procedures. Across EGS procedures, at least 12% of older people are discharged directly to a nursing home after their acute care hospitalization.[3] After cholecystectomy, 15% of people ages 65 years to 69 years and 40% of people over age 80 years have an adverse discharge outcome (ie, increased care at home or nonhome discharge). On an adjusted basis, studies report a 1.6-fold to 10-fold increase in odds of loss of independence or adverse discharge location related to advanced age.

Advanced Age and Delirium

Having surgery on an emergency basis is a strong predictor of postoperative delirium; however, few data are available describing delirium rates after EGS in older people.[17] The authors identify a single study that identified postoperative delirium in 18% of older EGS patients[18]; age greater than 75 years was associated with a 3-fold increase in the odds of developing postoperative delirium.

PREOPERATIVE RISK STRATIFICATION
Multivariable Prediction Models

Many multivariable risk prediction models relevant to EGS exist. Some were derived and validated across a variety of surgical procedures and urgency categories (such as the National Surgical Quality Improvement Program universal risk calculator[19] and the Portsmouth Physiological and Operative Severity Score for Enumeration of Mortality and Morbidity[20]) and, therefore, include procedural risk and urgency as predictor variables. Others were specifically derived and internally validated in EGS patients. Risk models derived and/or validated in EGS populations may be preferable to risk models derived and validated across a variety of urgency classes and procedures, because both procedure-related risk factors and urgency-related risk factors substantively drive the predictive performance of more general prediction models. In other words, some models may seem very accurate because they are able to rely on urgency status and procedure type to discriminate between high-risk and low-risk patients; however, when applied only to emergency patients having high-risk procedures, their predictive accuracy may decrease substantially because these strong risk factors are common to all patients.

Oliver and colleagues[21] and Havens and colleagues[22] both have systematically reviewed and evaluated mortality risk prediction scores for EGS patients. Oliver and colleagues[21] concluded that the Acute Physiology and Chronic Health Evaluation II (APACHE II) was the most discriminative model (area under the curve [AUC] 0.76 to 0.98), whereas Havens and colleagues[22] suggest that the Emergency Surgery Acuity Score (ESAS) may be an optimal tool based on its high level of discrimination (AUC 0.86 in internal validation) and reliance on objective variables available before surgery. Both tools, however, present significant barriers to meaningful use. Although risk prediction models often are judged based on their discrimination (ie, AUC or C statistic) this measure reflects only 1 aspect of prediction accuracy (ie, how well a model can determine which of 2 randomly selected patients is more likely to experience the outcome of interest).[23] In the clinical setting, practitioners more often are interested in calibration (ie, how accurately does the model predict the probability that the outcome of interest will occur) so that patients and families can be informed of expected outcomes.[23] Although the APACHE II model has been externally validated, it is unclear if it is adequately calibrated to meaningfully predict expected outcome probabilities.[21] Meanwhile, the ESAS tool has not been externally validated and no formal evaluation of calibration has been reported.[24] Recently, Eugene and colleagues[25] reported a novel mortality risk calculator derived and internally validated using National Emergency Laparotomy Audit (NELA) data from the United Kingdom. Although their model had good discrimination (AUC 0.86) and calibration across risk deciles, the NELA risk model has not been externally validated. Finally, validation of existing models specifically in older populations of EGS patients is needed to support accurate prognostication in this high-risk stratum of the surgical population.

Geriatric Syndromes as Predictors of Risk

Frailty and sarcopenia are related but distinct geriatric syndromes relevant to risk stratification of older EGS patients. The advantage of using geriatric syndromes for risk stratification in EGS surgery includes their ability to identify a relatively homogenous high-risk stratum within the older population of EGS patients, the relative simplicity of clinical or image-based assessment (as opposed to calculating a multivariable risk score), and linkage of these assessments to specific acute geriatric conditions (such as disability and delirium) and associated risk-modifying strategies.

Frailty is an aggregate expression of risk to adverse health outcomes due to the accumulation of age-related and disease-related deficits.[26,27] Operationally, frailty is a multidimensional construct that identifies older individuals inherently vulnerable to stressors. Although frailty is a strong predictor of adverse outcomes in chronic and acute conditions, it is especially relevant in the perioperative setting given the substantial physiologic stress induced by surgery. More than 1 in 3 older people with frailty die in the year after having an EGS procedure (a 14% increase in absolute risk and a 29% increase in relative risk compared with older people without frailty).[3] Importantly, many of these deaths occur early in the postoperative period (hazard ratio 23 on postoperative day 1),[3] which is consistent with the elective setting[28] and highlights the vulnerability to surgical stress faced by older individuals with frailty.

Frailty can be identified using a variety of instruments.[29–31] The most promising instruments for clinical use are likely the frailty phenotype[32] and frailty scales.[27] Studies of clinically applied frailty assessments in the EGS population, however, are limited; most recommendations must be extrapolated from the elective surgery setting and other fields of acute care medicine.

The frailty phenotype, typically diagnosed using the Fried index,[32] currently is recommended by the American College of Surgeons and the American Geriatrics Society.[33] Using the Fried index, an individual is considered frail if demonstrating 3 or more of 5 traits (unintentional weight loss, slow gait speed, easy fatigue, history of falls, and decreased grip strength [**Table 1**]).[32] Application of the Fried index in the EGS setting may be limited because acute illness may preclude participation in physical performance measures or activity questionnaires. Individual components (eg, grip strength) of the Fried index have been evaluated as predictors of frailty and outcomes; however, their ability to discriminate high-risk from low-risk patients is limited.[34]

The authors believe that the frailty scale with the most convincing data for use in surgery and acute care is the Clinical Frailty Scale (CFS),[35–37] a clinical application of the Canadian Study of Health and Aging Frailty Index that is highly corelated with this 80-variable index ($\rho = 0.80$).[27] After clinical assessment, the clinician determines an older individual's degree of frailty through consultation with an image and vignette-based tool (see **Table 1**). Frailty is present if a score of greater than or equal to 4 is assigned. Despite its seemingly subjective appearance, the CFS has high inter-rater reliability[35,38] and may be determined through proxy interview or chart review.[35]

Table 1
Description of fried phenotype and clinical frailty scale

Fried Phenotype	Clinical Frailty Scale
Weight loss: >10 lb unintentionally in prior year	1. *Very fit*: people who are robust, very active, and motivated. These people commonly exercise regularly. They are among the fittest of their age.
Grip strength: lowest 20% (by gender and body mass index)	2. *Well*: people who have no active disease symptoms but are less fit than those in category 1. Often, they exercise or are very active occasionally.
Exhaustion: self-report	3. *Managing well*: people whose medical problems are well controlled, but they are rarely active beyond walking.
Slowness: 15-ft walking speed (by gender and height)	4. *Vulnerable*: although not dependent on others for daily help, symptoms often limit activities. A common complaint is being "slowed up" and/or being tired during the day.
Low activity: kilocalories per week (men <383, women <270)	5. Mildly frail: these people often have more evident slowing and need help in high-order instrumental activities of daily living. Typically, this impairs shopping and walking outside alone, meal preparation, and housework.
	6. *Moderately frail*: people need help with all outside activities and with keeping house. Inside, they often have problems with stairs and need help with bathing and might need minimal help with dressing.
	7. *Severely frail*: completely dependent for all personal care from whatever cause (physical or cognitive). Even so, they seem stable and not at high risk of dying (within approximately 6 mo).
	8. *Very severely frail*: completely dependent, approaching the end of life. Typically, they could not recover from even a minor illness.
	9. *Terminally ill*: approaching the end of life. This category applies to people with a life expectancy <6 mo, who are not evidently frail.
Frailty present if ≥3 characteristics present	*Frailty present if category ≥4*

Adapted from Fried LP, Tangen CM, Walston J, et al. Frailty in older adults: evidence for a phenotype. J Gerontol A Biol Sci Med Sci 2001;56(3):M148; with permission.

Compared with the Fried index, anesthesiologists find the CFS faster and easier to use.[37] After EGS procedures, the CFS predicts death or readmission in older patients, with an adjusted odds ratio of 4.6 compared with older patients without frailty.[39]

Sarcopenia is a progressive and generalized skeletal muscle disorder characterized by low muscle mass, strength, and quality.[40] Poor muscle function, typically demonstrated through reduced strength, is highly suggestive of sarcopenia; however, the diagnosis is confirmed through imaging.[40] The prevalence of abdominal CT imaging in individuals with acute intra-abdominal conditions makes sarcopenia a particularly relevant condition in the EGS setting, where low muscle cross-sectional area predicts a 1.6-fold increase in complications and a 2-fold increase in mortality.[41]

PREOPERATIVE
Patient Optimization

The urgent nature of EGS often precludes significant time for patient optimization; however, some acute or acute-on-chronic conditions should be optimized in a goal-directed and time-limited fashion prior to proceeding to the operating room unless an immediately life-threatening condition is present. In addition to acute exacerbations of common comorbidities, such as heart failure or obstructive lung disease, many EGS patients have, or are at risk of, sepsis. For these patients clinicians, should consider guidelines for sepsis care.[42] The 2018 Surviving Sepsis Campaign bundle has consolidated previous recommendations for interventions within 3 hours and 6 hours into a single hour-1 bundle to support immediate initiation of resuscitation and sepsis management. This bundle includes blood cultures, serum lactate measurement, broad-spectrum antibiotic therapy, goal-directed fluid therapy, and early use of vasopressors to maintain a mean arterial pressure of 65 mm Hg or higher.[43]

Any acute optimization also must consider the potentially deleterious effect of surgical delay. Although a substantial evidence base demonstrates the risk of delayed surgery in emergency orthopedic (ie, hip fracture) surgery,[44] a growing collection of evidence suggests that similar mechanisms may exist for EGS procedures.[45–47] Therefore, any patient optimization should be balanced against the risk of delaying urgent and necessary surgery.

Communication

Urgent surgery presents challenges in risk communication. Although many aspects of communication are primarily in the domain of the surgical team, anesthesiologists play a key role in risk communication, particularly in relation to the intraoperative period. Anesthesiologists should bear in mind key recommendations for communication in the setting of acute disease and urgent need for surgery (**Box 2**)[48] as well as clarifying patient and family preferences related to goals of care.

For anesthesiologists, discussion of perioperative do-not-resuscitate (DNR) orders are particularly relevant. Patients or their surrogates may opt not to receive certain resuscitative procedures due to the unacceptable potential burden of resultant outcomes.[49] Many patients who express aspects of a DNR order, however, still have surgery, making it crucial to recognize that automatic suspension of such orders in the operating room disregards patient autonomy.[49] Instead, an individualized approach discussed with the patient or an appropriate surrogate is required. This approach is reflected in the American Society of Anesthesiologists "Ethical Guidelines for the Anesthesia Care of Patients with Do-Not-Resuscitate Orders or Other Directives that Limit Treatment."[50] These guidelines recommend that individual patients (or their surrogates) be provided options, such as choosing a blanket intraoperative

---

Box 2
Goals for structured communication

Place patient acute illness in the context of chronic conditions.

Elicit patient preferences regarding life-prolonging therapies.

Describe treatment options in context of patient goals and priorities.

Direct treatment to achieve patient goals and priorities; consider time-limited trials in context of uncertainty.

Affirm continued commitment to care of the individual.

Data from Cooper Z, Koritsanszky LA, Cauley CE, et al. Recommendations for best communication practices to facilitate goal-concordant care for seriously ill older patients with emergency surgical conditions. Ann Surg 2016;263(1):1–6.

---

suspension of DNR orders, a procedure-oriented and individualized approach that delineates the specific resuscitative interventions deemed acceptable, or a limited attempt at resuscitation that respects and aligns with patient goals and values. Given the complexities of such decisions and their operationalization, it also is critical that surgeons and nurses are informed of intraoperative goals of care.[49]

Multidisciplinary Comanagement

Accumulating evidence supports an important role for geriatric medicine comanagement of older EGS patients,[51] consistent with high-quality evidence in hip fracture supporting the role of orthogeriatric care in improving function, survival, and length of stay.[52,53] Recent guidelines recommend geriatric comanagement in people over 70 years of age having EGS procedures.[12]

INTRAOPERATIVE
Goal-directed Fluid Therapy

Goal-directed fluid therapy, a strategy in which intravenous fluids are administered to target continuously measured hemodynamic measurements, such as stroke volume, stroke volume variation, pulse pressure variation, and cardiac output,[54] is recommended by NELA guidelines,[12] based on expert consensus.[55–57] Goal-directed fluid therapy may reduce morbidity and length of stay, although it has not been shown to reduce mortality in noncardiac surgery.[58–61] The FLuid Optimisation in Emergency LAparotomy trial currently is under way to establish the effect of cardiac output monitoring in emergency laparotomy patients.[62]

Prevention of Intraoperative Hypotension

Increasing evidence links perioperative hypotension to postoperative complications, such as myocardial ischemia,[63] stroke,[64] and acute kidney injury.[65,66] This effect is seen with both absolute hypotension (eg, mean arterial pressure below 65 mm Hg) or relative hypotension (<10%–20% of baseline).[67,68] A recent systematic review determined that no solid conclusions could be made regarding choice of specific blood pressure targets and that further research is needed.[64,69]

Inhalational Versus Total Intravenous Anesthesia

Because most EGS procedures require general anesthesia, clinicians are faced with a choice between inhalational versus total intravenous anesthesia (TIVA) techniques; however, data specific to EGS procedures currently are not available. A Cochrane review of TIVA versus inhalational anesthesia in older people having noncardiac procedures of any urgency demonstrated significant uncertainty in terms of the impact of TIVA on outcomes.[70] The review found no evidence of a difference in delirium rates or mortality between techniques. Low-certainty evidence suggested a possible improvement in rates of postoperative cognitive dysfunction, but further high-quality trials are needed to inform the choice of TIVA versus inhalational agents for maintenance of general anesthesia in older people having EGS procedures.

Risk Restratification

Postoperative risk restratification should take place to determine appropriate disposition. Given the nature of EGS, the preoperative risk assessment may not be accurate due to changes in a patient's clinical status and planned/actual surgical procedure. An end-of-surgery bundle or checklist also may be useful.[71]

POSTOPERATIVE
Acute Postoperative Monitoring

Older people, especially those with frailty, are vulnerable to the physiologic stress caused by acute illness and surgery. Although patient-level randomized trial data to inform the provision of a high-dependency unit care after EGS procedures are lacking, a recent cluster randomized trial in acutely ill nonsurgical patients found no difference in mortality rates after introduction of systematic intensive care unit (ICU) admission criteria.[72] A further study of critical care admissions after elective surgery found no association between hospital-level postoperative ICU admissions and mortality.[73] After EGS procedures, however, observational evidence suggests that potentially inappropriate (based on acute illness) ward-based disposition (as opposed to a monitored setting) was associated with higher mortality than admission directly to the ICU.[74] In older EGS patients with frailty, the relative impact of frailty on mortality was most pronounced for procedures with low baseline rates of ICU admission.[3] Therefore, clinicians should carefully consider the merits of higher acuity monitored care in vulnerable and acutely ill older EGS patients after surgery.

Acute Rehabilitation

Healthy older adults on bed rest lose more than 1 lb of muscle per week,[75] a rate 3-times to 6-times higher than younger people.[76] Given the catabolic response to acute illness, this rate of muscle loss may be even more pronounced in older EGS patients. Although preoperative exercise and nutritional supplementation seem effective in elective surgery to improve postoperative function in high-risk older people,[77,78] this approach is not directly applicable to EGS patients. Emerging evidence suggests that simple, short course in-hospital postoperative rehabilitation can improve objective lower limb function in older EGS patients with frailty.[79]

AREAS FOR FUTURE CONSIDERATION

Overall, little robust epidemiologic or interventional literature is available to inform the care of older EGS patients, and high-priority knowledge gaps are present across the perioperative period. Preoperatively, accurate, and validated risk prediction models specifically calibrated for older people are lacking. Furthermore, few clinically oriented studies have assessed the utility of frailty and sarcopenia definitions in predicting risk or in guiding enhanced clinical care. Few data specific to the intraoperative period are available, and important questions regarding goal-directed hemodynamic management and choice of maintenance agents for general anesthesia remain unanswered.

The role and ideal make-up of multidisciplinary perioperative teams also require further study, as does the role of acute monitoring strategies and enhanced rehabilitation interventions.

REFERENCES

1. Scott JW, Olufajo OA, Brat GA, et al. Use of national burden to define operative emergency general surgery. JAMA Surg 2016;02115:e160480.
2. Ingraham AM, Cohen ME, Raval MV, et al. Variation in quality of care after emergency general surgery procedures in the elderly. J Am Coll Surg 2011;212: 1039–48.
3. McIsaac DI, Moloo H, Bryson GL, et al. The association of frailty with outcomes and resource use after emergency general surgery: a population-based cohort study. Anesth Analg 2017;124:1653–61.
4. Kuy S, Sosa JA, Roman SA, et al. Age matters: a study of clinical and economic outcomes following cholecystectomy in elderly Americans. Am J Surg 2011;201: 789–96.
5. Haider A, Obirieze A, Velopulos C, et al. Incremental cost of emergency versus elective surgery. Ann Surg 2015;262:260–6.
6. He W, Goodkind D, Kowal P. An aging world 2015. Washington, DC. Available at: https://www.census.gov/content/dam/Census/library/publications/2016/demo/p95-16-1.pdf. Accessed January 3, 2019.
7. Etzioni DA, Liu JH, Maggard MA, et al. The aging population and its impact on the surgery workforce. Ann Surg 2003;238:170–7.
8. Wohlgemut JM, Ramsay G, Jansen JO. The changing face of emergency general surgery. Ann Surg 2018. [Epub ahead of print].
9. Akpan A, Roberts C, Bandeen-Roche K, et al. Standard set of health outcome measures for older persons. BMC Geriatr 2018;18:36.
10. Cooper Z, Scott JW, Rosenthal RA, et al. Emergency major abdominal surgical procedures in older adults: a systematic review of mortality and functional outcomes. J Am Geriatr Soc 2015;63:2563–71.
11. Shah AA, Zafar SN, Kodadek LM, et al. Never giving up: outcomes and presentation of emergency general surgery in geriatric octogenarian and nonagenarian patients. Am J Surg 2016;212:211–20.e3.
12. NELA Project Team: Third patient report of the National emergency laparotomy Audit RCoA London, 2017. 2017. https://doi.org/10.1557/opl.2014.223.
13. Devlin N, Appelby J. Getting the most out of PROMs: putting health utcomes at the heart of NHS decision making 2010. London: Kings Fund.
14. Fried TR, Bradley EH, Towle VR, et al. Understanding the treatment preferences of seriously ill patients. N Engl J Med 2002;346:1061–6.
15. Fiore JF, Figueiredo S, Balvardi S, et al. How do we value postoperative recovery?: a systematic review of the measurement properties of patient-reported outcomes after abdominal surgery. Ann Surg 2018;267(4):656–69.
16. Berian J, Mohanty S, Ko CY, et al. Association of loss of independence with readmission and death after discharge in older patients after surgical procedures. JAMA Surg 2016;1–7. https://doi.org/10.1001/jamasurg.2016.1689.
17. Scholz AFM, Oldroyd C, McCarthy K, et al. Systematic review and meta-analysis of risk factors for postoperative delirium among older patients undergoing gastrointestinal surgery. Br J Surg 2016;103:e21–8.

18. Ansaloni L, Catena F, Chattat R, et al. Risk factors and incidence of postoperative delirium in elderly patients after elective and emergency surgery. Br J Surg 2010; 97:273–80.

19. Bilimoria KY, Liu Y, Paruch JL, et al. Development and evaluation of the universal ACS NSQIP surgical risk calculator: a decision aid and informed consent tool for patients and surgeons. J Am Coll Surg 2013;217:833–42.e1-3.

20. Richards CH, Leitch FE, Horgan PG, et al. A systematic review of POSSUM and its related models as predictors of post-operative mortality and morbidity in patients undergoing surgery for colorectal cancer. J Gastrointest Surg 2010;14: 1511–20.

21. Oliver CM, Walker E, Giannaris S, et al. Risk assessment tools validated for patients undergoing emergency laparotomy: a systematic review. Br J Anaesth 2015;115:849–60.

22. Havens JM, Columbus AB, Seshadri AJ, et al. Risk stratification tools in emergency general surgery. Trauma Surg Acute Care Open 2018;3:e000160.

23. Harrell FE, Lee KL, Mark DB. Multivariable prognostic models: issues in developing models, evaluating assumptions and adequacy, and measuring and reducing errors. Stat Med 1996;15:361–87.

24. Sangji NF, Bohnen JD, Ramly EP, et al. Derivation and validation of a novel Emergency Surgery Acuity Score (ESAS). J Trauma Acute Care Surg 2016;81:213–20.

25. Eugene N, Oliver CM, Bassett MG, et al. Development and internal validation of a novel risk adjustment model for adult patients undergoing emergency laparotomy surgery: the National Emergency Laparotomy Audit risk model. Br J Anaesth 2018;121:739–48.

26. Fried LP, Ferruci L, Darer J, et al. Untangling the concepts of disability, frailty and comorbidity: Implications for improved targeting and care. J Gerontol A Biol Sci Med Sci 2004;59:M255–63.

27. Rockwood K, Song X, MacKnight C, et al. A global clinical measure of fitness and frailty in elderly people. CMAJ 2005;173:489–95.

28. McIsaac DI, Bryson GL, van Walraven C. Association of frailty and 1-year postoperative mortality following major elective noncardiac surgery: a population-based cohort study. JAMA Surg 2016;151(6):538–45.

29. Lin H-S, Watts JN, Peel NM, et al. Frailty and post-operative outcomes in older surgical patients: a systematic review. BMC Geriatr 2016;16:157.

30. Beggs T, Sepehri A, Szwajcer A, et al. Frailty and perioperative outcomes: a narrative review. Can J Anaesth 2015;62:143–57.

31. Kim DH, Kim CA, Placide S, et al. Preoperative frailty assessment and outcomes at 6 months or later in older adults undergoing cardiac surgical procedures. Ann Intern Med 2016. https://doi.org/10.7326/M16-0652.

32. Fried LP, Tangen CM, Walston J, et al. Frailty in older adults : evidence for a phenotype. J Gerontol A Biol Sci Med Sci 2001;56:146–57.

33. Chow WB, Rosenthal RA, Merkow RP, et al. Optimal preoperative assessment of the geriatric surgical patient: a best practices guideline from the American College of Surgeons National Surgical Quality Improvement Program and the American Geriatrics Society. J Am Coll Surg 2012;215:453–66.

34. Revenig LM, Canter DJ, Kim S, et al. Report of a simplified frailty score predictive of short-term postoperative morbidity and mortality. J Am Coll Surg 2015;220(5): 904–11.e1.

35. Shears M, Takaoka A, Rochwerg B, et al. Assessing frailty in the intensive care unit: a reliability and validity study. J Crit Care 2018;45:197–203.

36. Bagshaw SM, Stelfox HT, McDermid RC, et al. Association between frailty and short- and long-term outcomes among critically ill patients: a multicentre prospective cohort study. Can Med Assoc J 2014;186:E95–102.
37. McIsaac DI, Taljaard M, Bryson GL, et al. Frailty as a predictor of death or new disability after surgery: a prospective cohort study. Ann Surg 2018. [Epub ahead of print].
38. Wallis SJ, Wall J, Biram RWS, et al. Association of the Clinical Frailty Scale (CFS) with hospital outcomes. QJM 2015. https://doi.org/10.1093/qjmed/hcv066.
39. Li Y, Pederson J, Churchill T, et al. Impact of frailty on outcomes after discharge in older surgical patients: a prospective cohort study. CMAJ 2018;190:184–90.
40. Cruz-Jentoft AJ, Bahat G, Bauer J, et al. Writing Group for the European Working Group on Sarcopenia in Older People 2 (EWGSOP2) and the EG for E: Sarcopenia: revised European consensus on definition and diagnosis. Age Ageing 2018. https://doi.org/10.1093/ageing/afy169.
41. Jones K, Gordon-Weeks A, Coleman C, et al. Radiologically determined sarcopenia predicts morbidity and mortality following abdominal surgery: a systematic review and meta-analysis. World J Surg 2017;41:2266–79.
42. Levy MM, Evans LE, Rhodes A. The surviving sepsis campaign bundle. Crit Care Med 2018;46:997–1000.
43. Ommundsen N, Wyller TB, Nesbakken A, et al. Frailty is an independent predictor of survival in older patients with colorectal cancer. Oncologist 2014;19(12): 1268–75.
44. Simunovic N, Devereaux PJ, Sprague S, et al. Effect of early surgery after hip fracture on mortality and complications: systematic review and meta-analysis. CMAJ 2010;182:1609–16.
45. McIsaac DI, Abdulla K, Yang H, et al. Association of delay of urgent or emergency surgery with mortality and use of health care resources: a propensity score–matched observational cohort study. Can Med Assoc J 2017;189: E905–12.
46. Buck DL, Vester-Andersen M, Møller MH. Surgical delay is a critical determinant of survival in perforated. Br J Surg 2013;100:1045–9.
47. Azuhata T, Kinoshita K, Kawano D, et al. Time from admission to initiation of surgery for source control is a critical determinant of survival in patients with gastrointestinal perforation with associated septic shock. Crit Care 2014;18:1–10.
48. Cooper Z, Koritsanszky LA, Cauley CE, et al. Recommendations for best communication practices to facilitate goal-concordant care for seriously ill older patients with emergency surgical conditions. Ann Surg 2016;263:1–6.
49. Azer SA. Social media channels in health care research and rising ethical issues. AMA J Ethics 2017;19:1061–9.
50. American Society of Anesthesiologists. Ethical guidelines for the anesthesia care of patients with do not resuscitate orders or other directives that limit treatment. Am Soc Anesthesiol 2016;1–3. House Deleg. Park Ridge. Available at: https://www.google.ca/url?sa=t&rct=j&q=&esrc=s&source=web&cd=1&ved=2ahUKEwjKmlvl-LviAhVloFkKHeYoDnEQFjAAegQIAhAC&url=https%3A%2F%2Fwww.asahq.org%2F~%2Fmedia%2Fsites%2Fasahq%2Ffiles%2Fpublic%2Fresources%2Fstandards-guidelines%2Fethical-guidelines-for-the-anesthesia-care-of-patients.pdf&usg=AOvVaw2yMuwbMuMRfWIqw1CSIi3H. Accessed May 27, 2019.
51. Oliver CM, Bassett MG, Poulton TE, et al. Organisational factors and mortality after an emergency laparotomy: multilevel analysis of 39 903 National Emergency Laparotomy Audit patients. Br J Anaesth 2018. https://doi.org/10.1016/j.bja.2018.07.040.

52. Grigoryan KV, Javedan H, Rudolph JL. Orthogeriatric care models and outcomes in hip fracture patients: a systematic review and meta-analysis. J Orthop Trauma 2014;28:e49–55.

53. Prestmo A, Hagen G, Sletvold O, et al. Comprehensive geriatric care for patients with hip fractures: a prospective, randomised, controlled trial. Lancet 2015;385: 1623–33.

54. Wrzosek A, Jakowicka-Wordliczek J, Zajaczkowska R, et al. Perioperative restrictive versus goal-directed fluid therapy for adults undergoing major non-cardiac surgery. Cochrane Database Syst Rev 2017;8:CD012767.

55. Navarro LHC, Bloomstone JA, Auler JOC, et al. Perioperative fluid therapy: a statement from the international Fluid Optimization Group. Perioper Med 2015; 4(1):3.

56. Richards T. An age old problem. BMJ 2007;335:698.

57. Powell-Tuck J, Gosling P, Lobo DN, et al. British consensus guidelines on intravenous fluid therapy for adult surgical patients GIFTASUP. Jics 2009;10:13–5. Available at: https://www.bapen.org.uk/resources-and-education/education-and-guidance/bapen-principles-of-good-nutritional-practice/giftasup. Accessed May 27, 2019.

58. Grocott MP, Dushianthan A, Hamilton MA, et al. Perioperative increase in global blood flow to explicit defined goals and outcomes following surgery. Cochrane Database Syst Rev 2012;(11):CD004082.

59. Som A, Maitra S, Bhattacharjee S, et al. Goal directed fluid therapy decreases postoperative morbidity but not mortality in major non-cardiac surgery: a meta-analysis and trial sequential analysis of randomized controlled trials. J Anesth 2017;31:66–81.

60. Xu C, Peng J, Liu S, et al. Goal-directed fluid therapy versus conventional fluid therapy in colorectal surgery: a meta analysis of randomized controlled trials. Int J Surg 2018;56:264–73.

61. Pearse RM, Harrison DA, MacDonald N, et al. Effect of a perioperative, cardiac output-guided hemodynamic therapy algorithm on outcomes following major gastrointestinal surgery a randomized clinical trial and systematic review. JAMA 2014;311:2181–90.

62. FLuid optimisation in emergency LAparotomy trial. Available at: https://floela.org/home?newsid=8. Accessed May 27, 2019.

63. Sessler DI, Meyhoff CS, Zimmerman NM, et al. Period-dependent associations between hypotension during and for four days after noncardiac surgery and a composite of myocardial infarction and death: a substudy of the pOISE-2 trial. Anesthesiology 2018;128:317–27.

64. Wesselink EM, Kappen TH, Torn HM, et al. Intraoperative hypotension and the risk of postoperative adverse outcomes: a systematic review. Br J Anaesth 2018;121:706–21.

65. Salmasi V, Maheshwari K, Yang D, et al. Relationship between intraoperative hypotension, defined by either reduction from baseline or absolute thresholds, and acute kidney and myocardial injury after noncardiac surgery. Anesthesiology 2017;126:47–65.

66. Outcomes M, Registration T. Effect of individualized vs standard blood pressure management strategies on postoperative organ dysfunction among high-risk patients undergoing major surgery - a randomized clinical trial. JAMA 2017;318: 1346–57.

67. Hallqvist L, Mårtensson J, Granath F, et al. Intraoperative hypotension is associated with myocardial damage in noncardiac surgery: an observational study. Eur J Anaesthesiol 2016;33:450–6.
68. Futier E, Lefrant J-Y, Guinot P-G, et al. Effect of individualized vs standard blood pressure management strategies on postoperative organ dysfunction among high-risk patients undergoing major surgery. JAMA 2017;318:1346.
69. Ke JXC, George RB, Beattie WS. Making sense of the impact of intraoperative hypotension: from populations to the individual patient. Br J Anaesth 2018;121: 689–91.
70. Miller D, Lewis SR, Pritchard MW, et al. Intravenous versus inhalational maintenance of anaesthesia for postoperative cognitive outcomes in elderly people undergoing non-cardiac surgery. Cochrane Database Syst Rev 2018;(8):CD012317.
71. The Royal College of Surgeons of England/Department of Health. The higher risk general surgical patient: towards improved care for a forgotten group. Report on the peri-operative care of the higher risk general surgical patient. London: RCSENG - Professional Standards and Regulation; 2011. Available at: https://www.google.ca/url?sa=t&rct=j&q=&esrc=s&source=web&cd=2&ved=2ahUK EwinxbDj97viAhUw1VkKHVbsD6AQFjABegQIBRAC&url=https%3A%2F%2Fwww. rcseng.ac.uk%2F-%2Fmedia%2Ffiles%2Frcs%2Flibrary-and-publications%2Fnon-journal-publications%2Fthe-higher-risk-general-surgical-patient–towards-improved-care-for-a-forgotten-group.pdf&usg=AOvVaw3xA7SAKsOSyuGQ8-aKyl60.   Accessed May 27, 2019.
72. Guidet B, Leblanc G, Simon T, et al. Effect of systematic intensive care unit triage on long-term mortality among critically ill elderly patients in france. JAMA 2017; 318:1450.
73. Kahan BC, Koulenti D, Arvaniti K, et al. Critical care admission following elective surgery was not associated with survival benefit: prospective analysis of data from 27 countries. Intensive Care Med 2017;43:971–9.
74. Vester-Andersen M, Lundstrom LH, Moller MH, et al. Mortality and postoperative care pathways after emergency gastrointestinal surgery in 2904 patients: a population-based cohort study. Br J Anaesth 2014;112:860–70.
75. Kortebein P, Ferrando A, Lombeida J, et al. Effect of 10 days of bed rest on skeletal muscle in healthy older adults. JAMA 2007;297:1772–4.
76. English KL, Paddon-Jones D. Protecting muscle mass and function in older adults during bed rest. Curr Opin Clin Nutr Metab Care 2010;13:34–9.
77. Minnella EM, Awasthi R, Gillis C, et al. Patients with poor baseline walking capacity are most likely to improve their functional status with multimodal prehabilitation. Surgery 2016;160:1070–9.
78. Barberan-Garcia A, Ubré M, Roca J, et al. Personalised prehabilitation in high-risk patients undergoing elective major abdominal surgery: a randomized blinded controlled trial. Ann Surg 2018;267:50–6.
79. McComb A, Warkentin LM, McNeely ML, et al. Development of a reconditioning program for elderly abdominal surgery patients: the Elder-friendly Approaches to the Surgical Environment-BEdside reconditioning for Functional ImprovemenTs (EASE-BE FIT) pilot study. World J Emerg Surg 2018;13:21.

Acute Pain in Older Adults

Recommendations for Assessment and Treatment

Jay Rajan, MD, Matthias Behrends, MD*

KEYWORDS

- Acute pain • Elderly • Geriatrics • Pain medicine • Anesthesia • Postsurgical care

KEY POINTS

- Older adults experience significant physiologic and psychosocial changes with aging that can affect pain assessment and treatment.
- Medication choice must be adjusted carefully in older adults with respect to comorbidities, cognitive function, and organ reserve.
- Pain should be treated as seriously in the elderly as in younger patients, because it can provoke consequences, such as delirium.
- If applicable, regional anesthesia should be considered a component of a multimodal pain management regimen.

INTRODUCTION

The treatment of acute pain requires special attention when focused on older adults, who are usually defined as those age 65 years or older. Various physiologic changes occur with increasing age that affect how pain is diagnosed and managed. In a population where the incidence of acute postoperative pain is very high,[1] it is important to remember these changes when assessing pain in the elderly and determining which treatments are appropriate. With effective acute pain management, especially in the perioperative setting, older adults experience decreased morbidity and mortality, faster recovery, shorter hospital stays, and decreased health care costs.[2]

AGE-RELATED CHANGES AND IMPLICATIONS IN PAIN MANAGEMENT
Physiologic Changes with Age

At the physiologic level, the sensation of pain changes with age. Proprioception is known to decrease with age[3]; it has been suggested that although C-fiber function

Disclosure Statement: The authors have nothing to disclose.
Department of Anesthesia and Perioperative Care, University of California, San Francisco, 513 Parnassus Avenue, S-455, San Francisco, CA 94143, USA
* Corresponding author.
E-mail address: matthias.behrends@ucsf.edu

Anesthesiology Clin 37 (2019) 507–520
https://doi.org/10.1016/j.anclin.2019.04.009   anesthesiology.theclinics.com
1932-2275/19/© 2019 Elsevier Inc. All rights reserved.

remains stable, A-delta pain transmissions also decrease with age.[4] These changes, however, do not translate into diminished central sensation of pain in the elderly.[5]

In addition to neurologic changes with age, numerous metabolic changes occur in older adults that affect the pharmacokinetics of various analgesic drugs. Significant changes in body composition with age, such as an increase in body fat combined with a decrease in muscle mass, also affect the pharmacokinetics of certain pain medications. In addition, plasma volume and intracellular water both decrease by as much as 20% to 30% by the age of 75.[6] These changes in body composition have important ramifications; lipid-soluble drugs like fentanyl may have a longer duration of action given a high volume of fat distribution, whereas less lipid-soluble drugs like morphine may be much more potent in their effects, owing to a smaller volume of distribution and decreased plasma volume. In addition, boluses of certain drugs may result in higher peak concentrations and may bring on a higher risk of unwanted side effects.

Hepatic size and blood flow begin to decrease beyond the age of 50, and there also are significant decreases in kidney size and with age.[7] With decrease in kidney size, the number of nephrons decreases in parallel, resulting in a reduction in glomerular filtration rate and functional renal reserve with advanced age. These decreases in metabolic function significantly alter the duration, potency, and clearance of various medications, requiring careful dose adjustments and clinical monitoring of elderly patients.

Functional and Clinical Changes

Elderly patients often have various comorbidities related to age, lifestyle, and genetics that affect pain assessment and treatment. Chronic conditions like hypertension and diabetes are common in patients above the age of 65 and result in patients being treated with numerous medications, a prescribing practice commonly referred to as *polypharmacy*. Polypharmacy is highly associated with an increased risk of delirium,[8] and being prescribed five drugs or more increases the risk of adverse drug reactions by 50%.[9] Prior to prescribing medications or offering interventions for the treatment of pain, these conditions and related medications need to be considered properly.

With increasing age, issues with cognitive function also are important to consider when treating pain. Many pain medications have central nervous system side effects, and the clinical effect profile of certain drugs or interventions may change drastically. The prevalence of dementia among people ages 65 years or older was approximately 11% as of the last US census.[10] Contributing factors to dementia and cognitive impairment can include the lack of cholinergic and dopaminergic reserves. Many pain medications alter these reserves or interact with other medications to cause unfavorable central nervous system effects, contributing to health care–associated delirium or further cognitive decline. Delirium and dementia also make pain assessment challenging, because patients with altered mental status are much more likely to underreport their pain.[11]

Physiologic changes with aging are summarized in **Table 1**.

CHALLENGES WITH PAIN TREATMENT IN THE ELDERLY
Cultural Changes in Pain Management

One of the most significant issues regarding acute pain in elderly patients is the undertreatment of pain. Although the lack of appropriate pain assessment in the cognitively impaired seems like a clear contributor, prior studies also have pointed out several cultural concerns impairing appropriate pain management.[12] Undertreated pain in the elderly can have troubling consequences, such as delirium or the development of

Table 1
Physiologic changes with aging and their clinical significance in pain management

Organ System	Changes with Aging	Clinical Impact on Pain Management
Cardiovascular	Decreased cardiac output, atherosclerosis	• Slower body distribution of drugs • Higher risk of adverse coronary or vascular event with uncontrolled pain
Nervous system	Cognitive impairment and cortical atrophy are common; decreased proprioception, altered peripheral nerve conductivity, diminished autonomic responses, higher risk for cerebrovascular disease, high risk of delirium	• Altered sensation of pain (but not diminished) • Increased risk for injury • Poor sympathetic response to pain • Varying presentations of pain (especially in setting of delirium)
Respiratory system	Diminished respiratory reserve	• Higher risk of respiratory decompensation from pain
Renal	Glomerulosclerosis, renal cortical atrophy, decreased glomerular filtration rate	• Decreased clearance of medications • Reduced renal reserve to recover from nephrotoxic medications
Gastrointestinal, hepatic	Fewer hepatocytes	• Decreased hepatic metabolism of drugs Risk of adverse drug interactions
Musculoskeletal	Muscular atrophy	• Decreased drug volume of distribution • Higher risk of drug toxicity and adverse interactions

chronic pain. Sensitivity to pain often is underestimated in elderly patients, and pain often is assumed an expected part of the aging process by both patients and care-givers.[13] Older adults often perceive themselves as high utilizers of health care services and may try to minimize their perceived burden on health care workers by under-reporting their pain.[12] Often in the face of multimorbidity and polypharmacy common among older adults, both patients and caregivers have misconceptions about the clinical effect of using pain medications. These misconceptions often are centered around the idea that pain medications are too dangerous to use in the elderly, causing addiction or unwanted side effects more often than working to treat pain effectively.[14] Although the sensation of pain may be different in the elderly, because of peripheral and central nervous system changes, the perception of pain should not be considered any less seriously from patients of other ages. Pain in elderly patients should be treated to the appropriate extent.

Assessment of Pain

The most common methods of pain assessment are the visual analog scale and the numerical pain scoring scale.[15] Given the high incidence of cognitive impairment along with peripheral neurologic changes that alter the sensation of pain, however, the assessment of pain in elderly patients may extend beyond these two methods. Most assessment of pain in younger patients is done according to numerical scoring, visual analog scale, or verbal descriptor scale, but these scales generally require intact cognitive function for patients to effectively verbalize their pain. For more severely impaired or nonverbal patients, the Critical Care Pain Observation Tool (CPOT) and the Faces Pain Scale (quantifying the level pain based on facial expression)[16] are more widely in use and are the primary methods of assessing pain in the cognitively impaired at the home institution of the authors (both in and out of the critical care setting). The Doloplus-2 scale has been suggested as another possible observational tool to assess pain in both acute and subacute settings,[16] but the evidence supporting its use is conflicting,[17] particularly because of its vulnerability to observer bias.[16] In addition to CPOT or Faces assessments, collateral information from close friends, family, or caregivers can definitely supplement information provided by the patient in cases of suspected cognitive impairment or difficulties with communication. To determine which pain scale is the most appropriate to use, a careful assessment of cognitive and verbal function is required.

Issues of Consent and Decision Making

With the increased incidence of cognitive dysfunction and comorbid illnesses, pain treatment in older adults can be complicated by issues related to informed consent, assent, and decision making. When patients lack the cognitive capacity to express or treat their pain, a significant amount of responsibility is placed on the health care provider or a patient's durable power of attorney to decide how pain can be treated. Issues relating to consent need to be addressed when patients are eligible for surgical procedures or interventional pain management options, such as nerve blocks or neuraxial analgesia. Although all acute pain should be assessed and treated in appropriate manner, important consideration should be paid to any advanced directive made by the patient about which treatment modalities are permissible. A thorough discussion should be made with the durable power of attorney about any modalities that may seem unclear.

Expert Consultation for Pain

With respect to treating pain in the acute setting, certain questions about the interaction of patient comorbidity, cognition, and care goals warrant specialty-specific consultation. Geriatric-specific care has led to significant decreases in postoperative delirium, mortality, and functional decline for geriatric trauma in the acute care setting.[18] Geriatrics consultation teams are able to provide valuable advice regarding pain management options with respect to patient age and clinical status, often resulting in lower pain scores during hospital stays.[18] For treatment of pain in the acute setting, a geriatric expert consultation is helpful in providing age-specific recommendations on pain management.

ANALGESIC INTERVENTIONS AND TREATMENTS
Introduction

The goal of pain management in older adults, as it is in younger adults, is to provide analgesic interventions that can achieve pain relief with minimal side effects. Older adults are at increased risk to develop delirium and cognitive decline in the postoperative period, and both are associated with increased morbidity and mortality.[19] Undertreating pain is known to promote delirium,[19] but overaggressive pain management also can result in cognitive dysfunction, delirium, sedation, or falls. In addition, many medications or interventions may have unfavorable side-effect profiles resulting in organ dysfunction. Achieving the right balance between good pain control and avoidance of adverse effects can be challenging.

Acetaminophen
Acetaminophen (also known as paracetamol), a centrally acting cyclooxygenase inhibitor, is a weak analgesic with an established track record for safety and tolerability.

Whereas monotherapy with acetaminophen usually is indicated for mild pain, scheduled acetaminophen has now become well established as a central component of multimodal analgesic regimens (discussed later). Scheduling acetaminophen reduces opioid requirements across a broad range of surgeries and has been shown to reduce the incidence of delirium in older adults after surgery.[20]

Despite the decreases in hepatic clearance and volume of distribution seen with increasing age,[21] acetaminophen usually is well tolerated by elderly patients. There are few contraindications, notably liver disease, in which cases daily total dosing may need to be reduced. With an otherwise healthy hepatic system, however, acetaminophen doses given to elderly patients do not need to be reduced.[22]

Nonsteroidal anti-inflammatory drugs

Nonsteroidal anti-inflammatory drugs (NSAIDS) are potent analgesic and anti-inflammatory drugs. Their mechanism of action is the inhibition of various isoforms of the enzyme cyclooxygenase that are responsible for the production of proinflammatory prostaglandins. The analgesic and opioid-sparing effects of NSAIDS in the treatment of acute pain are well documented.[23] The side-effect profile of this class of drugs, however, is of special concern in the elderly population.[24]

Adverse events related to NSAIDs predominantly affect the cardiovascular, renal, and gastrointestinal systems and are much more pronounced in elderly patients due to decreased organ reserve. NSAIDs are more likely to cause renal failure in the elderly.[25] The incidence of gastrointestinal bleeding from NSAIDs is nearly twice as high in patients over 65 years of age than in younger patients.[26] Furthermore, the Food and Drug Administration warns that nonaspirin NSAIDS can promote heart attacks or strokes due to their interference with the cardioprotective effect of low-dose aspirin. This increased risk is seen even with shorter treatments (several weeks) and seems dose dependent.[27] Although chronic pain treatment with NSAIDS is discouraged, cautious use of NSAIDS in the treatment of acute pain in older patients can be considered. NSAIDs have utility for their strong analgesic and opioid-sparing effects, but dose reductions (25%–50%) or increasing the time between doses is recommended. An estimated glomerular filtration rate of less than 60 mL/min is a contraindication to NSAID use in the postoperative period.[28] Topical NSAIDs have demonstrated efficacy similar to oral NSAIDs, with an incidence of adverse events similar to placebo and are a recommended treatment option in patients with localized pain.[29]

Gabapentinoids (gabapentin and pregabalin)

Gabapentinoids are established drugs in the treatment of neuropathic pain and increasingly are used in the treatment of acute postsurgical pain. They act by binding to the α-2δ subunit of presynaptic voltage-gated calcium channels, resulting in their inhibition and subsequent reduction of excitatory neurotransmitter release from activated nociceptors. Other discussed analgesic mechanisms are the stimulation of descending inhibition, inhibition of descending serotonergic facilitation, and inhibition of inflammatory mediators.[30]

The use of gabapentin and pregabalin in the treatment of acute postsurgical pain is supported by the American Pain Society[31] and beneficial effects also have been demonstrated in the older population.[32] Furthermore, perioperatively administered gabapentinoids reduce the likelihood for developing chronic pain.[33] Gabapentin also was believed to reduce the incidence of postoperative delirium in elderly patients after surgery, but a randomized trial did not support this hypothesis.[34]

The most common side effects of gabapentinoids are dizziness and somnolence. These side effects affect all age groups, are mostly seen when treatment is started, and are dose dependent. In older adults, however, this significantly raises the risk for falls and impaired cognitive function. One concern is that these central effects of gabapentinoids likely are synergistic with central opioid effects, resulting in increased rates of respiratory depression, especially in older patients.[35,36] Although the dosing regimen with the best benefit-to-risk ratio has not been identified yet,[37] careful dosing of gabapentinoids in elderly patients is advised,[38] especially in the presence of renal dysfunction.

α_2-Adrenergic receptor agonists

The α_2-adrenergic receptor agonist clonidine has a long history of being used as an analgesic adjunct[39] but its ability to improve postoperative pain control has recently been challenged.[40] The α_2-agonist and muscle relaxant tizanidine may be a useful drug in the treatment of acute pain[39,41] and may be safer than other muscle relaxants in older adults (many of which are on the Beers list of potentially inappropriate medications[42]), but the level of evidence is still low. The α_2-agonist dexmedetomidine is increasingly used with good success in intensive care units (ICUs) for sedation as well as pain management.[43]

Unfortunately, data on the effectiveness of α_2-agonists for pain control in the elderly population are largely absent, but there is reason to be cautious. The hemodynamic effects of α_2-agonists must be considered when using them in patients who are more likely to suffer from cardiovascular pathologies. The perioperative use of clonidine has shown to result in serious adverse events due to hypotension.[44] A recently published study of low-dose dexmedetomidine infusion in the ICU after major noncardiac surgery did not report pain-related outcomes but demonstrated a reduced incidence of delirium, increased survival up to 2 years, and improved cognitive function and quality of life in 3-year survivors.[45]

Although the use of clonidine in the treatment of acute pain in elderly patients cannot be recommended, the use of dexmedetomidine has the potential to improve patient outcomes, including pain. Unfortunately, the sedative/hypnotic effect of dexmedetomidine mostly excludes its use in patients on acute care floors.

Ketamine

Ketamine is well established as an anesthetic as well as an analgesic drug. Ketamine is known to have multiple mechanisms of action, the most relevant the blockade of the N-methyl-D-aspartate (NMDA) receptor. Continuous infusions of ketamine have shown to improve pain control and reduce opioid requirements in the treatment of acute pain.[46,47] But although the excellent analgesic properties of ketamine in elderly patients are well established,[48] concerns about psychogenic side effects have limited the acceptance of ketamine as an analgesic in a population that is already prone to develop delirium. Side effects of ketamine can include night terrors, confusion, hallucinations, and fear. Although there is no clinical evidence that elderly patients are more sensitive to the psychogenic side effects of ketamine,[49] it is known that animals display changes in composition of the NMDA receptor site and function with age.[50] Extrapolation from these animal experiments would suggest that elderly patients may be more sensitive to ketamine effects and that doses should be decreased. A recent large trial of intraoperative bolus-dose ketamine use in older adults found little evidence for preventative analgesia (discussed later) but an increased frequency of hallucinations and nightmares in the ketamine group.[51] Because elderly patients who are more sensitive to the adverse effects of opioids may particularly benefit from the use of ketamine, the cautious use of low-dose ketamine infusions is to be recommended whereas bolus administration of ketamine should be avoided as it has an unacceptable frequency of adverse psychogenic events.

Systemic lidocaine

Lidocaine is an amide local anesthetic that has systemic analgesic effects when administered via intravenous infusion.[52] The systemic administration of lidocaine does not produce local anesthetic concentrations that would be able to block signal transduction in peripheral nerves. The suggested mechanism of analgesia of intravenous lidocaine is hyperpolarization and decreased excitability of postsynaptic spinal dorsal horn neurons.[53] Other mechanisms are the suppression of spontaneous impulses generated from injured nerve fibers as well as anti-inflammatory and antihyperalgesic effects.[54] Postoperatively administered systemic lidocaine have been shown to effectively reduce postoperative pain scores as well as opioid requirements in colorectal or urologic surgery in older adults.[55] The most commonly reported dose ranges are from 1 mg kg^{-1} h^{-1} to 2 mg kg^{-1} h^{-1}. The optimal dose range or duration of infusions, however, has not been established yet. Dose reduction or shorter infusions seem advisable in elderly patients because lidocaine clearance may decrease by as much as 30% to 40% due to the decrease in hepatic blood flow in these patients.[56]

Regional anesthesia

When used appropriately, continuous peripheral regional anesthesia and neuraxial anesthesia techniques are the most powerful tools available for acute pain management. Their use is associated with improved pain and promises a reduction of morbidity and mortality in the general population.[57] Despite the widespread use of regional techniques in elderly patients, data on the impact of regional anesthesia on outcomes compared with younger patients are limited.[58]

Regional anesthesia can help reduce adverse effects seen more frequently with systemic drugs, such as cognitive dysfunction and sedation. But regional anesthesia can be more challenging to perform in the elderly due to anatomic and neurophysiological changes seen with aging.

Neuraxial blocks Neuraxial blocks frequently are more difficult to perform due to degenerative disk disease and vertebral joint changes. Intervertebral and epidural spaces decrease in size with aging, and needle advancement in an often-calcified ligamentum flavum can be more challenging. The superior pain control provided by postoperative epidural analgesia, however, compared with systemic opioid therapy is well documented,[59] and this effect is still seen in the older patient population.[60] Unfortunately, there is no evidence that the opioid-sparing effect of epidural analgesia results in a reduction in the incidence of postoperative delirium.[61] The reduction of the size of the epidural space with increasing age results in increased cephalad spread of the epidural solution.[62] This increased risk of cephalad epidural solution spread may result in adverse cardiovascular events, such as hypotension; therefore, a reduced epidural infusion dose may be required in older patients.

Opioids are known to have a synergistic effect with local anesthetics when applied epidurally. The coadministration of opioids improves pain control or allows for the reduction of local anesthetic thus reducing side effects, such as hypotension. Neuraxially administered opioids, however, have more pronounced central nervous system–depressant effects in elderly patients. Therefore, dose reductions up to 50% have been recommended.[63]

Peripheral nerve blocks Peripheral nerve blocks can provide excellent pain control when used appropriately while avoiding some of the adverse events frequently seen with opioid analgesia as well as neuraxial analgesia, such as sedation, cognitive impairment, urinary retention, and hypotension.[64] There is evidence supporting the effectiveness of peripheral nerve blocks to provide pain control while minimizing side effects in elderly patients.[65] Peripheral nerve blocks in elderly patients have a faster onset and a prolonged duration compared with in younger patients,[66,67] because nerves become more susceptible to the effects of local anesthetics with increasing age.[68] The risk for nerve damage increases with advanced age because the susceptibility to the neurotoxic drug effects of local anesthetics increases as well.[69]

Opioids
Due to the physiologic changes, described previously, opioids administered to older adults tend to be more potent and have a longer duration of action,[70] thus carrying a higher risk for adverse events in these patients. Nonetheless, opioids still are considered a mainstay in acute pain management in this patient population because the temporary use of opioids in the treatment of acute pain is known to improve pain scores effectively. Depending on the situation, however, nonopioid modalities can prove similarly effective.[71] Opioids should be used at the lowest dose possible and for the shortest duration possible when nonopioid medication and nonpharmacologic modalities for pain management do not provide sufficient pain relief.[72]

Opioid therapy in older adults follows in general the same principles in younger patients. Meperidine should be avoided in older adults due to the neurotoxic and deliriogenic effects of its metabolite normeperidine. The use of extended-release opioids in the treatment of acute pain generally is discouraged in opioid-naïve patients. The use of opioid with dual analgesic mechanisms, such as tramadol and tapentadol, potentially reduces the incidence of opioid-related side effects.

When using opioids for acute pain management in older adults, dose reduction by 25% to 50% compared with younger adults generally is recommended. Patient-controlled analgesia has been shown a feasible pain management option in cognitively intact elderly patients with severe acute pain.[73]

Multimodal analgesia
A multimodal approach to pain management describes the combined use of multiple analgesic drugs with different mechanisms of action to improve pain control or reduce opioid requirements while reducing side effects seen with larger doses of the individual drugs.[74] Multimodal analgesia can include any combination of any number of analgesics and offers the prospect of significant efficacy by combining analgesic drugs that may have only limited analgesic effects on their own. Despite that the concept of multimodal analgesia found wide acceptance and was incorporated in countless enhanced recovery after surgery pathways, there still is surprisingly on the efficacy of the concurrent use of multiple nonopioid analgesics. A recently published network meta-analysis demonstrated that morphine consumption reduction was greatest when multiple analgesics other than morphine were used.[23] The optimal number and choice of drugs for multimodal analgesia still need to be established because there may be a tipping point when additional interventions increase the risk for adverse events without further improving pain control. There currently are no recommended multimodal strategies that are specifically aimed at the geriatric population.

Preventive analgesia

As a general principle, perioperative pain management begins as early as possible and includes preoperative or intraoperative interventions aimed at reducing postoperative pain. Preventive analgesia is based on the concept that preventing central sensitization, that is, the amplification of pain signaling seen with trauma, such as surgery, is able to reduce acute postoperative pain and even potentially persistent postsurgical pain.[75] Intraoperative interventions that have been associated with reduced postoperative pain and opioid requirements include ketamine,[76] lidocaine,[77] magnesium,[78] and dexmedetomidine[79] infusions. The role of this attractive concept in pain management specifically for older adults currently is unclear.

Recommended dosing adjustments for medications in older adults are summarized in **Table 2**.

Table 2	
Recommended modifications to drug dosing in elderly patients	
Drug	**Recommended Changes to Drug Dosing**
Acetaminophen	• No age-related dose reduction is needed in absence of liver disease. • Maximum daily dose is 4 g/d. • Reduce dose or avoid in liver disease/dysfunction.
NSAIDs	• Dose reductions (25%–50%) are recommended. • Creatinine clearance <50 mL/min is a contraindication. • Avoid nonselective COX inhibitors in peptic ulcer disease. • Avoid selective COX-2 inhibitors in cardiovascular disease.
Gabapentinoids	• Side effects most likely are dose dependent. • Dose reduction in elderly patients may be advised. • Reduce dose or avoid in renal dysfunction.
Ketamine	• Unknown if older patients are more sensitive to the psychogenic side effects of ketamine. • Although ketamine does not promote delirium in older patients, its discontinuation is routinely requested in patients displaying any type of cognitive dysfunction.
α_2-Agonists	• Use of dexmedetomidine mostly is recommended but limited to settings of advanced care (postanesthetic care unit and ICU). • There are limited data on tizanidine but considered a safer option in older adults compared with other muscle relaxants. • Use of clonidine is not recommended.
Intravenous lidocaine	• Dose reduction or shorter infusions seem advisable; lidocaine clearance may decrease by as much as 30%–40% due to the decrease in hepatic blood flow.
Systemic opioids	• Dose reduction by 25%–50% is recommended.
Perineural local anesthetics	• Peripheral nerve blocks in elderly patients have faster onset and prolonged duration. • Consider dose reduction.
Epidural local anesthetics	• There is increased cephalad spread in the epidural space. • There is increased risk for hypotension. • Dose reduction may be required with epidural infusions in older patients.
Epidural opioids	• Dose reduction up to 50% has been recommended

SUMMARY

The assessment and treatment of pain requires special attention when working with older patients. Because of various changes in function and cognition, properly assessing pain in older patients requires special care with proper assessment tools. Due to various natural physiologic changes with aging, certain treatments may prove more optimal choices than others. In addition, understanding the comorbidities and social context around each patient will help inform which medications are more suitable than others. Geriatric consultation often is helpful to help address pain in older patients during acute stays in a health care setting. Although acetaminophen requires no adjustment to dosing in elderly patients, most other medications and interventions for pain require a decrease in dosing compared with younger patients. Multimodal and preventive analgesia are promising approaches that merit further research in the older population; this remains an active, vibrant, and rapidly evolving field of research as more older adults seek care for surgery and other conditions of acute pain.

REFERENCES

1. Bugliosi TF, Meloy TD, Vukov LF. Acute abdominal pain in the elderly. Ann Emerg Med 1990;19(12):1383–6.
2. Jin F, Chung F. Minimizing perioperative adverse events in the elderly. Br J Anaesth 2001;87(4):608–24.
3. Kaye AD, Baluch A, Scott JT. Pain management in the elderly population: a review. Ochsner J 2010;10(3):179–87.
4. Chakour MC, Gibson SJ, Bradbeer M, et al. The effect of age on A delta- and C-fibre thermal pain perception. Pain 1996;64(1):143–52.
5. McKeown JL. Pain management issues for the geriatric surgical patient. Anesthesiol Clin 2015;33(3):563–76.
6. Turnheim K. When drug therapy gets old: pharmacokinetics and pharmacodynamics in the elderly. Exp Gerontol 2003;38(8):843–53.
7. Denic A, Glassock RJ, Rule AD. Structural and functional changes with the aging kidney. Adv Chronic Kidney Dis 2016;23(1):19–28.
8. Hein C, Forgues A, Piau A, et al. Impact of polypharmacy on occurrence of delirium in elderly emergency patients. J Am Med Dir Assoc 2014;15(11): 850.e11-5.
9. Field TS, Gurwitz JH, Avorn J, et al. Risk factors for adverse drug events among nursing home residents. Arch Intern Med 2001;161(13):1629–34.
10. Hebert LE, Weuve J, Scherr PA, et al. Alzheimer disease in the United States (2010-2050) estimated using the 2010 census. Neurology 2013;80(19):1778–83.
11. Jones J, Sim TF, Hughes J. Pain assessment of elderly patients with cognitive impairment in the emergency department: implications for pain management-a narrative review of current practices. Pharmacy (Basel) 2017;5(2) [pii:E30].
12. Weiner DK, Rudy TE. Attitudinal barriers to effective treatment of persistent pain in nursing home residents. J Am Geriatr Soc 2002;50(12):2035–40.
13. Catananti C, Gambassi G. Pain assessment in the elderly. Surg Oncol 2010; 19(3):140–8.
14. Thielke S, Sale J, Reid MC. Aging: are these 4 pain myths complicating care? J Fam Pract 2012;61(11):666–70.
15. Hjermstad MJ, Fayers PM, Haugen DF, et al. Studies comparing numerical rating scales, verbal rating scales, and visual analogue scales for assessment of pain intensity in adults: a systematic literature review. J Pain Symptom Manage 2011;41(6):1073–93.

16. Torvik K, Kaasa S, Kirkevold Ø, et al. Validation of Doloplus-2 among nonverbal nursing home patients–an evaluation of Doloplus-2 in a clinical setting. BMC Geriatr 2010;10:9.
17. Rostad HM, Utne I, Grov EK, et al. Measurement properties, feasibility and clinical utility of the Doloplus-2 pain scale in older adults with cognitive impairment: a systematic review. BMC Geriatr 2017;17(1):257.
18. Fallon WF, Rader E, Zyzanski S, et al. Geriatric outcomes are improved by a geriatric trauma consultation service. J Trauma 2006;61(5):1040–6.
19. Inouye SK, Westendorp RG, Saczynski JS. Delirium in elderly people. Lancet 2014;383(9920):911–22.
20. Subramaniam B, Shankar P, Shaefi S, et al. Effect of intravenous acetaminophen vs placebo combined with propofol or dexmedetomidine on postoperative delirium among older patients following cardiac surgery: the DEXACET randomized clinical trial. JAMA 2019;321(7):686–96.
21. Liukas A, Kuusniemi K, Aantaa R, et al. Pharmacokinetics of intravenous paracetamol in elderly patients. Clin Pharmacokinet 2011;50(2):121–9.
22. Mian P, Allegaert K, Spriet I, et al. Paracetamol in older people: towards evidence-based dosing? Drugs Aging 2018;35(7):603–24.
23. Martinez V, Beloeil H, Marret E, et al. Non-opioid analgesics in adults after major surgery: systematic review with network meta-analysis of randomized trials. Br J Anaesth 2017;118(1):22–31.
24. Barkin RL, Beckerman M, Blum SL, et al. Should nonsteroidal anti-inflammatory drugs (NSAIDs) be prescribed to the older adult? Drugs Aging 2010;27(10):775–89.
25. Ailabouni W, Eknoyan G. Nonsteroidal anti-inflammatory drugs and acute renal failure in the elderly. A risk-benefit assessment. Drugs Aging 1996;9(5):341–51.
26. Sostres C, Gargallo CJ, Lanas A. Nonsteroidal anti-inflammatory drugs and upper and lower gastrointestinal mucosal damage. Arthritis Res Ther 2013;15(Suppl 3):S3.
27. Administration USFaD. FDA Drug Safety Communication: FDA strengthens warning that non-aspirin nonsteroidal anti-inflammatory drugs (NSAIDs) can cause heart attacks or strokes. 2015. Available at: https://www.fda.gov/drugs/drugsafety/ucm451800.htm. Accessed March 13, 2019.
28. Tawfic QA, Bellingham G. Postoperative pain management in patients with chronic kidney disease. J Anaesthesiol Clin Pharmacol 2015;31(1):6–13.
29. Rannou F, Pelletier JP, Martel-Pelletier J. Efficacy and safety of topical NSAIDs in the management of osteoarthritis: Evidence from real-life setting trials and surveys. Semin Arthritis Rheum 2016;45(4 Suppl):S18–21.
30. Chincholkar M. Analgesic mechanisms of gabapentinoids and effects in experimental pain models: a narrative review. Br J Anaesth 2018;120(6):1315–34.
31. Chou R, Gordon DB, de Leon-Casasola OA, et al. Management of postoperative pain: a clinical practice guideline from the American Pain Society, the American Society of Regional Anesthesia and Pain Medicine, and the American Society of Anesthesiologists' Committee on Regional Anesthesia, Executive Committee, and Administrative Council. J Pain 2016;17(2):131–57.
32. Pesonen A, Suojaranta-Ylinen R, Hammarén E, et al. Pregabalin has an opioid-sparing effect in elderly patients after cardiac surgery: a randomized placebo-controlled trial. Br J Anaesth 2011;106(6):873–81.
33. Schmidt PC, Ruchelli G, Mackey SC, et al. Perioperative gabapentinoids: choice of agent, dose, timing, and effects on chronic postsurgical pain. Anesthesiology 2013;119(5):1215–21.

34. Leung JM, Sands LP, Chen N, et al. Perioperative gabapentin does not reduce postoperative delirium in older surgical patients: a randomized clinical trial. Anesthesiology 2017;127(4):633–44.
35. Cavalcante AN, Sprung J, Schroeder DR, et al. Multimodal analgesic therapy with gabapentin and its association with postoperative respiratory depression. Anesth Analg 2017;125(1):141–6.
36. Weingarten TN, Jacob AK, Njathi CW, et al. Multimodal analgesic protocol and postanesthesia respiratory depression during phase I recovery after total joint arthroplasty. Reg Anesth Pain Med 2015;40(4):330–6.
37. Verret M, Lauzier F, Zarychanski R, et al. Perioperative use of gabapentinoids for the management of postoperative acute pain: protocol of a systematic review and meta-analysis. Syst Rev 2019;8(1):24.
38. Fleet JL, Dixon SN, Kuwornu PJ, et al. Gabapentin dose and the 30-day risk of altered mental status in older adults: a retrospective population-based study. PLoS One 2018;13(3):e0193134.
39. Chan AK, Cheung CW, Chong YK. Alpha-2 agonists in acute pain management. Expert Opin Pharmacother 2010;11(17):2849–68.
40. Turan A, Babazade R, Kurz A, et al. Clonidine does not reduce pain or opioid consumption after noncardiac surgery. Anesth Analg 2016;123(3):749–57.
41. Yazicioğlu D, Caparlar C, Akkaya T, et al. Tizanidine for the management of acute postoperative pain after inguinal hernia repair: a placebo-controlled double-blind trial. Eur J Anaesthesiol 2016;33(3):215–22.
42. American Geriatrics Society Beers Criteria Update Expert Panel. American Geriatrics Society 2019 updated beers criteria for potentially inappropriate medication use in older adults. J Am Geriatr Soc 2019. https://doi.org/10.1111/jgs.15767.
43. Morad A, Farrokh S, Papangelou A. Pain management in neurocritical care; an update. Curr Opin Crit Care 2018;24(2):72–9.
44. Devereaux PJ, Sessler DI, Leslie K, et al. Clonidine in patients undergoing noncardiac surgery. N Engl J Med 2014;370(16):1504–13.
45. Zhang DF, Su X, Meng ZT, et al. Impact of dexmedetomidine on long-term outcomes after noncardiac surgery in elderly: 3-year follow-up of a randomized controlled trial. Ann Surg 2018. [Epub ahead of print].
46. Bell RF, Kalso EA. Ketamine for pain management. Pain Rep 2018;3(5):e674.
47. Brinck EC, Tiippana E, Heesen M, et al. Perioperative intravenous ketamine for acute postoperative pain in adults. Cochrane Database Syst Rev 2018;(12):CD012033.
48. Motov S, Mann S, Drapkin J, et al. Intravenous subdissociative-dose ketamine versus morphine for acute geriatric pain in the Emergency Department: a randomized controlled trial. Am J Emerg Med 2019;37(2):220–7.
49. Rasmussen KG. Psychiatric side effects of ketamine in hospitalized medical patients administered subanesthetic doses for pain control. Acta Neuropsychiatr 2014;26(4):230–3.
50. Zhao X, Rosenke R, Kronemann D, et al. The effects of aging on N-methyl-D-aspartate receptor subunits in the synaptic membrane and relationships to long-term spatial memory. Neuroscience 2009;162(4):933–45.
51. Avidan MS, Maybrier HR, Abdallah AB, et al. Intraoperative ketamine for prevention of postoperative delirium or pain after major surgery in older adults: an international, multicentre, double-blind, randomised clinical trial. Lancet 2017; 390(10091):267–75.
52. Eipe N, Gupta S, Penning J. Intravenous lidocaine for acute pain: an evidence-based clinical update. BJA Educ 2016;16(9):292–8.

53. Kurabe M, Furue H, Kohno T. Intravenous administration of lidocaine directly acts on spinal dorsal horn and produces analgesic effect: an in vivo patch-clamp analysis. Sci Rep 2016;6:26253.

54. Koppert W, Ostermeier N, Sittl R, et al. Low-dose lidocaine reduces secondary hyperalgesia by a central mode of action. Pain 2000;85(1–2):217–24.

55. Daykin H. The efficacy and safety of intravenous lidocaine for analgesia in the older adult: a literature review. Br J Pain 2017;11(1):23–31.

56. Rivera R, Antognini JF. Perioperative drug therapy in elderly patients. Anesthesiology 2009;110(5):1176–81.

57. Bugada D, Ghisi D, Mariano ER. Continuous regional anesthesia: a review of perioperative outcome benefits. Minerva Anestesiol 2017;83(10):1089–100.

58. Tsui BC, Wagner A, Finucane B. Regional anaesthesia in the elderly: a clinical guide. Drugs Aging 2004;21(14):895–910.

59. Wu CL, Cohen SR, Richman JM, et al. Efficacy of postoperative patient-controlled and continuous infusion epidural analgesia versus intravenous patient-controlled analgesia with opioids: a meta-analysis. Anesthesiology 2005;103(5):1079–88 [quiz: 1109-10].

60. Mann C, Pouzeratte Y, Boccara G, et al. Comparison of intravenous or epidural patient-controlled analgesia in the elderly after major abdominal surgery. Anesthesiology 2000;92(2):433–41.

61. Fong HK, Sands LP, Leung JM. The role of postoperative analgesia in delirium and cognitive decline in elderly patients: a systematic review. Anesth Analg 2006;102(4):1255–66.

62. Hirabayashi Y, Shimizu R, Matsuda I, et al. Effect of extradural compliance and resistance on spread of extradural analgesia. Br J Anaesth 1990;65(4):508–13.

63. Sadean MR, Glass PS. Pharmacokinetics in the elderly. Best Pract Res Clin Anaesthesiol 2003;17(2):191–205.

64. Zaric D, Boysen K, Christiansen C, et al. A comparison of epidural analgesia with combined continuous femoral-sciatic nerve blocks after total knee replacement. Anesth Analg 2006;102(4):1240–6.

65. Halaszynski TM. Pain management in the elderly and cognitively impaired patient: the role of regional anesthesia and analgesia. Curr Opin Anaesthesiol 2009;22(5):594–9.

66. Paqueron X, Boccara G, Bendahou M, et al. Brachial plexus nerve block exhibits prolonged duration in the elderly. Anesthesiology 2002;97(5):1245–9.

67. Hanks RK, Pietrobon R, Nielsen KC, et al. The effect of age on sciatic nerve block duration. Anesth Analg 2006;102(2):588–92.

68. Dorfman LJ, Bosley TM. Age-related changes in peripheral and central nerve conduction in man. Neurology 1979;29(1):38–44.

69. Neal JM, Barrington MJ, Brull R, et al. The second ASRA practice advisory on neurologic complications associated with regional anesthesia and pain medicine: executive summary 2015. Reg Anesth Pain Med 2015;40(5):401–30.

70. Chau DL, Walker V, Pai L, et al. Opiates and elderly: use and side effects. Clin Interv Aging 2008;3(2):273–8.

71. Chang AK, Bijur PE, Esses D, et al. Effect of a single dose of oral opioid and non-opioid analgesics on acute extremity pain in the emergency department: a randomized clinical trial. JAMA 2017;318(17):1661–7.

72. Shah A, Hayes CJ, Martin BC. Factors influencing long-term opioid use among opioid naive patients: an examination of initial prescription characteristics and pain etiologies. J Pain 2017;18(11):1374–83.

73. Mann C, Pouzeratte Y, Eledjam JJ. Postoperative patient-controlled analgesia in the elderly: risks and benefits of epidural versus intravenous administration. Drugs Aging 2003;20(5):337–45.
74. Wick EC, Grant MC, Wu CL. Postoperative multimodal analgesia pain management with nonopioid analgesics and techniques: a review. JAMA Surg 2017; 152(7):691–7.
75. Dahl JB, Kehlet H. Preventive analgesia. Curr Opin Anaesthesiol 2011;24(3): 331–8.
76. Laskowski K, Stirling A, McKay WP, et al. A systematic review of intravenous ketamine for postoperative analgesia. Can J Anaesth 2011;58(10):911–23.
77. Barreveld A, Witte J, Chahal H, et al. Preventive analgesia by local anesthetics: the reduction of postoperative pain by peripheral nerve blocks and intravenous drugs. Anesth Analg 2013;116(5):1141–61.
78. De Oliveira GS, Castro-Alves LJ, Khan JH, et al. Perioperative systemic magnesium to minimize postoperative pain: a meta-analysis of randomized controlled trials. Anesthesiology 2013;119(1):178–90.
79. Le Bot A, Michelet D, Hilly J, et al. Efficacy of intraoperative dexmedetomidine compared with placebo for surgery in adults: a meta-analysis of published studies. Minerva Anestesiol 2015;81(10):1105–17.

Special Considerations for the Aging Brain and Perioperative Neurocognitive Dysfunction

Kimberly F. Rengel, MD*, Pratik P. Pandharipande, MD,
Christopher G. Hughes, MD

KEYWORDS

- Postoperative delirium • Postoperative cognitive dysfunction • Neuroinflammation
- Long-term cognitive impairment • Geriatric anesthesia

KEY POINTS

- Millions of surgical procedures are performed each year in older adults who are at a higher risk for perioperative neurocognitive changes, including postoperative delirium and postoperative cognitive dysfunction (POCD).
- Delirium is a syndrome of acute brain dysfunction and is associated with long-term cognitive impairment.
- The risk factor most strongly associated with postoperative delirium and cognitive dysfunction is increasing age. Other risks that increase vulnerability include baseline cognitive impairment, frailty and high comorbidity burden, benzodiazepines, anticholinergic medications, and poorly controlled postoperative pain.
- A proposed common mechanism for postoperative delirium and POCD is a neuroinflammatory state that results from the systemic inflammatory response to the stress of surgery.
- Perioperative interventions to minimize delirium include optimizing anesthetic depth, avoiding deliriogenic medications, controlling postoperative pain, and use of dexmedetomidine for postoperative sedation.

Disclosure: Dr Pandharipande received support from the National Institutes of Health (HL111111, GM120484). Dr Hughes received support from American Geriatrics Society Jahnigen Career Development Award and the National Institutes of Health (HL111111, AG045085, GM120484).

Department of Anesthesiology, Division of Anesthesiology Critical Care Medicine, Vanderbilt University School of Medicine, 1211 21st Avenue South, 422 MAB, Nashville, TN 37212, USA
* Corresponding author.
E-mail address: kimberly.rengel@vumc.org

Anesthesiology Clin 37 (2019) 521–536
https://doi.org/10.1016/j.anclin.2019.04.010
1932-2275/19/© 2019 Elsevier Inc. All rights reserved.

anesthesiology.theclinics.com

INTRODUCTION

A substantial number of surgeries are performed annually in older adults, leading to increasing awareness of their susceptibility to postoperative neuropsychiatric complications, including postoperative delirium and postoperative cognitive dysfunction (POCD). Preservation of cognitive and functional status is highly important to patients and was found to be more meaningful than survival in a survey of older adults with limited life expectancy.[1] Originally thought to be a transient phenomenon, developing delirium in the early postoperative course is associated with long-term consequences, including increased mortality, prolonged hospitalization, discharge to an institution, and long-term cognitive decline and dementia.[2–6] POCD, recently recategorized into delayed neurocognitive recovery or postoperative neurocognitive disorder, depending on duration, has also been associated with higher mortality, an inability to return to previous function, and dementia.[7,8] This article outlines the diagnosis and proposed mechanisms that contribute to delirium and cognitive decline after surgery, as well as strategies to minimize or prevent the occurrence of these two important perioperative neurologic complications.

THE AGING BRAIN

The normal aging process includes physiologic changes in the brain that predispose older adults to developing neurocognitive dysfunction. Older adults have depressed physiologic reserve in many organ systems (renal, pulmonary, cardiac) that increases vulnerability to systemic stressors such as surgery; this is equally true for the brain.[9] Brain volume and white matter integrity decline with increasing age,[10] which is coupled with loss of neuronal tissue over time.[11] In addition, cerebral blood flow declines with aging,[12] decreasing oxygen delivery, slowing metabolism, and altering neurotransmitter activity and production.[11] Endothelial cell function declines[13] and blood-brain barrier (BBB) permeability increases with age,[14] increasing the brain's susceptibility to systemic insults. These physiologic changes share similarities to the perturbations observed in patients with delirium and POCD and may provide insight into the increased incidence of neurocognitive dysfunction after surgery in older adults.

POSTOPERATIVE DELIRIUM
Definition and Diagnosis

Delirium is defined as a state of acute cerebral dysfunction. The Diagnostic and Statistical Manual of Mental Disorders, Fifth Edition (DSM-5) identifies 5 distinct criteria for presence of delirium: disturbance in attention and awareness, impaired cognition, acute presentation with fluctuation throughout the day, absence of a preexisting neurocognitive disorder, and evidence that changes are related to an ongoing medical condition.[15] It can be separated into clinical phenotypes based upon concurrent clinical factors such as surgery, sepsis, sedation, and hypoxemia. Delirium may be further classified into 3 motoric subtypes (hyperactive, hypoactive, or mixed) based on the patient's psychomotor symptoms.[16,17] In contrast with the easily identifiable restlessness and agitation associated with hyperactive delirium, patients with hypoactive delirium are lethargic with slowed mobility and mentation. Hypoactive delirium is often the most common subtype observed, followed by mixed; pure hyperactive delirium is rare.[18] In the immediate postoperative period, hypoactive delirium may be difficult to differentiate from prolonged emergence from anesthesia, is frequently missed by providers,[19] and is associated with poorer outcomes.[18,20]

The gold standard for diagnosis of delirium is a formal evaluation by a psychiatric professional for presence of the DSM-5 criteria.[15] Validated instruments for bedside delirium assessment have been developed including the Nursing Delirium Symptom Checklist (NuDESC)[21] and the Confusion Assessment Method (CAM) for Intensive Care Unit (CAM-ICU).[22] Applied in the early postoperative period, the NuDESC and CAM-ICU showed greater than 90% specificity in identifying delirium, although neither tool showed sensitivity for postanesthesia care unit (PACU) delirium.[23] **Box 1** lists the key features of these diagnostic tools.

Epidemiology

The reported prevalence of postoperative delirium (POD) is variable with type of surgery, delirium assessment method, and patient comorbidities.[24] It is often considered the most common surgical complication. Delirium prevalence is frequently underestimated in clinical practice because the clinical presentations of delirium and emergence from anesthesia may overlap and many patients present with hypoactive symptoms. However, among older patients who meet PACU discharge criteria after recovering from general anesthesia, up to 45% remain positive for delirium.[2] Up to 50% of older adults may experience postoperative delirium[25]; reported prevalence is highest after orthopedic (12%–51%)[26,27] and cardiac (11%–52%) surgery.[3,28] Of note, delirium prevalence increases for patients requiring postoperative ICU management, where up to 80% of patients on mechanical ventilation develop delirium.[29]

Pathophysiology

Delirium development is a multifactorial process with proposed mechanisms including neuroinflammation, oxidative stress, endothelial dysfunction, BBB disruption, decreased cholinergic function, neurotransmitter imbalance, and altered cerebral structural integrity.[30] Aging decreases cognitive reserve and increases susceptibility to many of the potential mechanisms of delirium. Surgical insult prompts a release of peripheral inflammatory mediators that induce a neuroinflammatory cascade mediated by microglial cells (**Fig. 1**).[11,31] Normally in a quiescent state, activated microglial cells upregulate production of proinflammatory cytokines and promote neuronal apoptosis leading to a disturbance in cognitive function.[30,32] Systemic inflammatory mediators also cause dysfunction in endothelial cells, including those of the BBB. Increases in the levels of biomarkers associated with BBB permeability and endothelial

---

Box 1
Delirium diagnosis

CAM-ICU[27]
- Acute change in mental status or fluctuation in the past 24 hours (feature 1)
- Inability to sustain attention (feature 2)
- Presence of altered consciousness (feature 3)
- Disorganized thinking (feature 4)

Diagnosis requires the presence of both features 1 and 2, plus either of feature 3 or 4

NuDESC[26]

Patients are screened by nursing staff and given a score ranging from 0 to 2 for the severity in each of the following categories:
- Disorientation
- Psychomotor agitation
- Inability to communicate clearly
- Altered perception or visual hallucination
- Depressed psychomotor activity

A score greater than or equal to 2 indicates delirium

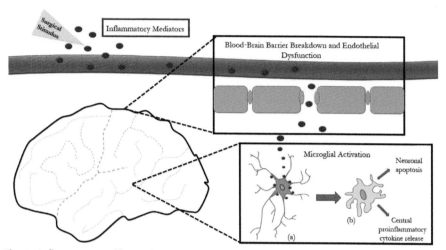

Fig. 1. Inflammatory effects of surgical stress on the brain. (a) Resting Microglia. (b) Activated Microglia

dysfunction, such as S100B, E-selectin, and plasminogen activator-1, have been associated with prolonged delirium in critical illness.[33] Neurotransmitter imbalances have also been shown to contribute to delirium development, including acetylcholine, dopamine, serotonin, norepinephrine, and gamma-aminobutyric acid.[11,30]

Risk Factors

It is helpful to classify delirium risk factors into preoperative, intraoperative, and postoperative periods (**Box 2**). The 2 preoperative factors most commonly cited are advancing age and baseline cognitive impairment.[34–37] Even in the absence of cognitive impairment, baseline microstructural changes of cerebral white matter increase the risk of developing POD.[38] Preoperative physical function and health also affect outcomes after surgery. Increased burden of comorbidities (eg, sleep apnea, heart

---

Box 2
Risk factors for perioperative delirium

Preoperative
- Advancing age
- Baseline cognitive impairment
- Cerebral white matter changes
- Frailty
- High comorbidity burden
- High severity of illness

Intraoperative
- Benzodiazepine administration
- Morphine and meperidine
- Perioperative steroid administration
- Anticholinergic medications

Postoperative
- Postoperative mechanical ventilation
- Poorly controlled postoperative pain
- Deep sedation

failure, and diabetes),[39] preoperative frailty,[40] and high severity of illness indicated by American Society of Anesthesiologists score greater than or equal to 3[41] all increase risk of POD. Poor physical and cognitive reserve likely interferes with the body's homeostatic ability to maintain normal brain function after the acute stress insult of surgery and hospitalization.

Intraoperative and postoperative risk factors are important targets for modification that may reduce delirium occurrence. Certain sedating and analgesic medications used in the perioperative period, including lorazepam, midazolam, morphine, and meperidine, are more strongly associated with delirium than alternative agents such as propofol, dexmedetomidine, and fentanyl.[42–45] Patients may receive perioperative steroids, which are associated with transition to delirium during critical illness.[46] In addition, strongly anticholinergic medications (eg, diphenhydramine and promethazine) may precipitate delirium.[47] Patients with a higher severity of illness requiring postoperative mechanical ventilation are more likely to develop POD than those undergoing lower risk operations. In addition, poorly controlled pain is thought to increase the systemic stress response to surgery,[47] which may help explain why worsening pain scores are associated with postoperative delirium development.[48]

Perioperative Management

Studies examining rates of POD after general, regional, or neuraxial anesthetics have not found a significant difference in rates of delirium or postoperative confusion between the various anesthetic techniques.[49–52] Anesthetic agent selection during general anesthesia does not seem to affect delirium development either. Total intravenous propofol anesthetic did not lower risk of delirium development compared with desflurane[53,54] or sevoflurane,[55] and no difference was found when comparing desflurane to sevoflurane.[56] Application of intraoperative processed electroencephalography to monitor depth of anesthesia during a general anesthetic may be associated with less POD.[57–59] Use of EEG-based management, in addition to close monitoring of age-adjusted end-tidal minimum alveolar concentration fraction and optimization of cerebral perfusion, was endorsed in the latest best-practices recommendations from the Perioperative Neurotoxicity Working Group.[60] Use of electroencephalography criteria for targeted light sedation has also shown a reduction in POD for patients receiving propofol sedation during neuraxial anesthesia,[51] although findings were not replicated in a subsequent larger trial that targeted depth of sedation to a modified observer's assessment of alertness/sedation score (and also obtained separation in blinded electroencephalography sedation scores).[61] Anesthetic adjuncts, such as ketamine and dexmedetomidine, have not decreased postoperative delirium in recent randomized controlled trials.[62,63] Perioperative pain control is an important intervention for delirium prevention, because higher baseline and postoperative pain scores are associated with postoperative delirium.[48,64] Opioids are a mainstay of postoperative pain management but may be deliriogenic; multimodal medications, regional anesthesia, and application of opioid-sparing enhanced recovery after surgery protocols are beneficial alternatives.[65,66] However, a recent trial of perioperative gabapentin administration did not find a lower incidence of delirium despite reduction in opioid administration.[67]

Multicomponent prevention protocols that include reorientation, continuity of caregivers, decreased use of restraints, removal of catheters, providing hearing aids and eye glasses, and geriatrics consultation have been found to reduce delirium incidence and the total number of days of delirium in multiple studies of surgical and medical non-ICU patients.[68] Similarly, the Hospital Elder Life Program (hospitalelderlife.org) in the perioperative setting has been shown to reduce delirium and length of stay.[69]

ICU bundles involving pain assessment and control, awakening and breathing trials, minimizing sedation, delirium management, early mobility, and family participation (the ABCDEF bundle) are associated with improved delirium outcomes.[70] Prophylactic medications, including antipsychotics and cholinesterase inhibitors, administered to prevent delirium in the postoperative period have largely been ineffective.[71–73]

Treatment

Specific pharmacologic agents for the treatment of delirium should be restricted to patients who have failed prevention strategies and who are a risk to self or others. The most popular pharmacologic treatments are antipsychotic medications (eg, haloperidol, olanzapine, quetiapine) and dexmedetomidine. However, none of those agents are US Food and Drug Administration approved for the treatment of delirium. A recent large multicenter study that randomized delirious patients to haloperidol, ziprasidone, or placebo found no difference across the groups in delirium, length of stay, or survival.[74] Patients with hyperactive delirium have been shown to benefit from dexmedetomidine compared with haloperidol in nonintubated patients[75] or placebo in patients weaning on mechanical ventilation.[76] Overall, the treatment strategies for delirium are sparse, and the evidence is lacking for a single pharmacologic approach. Importantly, agents that tend to be used to prevent or treat delirium affect the sensorium and have significant side effects that may overall worsen outcomes.

POSTOPERATIVE COGNITIVE DYSFUNCTION
Definition and Diagnosis

POCD is characterized by a decline in cognitive performance, including memory, concentration, and the ability to process information.[77,78] POCD has been identified within 1 week of surgery (early), but may persist up to 3 months (late) or 1 year (long-term or persistent) after an operation. Initially, POCD was a research construct used to study neurocognitive decline after surgery. However, recent consensus recommendations now align cognitive changes in the postoperative period with nomenclature for mild and major neurocognitive disorders (NCDs) from the DSM-5, developing a clinical diagnosis. Terminology has been developed to reflect the time at which changes become apparent:

- Neurocognitive disorder (diagnosed preoperatively)
- Postoperative delirium (acute postoperative event)
- Delayed neurocognitive recovery (decline diagnosed up to 30 days postoperatively)
- Postoperative neurocognitive disorder (decline after 30 days up to 12 months postoperatively)[79]

By this standard, a diagnosis of POCD includes the 3 criteria for NCDs:

- Subjective complaint of a cognitive change from patients, families, or clinicians
- Objective impairment or change in neurocognitive testing
- Assessment of activities of daily living in which impairment indicates major NCD[15]

It is important to note that the 'postoperative' term is an indicator of the temporal association and not a causal relationship. A key feature of identifying POCD is comparison of neuropsychological testing performed before and after an operation; however, a consistent battery of neurocognitive testing is currently lacking. The initial consensus-recommended battery of tests was published in 1995,[80] followed by an updated battery from the International Study of Postoperative Cognitive Dysfunction

Table 1	
International study of postoperative cognitive dysfunction testing battery	
Test	Feature
Mini Mental State Examination	Screening for dementia
Visual Verbal Learning (based on Rey's auditive recall of words)[114]	Short-term auditory-verbal memory
Concept Shifting Task (based on the Trail Making Test)[115]	Visual attention and task switching
Stroop Color Word Test	Selective attention, cognitive flexibility, and processing speed
Memory Scanning Task	Short-term or working memory
Letter-digit coding (based on the Symbol Digit Substitution Task from the Wechsler Adult Intelligence Scale)	Processing speed
Four Boxes Test	Reaction time

Data from Rasmussen LS, Larsen K, Houx P, et al. The assessment of postoperative cognitive function. Acta Anaesthesiol Scand 2001;45(3):275-89.

(ISPOCD) research group that assesses cognitive flexibility, sensorimotor speed, memory, and attention (**Table 1**).[81] The variation in prevalence and severity of POCD is further confounded by a lack of agreement on the threshold standard deviations below normal that indicate cognitive decline and the timing interval of assessments in the postoperative period.[82] In addition, the real-world implications of changes in cognitive testing scores to patients have not been established.

Epidemiology

One of the earliest control-matched, multicenter trials identified POCD in 25.8% of patients more than 60 years old at 1 week and 9.9% of patients at 3 months after noncardiac surgery and found an association between increasing age and development of POCD.[83] In a longitudinal study of patients more than 18 years old, 30% to 41% of patients showed POCD 1 week after surgery, which declined to about 5% in patients less than 60 years old at 3 months, but remained at 12.7% for patients more than 60 years old.[84] POCD rates in older adults have been cited as high as 54.3% at 6 weeks and 46.1% at 1 year.[85] Coronary artery bypass grafting (CABG) surgery is associated with higher rates of POCD. In one longitudinal study after on-pump CABG, POCD was present in 53% of patients at discharge, 36% at 6 weeks, 24% at 6 months, and 42% at 5 years.[86] This finding has raised interest in a possible delayed cognitive decline presenting years after CABG, despite initial short-term improvement, that may be related more to the vascular disease process than exposure to cardiopulmonary bypass.[87]

Pathophysiology

The mechanisms resulting in POCD development are multifactorial and have not been well defined. POCD may share a similar pathophysiology to postoperative delirium and long-term cognitive impairment observed after critical illness; the leading common proposed mechanism is a neuroinflammatory cascade. Eckenhoff and Laudansky[88] developed a model similar to that of delirium discussed earlier, in which surgery induces an inflammatory response that is transmitted to the central nervous system via afferent nerve signaling or through a compromised BBB. The resulting neuroinflammation may lead to neurocognitive dysfunction (see **Fig. 1**). Supporting this theory, a recent meta-analysis found patients with POCD had significantly increased levels of C-reactive protein and interleukin-6.[89] In addition, Hughes and colleagues[90] recently found that increased levels of S100B and E-selectin, markers of BBB compromise and endothelial injury, were associated with long-term cognitive impairment after critical illness, which may suggest a role for BBB injury in long-term POCD.

Risk Factors

As awareness and interest regarding POCD have increased, multiple studies have evaluated the risk factors associated with POCD and, similar to POD, may be classified into preoperative, intraoperative, and postoperative categories (**Box 3**). Across multiple studies, advancing age has been the preoperative factor most frequently associated with POCD.[78,83,84,91] Lower education levels, history of cerebrovascular disease, and baseline cognitive impairment are also associated with POCD.[5,83,84,91]

Intraoperative factors are less well defined in current literature. The earliest study from ISPOCD identified an association between duration of anesthesia and POCD.[83] However, further investigation indicates no difference in POCD occurrence when comparing general with regional[92] or neuraxial anesthesia (without sedation).[93] Studies of community-dwelling older adults have found little or no difference in cognitive trajectory between participants requiring general anesthesia and those who do not, raising the question as to whether anesthesia exposure or the natural course of aging and illness have a stronger influence on cognitive health.[94–96] Intraoperative hemodynamic factors, including hypoxia and hypotension, were not found to alter rates of POCD.[83,97] Ongoing investigation is needed to further characterize whether components of surgery or anesthesia influence the development of POCD, although current evidence suggests there is not an association.

During the postoperative period, delirium development is a potential harbinger of prolonged cognitive dysfunction. In cardiac surgery patients, those that developed postoperative delirium were more likely to show cognitive decline at 1 year[3] and 5 years[5] after surgery compared with patients who did not experience delirium. Among older adults undergoing elective noncardiac surgery, those who developed postoperative delirium were more likely to later show mild cognitive impairment or dementia[98] and may experience a secondary decline up to 3 years later.[4] Further, in critical illness, increased duration of delirium was one of the primary risk factors for worse cognition up to 12 months after discharge,[6] and increased severity of postoperative delirium is associated with worse long-term cognitive function.[99] Postoperative

---

Box 3
Risk factors for postoperative cognitive dysfunction

Preoperative
- Advancing age
- Lower education levels
- History of cerebrovascular disease
- Baseline cognitive impairment

Intraoperative
- Lack of monitoring depth of anesthetic
- Deep planes of anesthesia

Postoperative
- Postoperative delirium
- Poorly controlled postoperative pain[105]
- Intravenous opioid medication[105]

delirium is reproducibly associated with an increased risk of longer-term cognitive dysfunction, and there are likely mechanistic similarities or progression between these syndromes, but whether delirium itself causes POCD remains unknown.

Management Strategies to Reduce the Risk of Postoperative Cognitive Dysfunction

Studies in POCD up to this point have predominantly focused on incidence and risk factors, with limited direct evidence regarding optimal prevention strategies. Understanding known risk factors, identifying patients at highest risk for developing POCD, and discussing risk with patients and families before an operation are important first steps. Intraoperatively, monitoring depth of anesthesia and cerebral oxygenation and adjusting the anesthetic to optimize cerebral perfusion and avoid deep planes of anesthesia were shown to reduce POCD in 1 study.[100] One trial using processed electroencephalography to guide depth of anesthesia found no difference in cognitive scores 3 months after surgery[57]; however, reducing anesthesia exposure using targeted bispectral index reduced cognitive dysfunction at 3 months in a different study.[58] Efforts to reduce the inflammatory response to surgery and, thus, reduce risk of POCD have gained interest. A recent trial that randomized patients to receive dexamethasone or placebo before elective cardiac surgery showed a reduction in the incidence of POCD and a reduction in postoperative C-reactive protein levels.[101] Similarly, a trial that randomized patients to the COX-2 inhibitor parecoxib or placebo for total knee arthroplasty found a lower incidence of POCD at 1 week in the intervention group.[102] Dexmedetomidine has shown promising antiinflammatory and immunomodulatory effects in animal models; however, data do not currently support its use for prevention of POCD.[63,103] Because postoperative delirium is a risk factor for developing POCD, applying strategies to minimize the risk of delirium outlined previously may be beneficial in preventing long-term cognitive dysfunction. Postoperative pain management strategies that use nonopioid medications, emphasize oral narcotic formulations rather than intravenous, and avoid morphine have also been associated with a reduction in POCD.[104,105]

An emerging concept in the prevention of postoperative cognitive and physical dysfunction is prehabilitation, a process of enhancing function and reserve before a stressor (eg, surgery) to minimize decline and speed recovery. Physical prehabilitation programs have improved recovery to baseline after major operations across a variety of surgical specialties.[106–108] Beyond functional recovery, there is interest in the effects of prehabilitation on cognitive outcomes because an increasing body of evidence has shown structural changes and improved cognition in physically active seniors.[109–111] Cognitive therapies have been applied successfully to improve outcomes in survivors of traumatic brain injury,[112] and combined cognitive and physical rehabilitation interventions have shown improved executive function and functional status in ICU survivors[113] but have not yet been studied as a prehabilitation intervention. Perhaps a combined physical and cognitive prehabilitation program may be beneficial in the perioperative setting; however, further research is needed to explore the effects of prehabilitation on long-term cognitive outcomes.

SUMMARY

Surgical stress often leads to cognitive changes in older adults, including delirium and POCD, which may persist for months to years after surgery. Precise mechanisms are unclear but likely overlap. An inflammatory state caused by surgical stress leading to neuroinflammation and neuronal damage is likely a central factor. Increasing age is strongly associated with delirium and POCD and is often coupled with baseline factors that increase cognitive vulnerability. Postoperative delirium is also strongly associated with developing POCD and subsequent dementia; thus, applying techniques to prevent delirium may prove to be an important perioperative strategy. Future research will need to standardize the diagnosis of POCD, further characterize the mechanisms that contribute to neurocognitive changes in the perioperative setting, and identify strategies and interventions to minimize the occurrence of delirium and cognitive dysfunction in older adults.

REFERENCES

1. Fried TR, Bradley EH, Towle VR, et al. Understanding the treatment preferences of seriously ill patients. N Engl J Med 2002;346(14):1061–6.
2. Neufeld KJ, Leoutsakos JM, Sieber FE, et al. Outcomes of early delirium diagnosis after general anesthesia in the elderly. Anesth Analg 2013;117(2):471–8.
3. Saczynski JS, Marcantonio ER, Quach L, et al. Cognitive trajectories after postoperative delirium. N Engl J Med 2012;367(1):30–9.
4. Inouye SK, Marcantonio ER, Kosar CM, et al. The short-term and long-term relationship between delirium and cognitive trajectory in older surgical patients. Alzheimers Dement 2016;12(7):766–75.
5. Lingehall HC, Smulter NS, Lindahl E, et al. Preoperative cognitive performance and postoperative delirium are independently associated with future dementia in older people who have undergone cardiac surgery: a longitudinal cohort study. Crit Care Med 2017;45(8):1295–303.
6. Hughes CG, Patel MB, Jackson JC, et al. Surgery and anesthesia exposure is not a risk factor for cognitive impairment after major noncardiac surgery and critical illness. Ann Surg 2016;265(6):1126–33.
7. Steinmetz J, Christensen KB, Lund T, et al. Long-term consequences of postoperative cognitive dysfunction. Anesthesiology 2009;110(3):548–55.
8. Steinmetz J, Siersma V, Kessing LV, et al. Is postoperative cognitive dysfunction a risk factor for dementia? A cohort follow-up study. Br J Anaesth 2013; 110(Suppl 1):i92–7.
9. Cunningham C, Maclullich AM. At the extreme end of the psychoneuroimmunological spectrum: delirium as a maladaptive sickness behaviour response. Brain Behav Immun 2013;28:1–13.
10. Kochunov P, Ramage AE, Lancaster JL, et al. Loss of cerebral white matter structural integrity tracks the gray matter metabolic decline in normal aging. Neuroimage 2009;45(1):17–28.
11. Maldonado JR. Neuropathogenesis of delirium: review of current etiologic theories and common pathways. Am J Geriatr Psychiatry 2013;21(12):1190–222.
12. Martin AJ, Friston KJ, Colebatch JG, et al. Decreases in regional cerebral blood flow with normal aging. J Cereb Blood Flow Metab 1991;11(4):684–9.
13. Versari D, Daghini E, Virdis A, et al. The ageing endothelium, cardiovascular risk and disease in man. Exp Physiol 2009;94(3):317–21.
14. Farrall AJ, Wardlaw JM. Blood-brain barrier: ageing and microvascular disease–systematic review and meta-analysis. Neurobiol Aging 2009;30(3):337–52.
15. Association AP. Diagnostic and statistical manual of mental disorders. 5th edition. Washington, DC: American Psychiatric Association; 2013.
16. Lipowski ZJ. Transient cognitive disorders (delirium, acute confusional states) in the elderly. Am J Psychiatry 1983;140(11):1426–36.
17. Lipowski ZJ. Delirium in the elderly patient. N Engl J Med 1989;320(9):578–82.

18. van den Boogaard M, Schoonhoven L, van der Hoeven JG, et al. Incidence and short-term consequences of delirium in critically ill patients: a prospective observational cohort study. Int J Nurs Stud 2012;49(7):775–83.

19. Peterson JF, Pun BT, Dittus RS, et al. Delirium and its motoric subtypes: a study of 614 critically ill patients. J Am Geriatr Soc 2006;54(3):479–84.

20. Stransky M, Schmidt C, Ganslmeier P, et al. Hypoactive delirium after cardiac surgery as an independent risk factor for prolonged mechanical ventilation. J Cardiothorac Vasc Anesth 2011;25(6):968–74.

21. Gaudreau JD, Gagnon P, Harel F, et al. Fast, systematic, and continuous delirium assessment in hospitalized patients: the nursing delirium screening scale. J Pain Symptom Manage 2005;29(4):368–75.

22. Ely EW, Inouye SK, Bernard GR, et al. Delirium in mechanically ventilated patients: validity and reliability of the confusion assessment method for the intensive care unit (CAM-ICU). JAMA 2001;286(21):2703–10.

23. Neufeld KJ, Leoutsakos JS, Sieber FE, et al. Evaluation of two delirium screening tools for detecting post-operative delirium in the elderly. Br J Anaesth 2013;111(4):7.

24. Brown CHt, Dowdy D. Risk factors for delirium: are systematic reviews enough? Crit Care Med 2015;43(1):232–3.

25. Inouye SK, Westendorp RG, Saczynski JS. Delirium in elderly people. Lancet 2014;383(9920):911–22.

26. Brown CHt, LaFlam A, Max L, et al. Delirium after spine surgery in older adults: incidence, risk factors, and outcomes. J Am Geriatr Soc 2016;64(10):2101–8.

27. Yang Y, Zhao X, Dong T, et al. Risk factors for postoperative delirium following hip fracture repair in elderly patients: a systematic review and meta-analysis. Aging Clin Exp Res 2017;29(2):115–26.

28. Rudolph JL, Jones RN, Levkoff SE, et al. Derivation and validation of a preoperative prediction rule for delirium after cardiac surgery. Circulation 2009;119(2): 229–36.

29. Ely EW, Siegel MD, Inouye SK. Delirium in the intensive care unit: an underrecognized syndrome of organ dysfunction. Semin Respir Crit Care Med 2001;22(2):115–26.

30. Hughes CG, Patel MB, Pandharipande PP. Pathophysiology of acute brain dysfunction: what's the cause of all this confusion? Curr Opin Crit Care 2012; 18(5):518–26.

31. Vasunilashorn SM, Ngo L, Inouye SK, et al. Cytokines and postoperative delirium in older patients undergoing major elective surgery. J Gerontol A Biol Sci Med Sci 2015;70(10):1289–95.

32. Cerejeira J, Firmino H, Vaz-Serra A, et al. The neuroinflammatory hypothesis of delirium. Acta Neuropathol 2010;119(6):737–54.

33. Hughes CG, Pandharipande PP, Thompson JL, et al. Endothelial activation and blood-brain barrier injury as risk factors for delirium in critically ill patients. Crit Care Med 2016;44(9):e809–17.

34. Vasilevskis EE, Han JH, Hughes CG, et al. Epidemiology and risk factors for delirium across hospital settings. Best Pract Res Clin Anaesthesiol 2012;26(3): 277–87.

35. Booka E, Kamijo T, Matsumoto T, et al. Incidence and risk factors for postoperative delirium after major head and neck cancer surgery. J Craniomaxillofac Surg 2016;44(7):890–4.

36. van der Sluis FJ, Buisman PL, Meerdink M, et al. Risk factors for postoperative delirium after colorectal operation. Surgery 2017;161(3):704–11.

37. Culley DJ, Flaherty D, Fahey MC, et al. Poor performance on a preoperative cognitive screening test predicts postoperative complications in older orthopedic surgical patients. Anesthesiology 2017;127(5):765–74.

38. Cavallari M, Dai W, Guttmann CR, et al. Neural substrates of vulnerability to postsurgical delirium as revealed by presurgical diffusion MRI. Brain 2016; 139(Pt 4):1282–94.

39. Ansaloni L, Catena F, Chattat R, et al. Risk factors and incidence of postoperative delirium in elderly patients after elective and emergency surgery. Br J Surg 2010;97(2):273–80.

40. Jung P, Pereira MA, Hiebert B, et al. The impact of frailty on postoperative delirium in cardiac surgery patients. J Thorac Cardiovasc Surg 2015;149(3): 869–75.e1-2.

41. Raats JW, van Eijsden WA, Crolla RM, et al. Risk factors and outcomes for postoperative delirium after major surgery in elderly patients. PLoS One 2015;10(8): e0136071.

42. Pandharipande P, Cotton BA, Shintani A, et al. Prevalence and risk factors for development of delirium in surgical and trauma intensive care unit patients. J Trauma 2008;65(1):34–41.

43. Morrison RS, Magaziner J, Gilbert M, et al. Relationship between pain and opioid analgesics on the development of delirium following hip fracture. J Gerontol A Biol Sci Med Sci 2003;58(1):76–81.

44. Sieber FE, Mears S, Lee H, et al. Postoperative opioid consumption and its relationship to cognitive function in older adults with hip fracture. J Am Geriatr Soc 2011;59(12):2256–62.

45. Van Rompaey B, Schuurmans MJ, Shortridge-Baggett LM, et al. Risk factors for intensive care delirium: a systematic review. Intensive Crit Care Nurs 2008; 24(2):98–107.

46. Schreiber MP, Colantuoni E, Bienvenu OJ, et al. Corticosteroids and transition to delirium in patients with acute lung injury. Crit Care Med 2014;42(6):1480–6.

47. Hayhurst CJ, Pandharipande PP, Hughes CG. Intensive care unit delirium: a review of diagnosis, prevention, and treatment. Anesthesiology 2016;125(6): 1229–41.

48. Vaurio LE, Sands LP, Wang Y, et al. Postoperative delirium: the importance of pain and pain management. Anesth Analg 2006;102(4):1267–73.

49. Guay J, Parker MJ, Gajendragadkar PR, et al. Anaesthesia for hip fracture surgery in adults. Cochrane Database Syst Rev 2016;(2):CD000521.

50. Slor CJ, de Jonghe JF, Vreeswijk R, et al. Anesthesia and postoperative delirium in older adults undergoing hip surgery. J Am Geriatr Soc 2011;59(7):1313–9.

51. Sieber FE, Zakriya KJ, Gottschalk A, et al. Sedation depth during spinal anesthesia and the development of postoperative delirium in elderly patients undergoing hip fracture repair. Mayo Clin Proc 2010;85(1):18–26.

52. Mason SE, Noel-Storr A, Ritchie CW. The impact of general and regional anesthesia on the incidence of post-operative cognitive dysfunction and postoperative delirium: a systematic review with meta-analysis. J Alzheimers Dis 2010;22(Suppl 3):67–79.

53. Royse CF, Andrews DT, Newman SN, et al. The influence of propofol or desflurane on postoperative cognitive dysfunction in patients undergoing coronary artery bypass surgery. Anaesthesia 2011;66(6):455–64.

54. Tanaka P, Goodman S, Sommer BR, et al. The effect of desflurane versus propofol anesthesia on postoperative delirium in elderly obese patients undergoing

total knee replacement: a randomized, controlled, double-blinded clinical trial. J Clin Anesth 2017;39:17–22.

55. Oh CS, Rhee KY, Yoon TG, et al. Postoperative delirium in elderly patients undergoing hip fracture surgery in the sugammadex era: a retrospective study. Biomed Res Int 2016;2016:1054597.

56. Meineke M, Applegate RL 2nd, Rasmussen T, et al. Cognitive dysfunction following desflurane versus sevoflurane general anesthesia in elderly patients: a randomized controlled trial. Med Gas Res 2014;4(1):6.

57. Radtke FM, Franck M, Lendner J, et al. Monitoring depth of anaesthesia in a randomized trial decreases the rate of postoperative delirium but not postoperative cognitive dysfunction. Br J Anaesth 2013;110(Suppl 1):i98–105.

58. Chan MT, Cheng BC, Lee TM, et al. BIS-guided anesthesia decreases postoperative delirium and cognitive decline. J Neurosurg Anesthesiol 2013;25(1): 33–42.

59. Whitlock EL, Torres BA, Lin N, et al. Postoperative delirium in a substudy of cardiothoracic surgical patients in the BAG-RECALL clinical trial. Anesth Analg 2014;118(4):809–17.

60. Berger M, Schenning KJ, Brown CHt, et al. Best practices for postoperative brain health: recommendations from the Fifth International Perioperative Neurotoxicity Working Group. Anesth Analg 2018;127(6):1406–13.

61. Sieber FE, Neufeld KJ, Gottschalk A, et al. Effect of depth of sedation in older patients undergoing hip fracture repair on postoperative delirium: the STRIDE randomized clinical trial. JAMA Surg 2018;153(11):987–95.

62. Avidan MS, Maybrier HR, Abdallah AB, et al. Intraoperative ketamine for prevention of postoperative delirium or pain after major surgery in older adults: an international, multicentre, double-blind, randomised clinical trial. Lancet 2017; 390(10091):267–75.

63. Deiner S, Luo X, Lin HM, et al. Intraoperative infusion of dexmedetomidine for prevention of postoperative delirium and cognitive dysfunction in elderly patients undergoing major elective noncardiac surgery: a randomized clinical trial. JAMA Surg 2017;152(8):e171505.

64. Lynch EP, Lazor MA, Gellis JE, et al. The impact of postoperative pain on the development of postoperative delirium. Anesth Analg 1998;86(4):781–5.

65. Krenk L, Rasmussen LS, Hansen TB, et al. Delirium after fast-track hip and knee arthroplasty. Br J Anaesth 2012;108(4):607–11.

66. Kurbegovic S, Andersen J, Krenk L, et al. Delirium in fast-track colonic surgery. Langenbecks Arch Surg 2015;400(4):513–6.

67. Leung JM, Sands LP, Chen N, et al. Perioperative gabapentin does not reduce postoperative delirium in older surgical patients: a randomized clinical trial. Anesthesiology 2017;127(4):633–44.

68. Siddiqi N, Harrison JK, Clegg A, et al. Interventions for preventing delirium in hospitalised non-ICU patients. Cochrane Database Syst Rev 2016;(3):CD005563.

69. Chen CC, Li HC, Liang JT, et al. Effect of a modified hospital elder life program on delirium and length of hospital stay in patients undergoing abdominal surgery: a cluster randomized clinical trial. JAMA Surg 2017;152(9):827–34.

70. Barnes-Daly MA, Phillips G, Ely EW. Improving hospital survival and reducing brain dysfunction at seven California Community Hospitals: implementing PAD guidelines via the ABCDEF bundle in 6,064 patients. Crit Care Med 2017; 45(2):171–8.

71. Neufeld KJ, Yue J, Robinson TN, et al. Antipsychotic medication for prevention and treatment of delirium in hospitalized adults: a systematic review and meta-analysis. J Am Geriatr Soc 2016;64(4):705–14.

72. Gamberini M, Bolliger D, Lurati Buse GA, et al. Rivastigmine for the prevention of postoperative delirium in elderly patients undergoing elective cardiac surgery–a randomized controlled trial. Crit Care Med 2009;37(5):1762–8.

73. van den Boogaard M, Slooter AJC, Bruggemann RJM, et al. Effect of haloperidol on survival among critically ill adults with a high risk of delirium: the REDUCE randomized clinical trial. JAMA 2018;319(7):680–90.

74. Girard TD, Thompson JL, Pandharipande PP, et al. Clinical phenotypes of delirium during critical illness and severity of subsequent long-term cognitive impairment: a prospective cohort study. Lancet Respir Med 2018;6(3):213–22.

75. Carrasco G, Baeza N, Cabre L, et al. Dexmedetomidine for the treatment of hyperactive delirium refractory to haloperidol in nonintubated ICU patients: a nonrandomized controlled trial. Crit Care Med 2016;44(7):1295–306.

76. Reade MC, Eastwood GM, Bellomo R, et al. Effect of dexmedetomidine added to standard care on ventilator-free time in patients with agitated delirium: a randomized clinical trial. JAMA 2016;315(14):1460–8.

77. Brown Ct, Deiner S. Perioperative cognitive protection. Br J Anaesth 2016; 117(suppl 3):iii52–61.

78. Monk TG, Price CC. Postoperative cognitive disorders. Curr Opin Crit Care 2011;17(4):376–81.

79. Evered L, Silbert B, Knopman DS, et al. Recommendations for the nomenclature of cognitive change associated with anaesthesia and surgery-2018. Br J Anaesth 2018;121(5):1005–12.

80. Murkin JM, Newman SP, Stump DA, et al. Statement of consensus on assessment of neurobehavioral outcomes after cardiac surgery. Ann Thorac Surg 1995;59(5):1289–95.

81. Rasmussen LS, Larsen K, Houx P, et al. The assessment of postoperative cognitive function. Acta Anaesthesiol Scand 2001;45(3):275–89.

82. Berger M, Nadler JW, Browndyke J, et al. Postoperative cognitive dysfunction: minding the gaps in our knowledge of a common postoperative complication in the elderly. Anesthesiol Clin 2015;33(3):517–50.

83. Moller JT, Cluitmans P, Rasmussen LS, et al. Long-term postoperative cognitive dysfunction in the elderly ISPOCD1 study. ISPOCD investigators. International Study of Post-Operative Cognitive Dysfunction. Lancet 1998;351(9106):857–61.

84. Monk TG, Weldon BC, Garvan CW, et al. Predictors of cognitive dysfunction after major noncardiac surgery. Anesthesiology 2008;108(1):18–30.

85. McDonagh DL, Mathew JP, White WD, et al. Cognitive function after major noncardiac surgery, apolipoprotein E4 genotype, and biomarkers of brain injury. Anesthesiology 2010;112(4):852–9.

86. Newman MF, Kirchner JL, Phillips-Bute B, et al. Longitudinal assessment of neurocognitive function after coronary-artery bypass surgery. N Engl J Med 2001; 344(6):395–402.

87. Selnes OA, Gottesman RF, Grega MA, et al. Cognitive and neurologic outcomes after coronary-artery bypass surgery. N Engl J Med 2012;366(3):250–7.

88. Eckenhoff RG, Laudansky KF. Anesthesia, surgery, illness and Alzheimer's disease. Prog Neuropsychopharmacol Biol Psychiatry 2013;47:162–6.

89. Liu X, Yu Y, Zhu S. Inflammatory markers in postoperative delirium (POD) and cognitive dysfunction (POCD): a meta-analysis of observational studies. PLoS One 2018;13(4):e0195659.

90. Hughes CG, Patel MB, Brummel NE, et al. Relationships between markers of neurologic and endothelial injury during critical illness and long-term cognitive impairment and disability. Intensive Care Med 2018;44(3):345–55.
91. Neerland BE, Krogseth M, Juliebo V, et al. Perioperative hemodynamics and risk for delirium and new onset dementia in hip fracture patients; a prospective follow-up study. PLoS One 2017;12(7):e0180641.
92. Guay J. General anaesthesia does not contribute to long-term post-operative cognitive dysfunction in adults: a meta-analysis. Indian J Anaesth 2011;55(4): 358–63.
93. Silbert BS, Evered LA, Scott DA. Incidence of postoperative cognitive dysfunction after general or spinal anaesthesia for extracorporeal shock wave lithotripsy. Br J Anaesth 2014;113(5):784–91.
94. Avidan MS, Searleman AC, Storandt M, et al. Long-term cognitive decline in older subjects was not attributable to noncardiac surgery or major illness. Anesthesiology 2009;111(5):964–70.
95. Dokkedal U, Hansen TG, Rasmussen LS, et al. Cognitive functioning after surgery in middle-aged and elderly Danish twins. J Neurosurg Anesthesiol 2016; 28(3):275.
96. Schulte PJ, Martin DP, Deljou A, et al. Effect of cognitive status on the receipt of procedures requiring anesthesia and critical care admissions in older adults. Mayo Clin Proc 2018;93(11):1552–62.
97. Langer T, Santini A, Zadek F, et al. Intraoperative hypotension is not associated with postoperative cognitive dysfunction in elderly patients undergoing general anesthesia for surgery: results of a randomized controlled pilot trial. J Clin Anesth 2018;52:111–8.
98. Sprung J, Roberts RO, Weingarten TN, et al. Postoperative delirium in elderly patients is associated with subsequent cognitive impairment. Br J Anaesth 2017;119(2):316–23.
99. Vasunilashorn SM, Fong TG, Albuquerque A, et al. Delirium severity post-surgery and its relationship with long-term cognitive decline in a cohort of patients without dementia. J Alzheimers Dis 2018;61(1):347–58.
100. Ballard C, Jones E, Gauge N, et al. Optimised anaesthesia to reduce post operative cognitive decline (POCD) in older patients undergoing elective surgery, a randomised controlled trial. PLoS One 2012;7(6):e37410.
101. Glumac S, Kardum G, Sodic L, et al. Effects of dexamethasone on early cognitive decline after cardiac surgery: a randomised controlled trial. Eur J Anaesthesiol 2017;34(11):776–84.
102. Zhu YZ, Yao R, Zhang Z, et al. Parecoxib prevents early postoperative cognitive dysfunction in elderly patients undergoing total knee arthroplasty: a double-blind, randomized clinical consort study. Medicine (Baltimore) 2016;95(28): e4082.
103. Carr ZJ, Cios TJ, Potter KF, et al. Does dexmedetomidine ameliorate postoperative cognitive dysfunction? a brief review of the recent literature. Curr Neurol Neurosci Rep 2018;18(10):64.
104. Zywiel MG, Prabhu A, Perruccio AV, et al. The influence of anesthesia and pain management on cognitive dysfunction after joint arthroplasty: a systematic review. Clin Orthop Relat Res 2014;472(5):1453–66.
105. Wang Y, Sands LP, Vaurio L, et al. The effects of postoperative pain and its management on postoperative cognitive dysfunction. Am J Geriatr Psychiatry 2007; 15(1):50–9.

106. Gillis C, Li C, Lee L, et al. Prehabilitation versus rehabilitation: a randomized control trial in patients undergoing colorectal resection for cancer. Anesthesiology 2014;121(5):937–47.
107. Topp R, Swank AM, Quesada PM, et al. The effect of prehabilitation exercise on strength and functioning after total knee arthroplasty. PM R 2009;1(8):729–35.
108. Nielsen PR, Jorgensen LD, Dahl B, et al. Prehabilitation and early rehabilitation after spinal surgery: randomized clinical trial. Clin Rehabil 2010;24(2):137–48.
109. ten Brinke LF, Bolandzadeh N, Nagamatsu LS, et al. Aerobic exercise increases hippocampal volume in older women with probable mild cognitive impairment: a 6-month randomised controlled trial. Br J Sports Med 2015;49(4):248–54.
110. Hillman CH, Erickson KI, Kramer AF. Be smart, exercise your heart: exercise effects on brain and cognition. Nat Rev Neurosci 2008;9(1):58–65.
111. Middleton L, Kirkland S, Rockwood K. Prevention of CIND by physical activity: different impact on VCI-ND compared with MCI. J Neurol Sci 2008; 269(1–2):80–4.
112. Park HY, Maitra K, Martinez KM. The effect of occupation-based cognitive rehabilitation for traumatic brain injury: a meta-analysis of randomized controlled trials. Occup Ther Int 2015;22(2):104–16.
113. Jackson JC, Ely EW, Morey MC, et al. Cognitive and physical rehabilitation of intensive care unit survivors: results of the RETURN randomized controlled pilot investigation. Crit Care Med 2012;40(4):1088–97.
114. Brand N, Jolles J. Learning and retrieval rate of words presented auditory and visually. J Gen Psychol 1985;112(2):201–10.
115. Reitan RM. Validity of the Trail Making Test as an indicator of organic brain damage. Percept Mot Skills 1958;8(3):271–6.

Supporting the Geriatric Critical Care Patient

Decision Making, Understanding Outcomes, and the Role of Palliative Care

Aaron Mittel, MD[a],*, May Hua, MD, MSc[b]

KEYWORDS

- Critical care • Quality of life • Uncertainty • Risk assessment

KEY POINTS

- Increasing age is associated with an increased disease burden and reduced life expectancy. As long-term outcomes of critical illness are worse for older adults, the risks and benefits of intensive care unit (ICU) admission must be considered on an individual basis.
- In many patients, it is reasonable to consider a "trial of ICU" to determine if the patient has a chance at meaningful recovery from critical illness.
- "Meaningful recovery" is unique to all patients, and may center on outcomes other than survival, such as functional independence and quality of life.

SPECIAL CHALLENGES OF THE GERIATRIC CRITICAL CARE PATIENT
Introduction

Geriatric patients, commonly defined as those aged 65 and older, are a rapidly growing portion of the US population and a challenge for the health care system. As the population has aged, older adults now represent a large percentage of patients admitted to intensive care units (ICUs).[1] This review focuses on issues particular to caring for this challenging patient population, with particular emphasis on the potential benefit of ICU care in older adults, the decision to pursue care in context of individualized risk-benefit analysis, the need to consider outcomes other than mortality, and long-term outcomes after critical illness in older adults.

Disclosure Statement: Dr M. Hua is supported by a Paul B. Beeson Career Development Award K08AG051184 from the National Institute on Aging and the American Federation for Aging Research.
[a] Department of Anesthesiology, Columbia University Medical Center, 622 West 168th Street, PH505-C, New York, NY 10032, USA; [b] Department of Anesthesiology, Columbia University Medical Center, 622 West 168th Street, PH5, Room 527D, New York, NY 10032, USA
* Corresponding author.
E-mail address: am4656@cumc.columbia.edu

Anesthesiology Clin 37 (2019) 537–546
https://doi.org/10.1016/j.anclin.2019.04.011
1932-2275/19/© 2019 Elsevier Inc. All rights reserved.

anesthesiology.theclinics.com

Epidemiology of Geriatric Intensive Care Unit Admissions

Geriatric ICU admissions are a common occurrence, with older adults currently comprising half of all critically ill patients.[2] The indications for admission to the ICU are similar to those of nongeriatric patients, with typical diagnoses consisting of septic shock, acute respiratory failure, pneumonia, heart failure, and trauma.[3,4] Although rates of these diagnoses among older critically ill patients are comparable to those of younger patients, the implications of ICU admission differ. In comparison with their younger counterparts, older patients are prone to longer stays, and thus constitute most of all patient days spent in the ICU.[5] Likewise, the mortality rates of older ICU populations are higher than in comparable, younger groups,[6] with approximately 30% of all older adults being admitted to the ICU in the last 30 days of their life.[7] Although this statistic is often cited to underscore the potential for overuse of aggressive care in the older adult population, it is important to recognize that mortality after ICU admission is not inevitable. In fact, even the very old (age >90 years) have been found to have reasonable post-ICU survival rates, with nearly 70% of patients surviving to hospital discharge, and more than 50% survival at 1 year.[6] Although the older adult population is certainly at high risk for mortality, these numbers highlight that the ICU has the potential to benefit many individuals.

Risk Scoring Specific to the Geriatric Population

There are several risk scoring systems designed to predict clinical outcomes following severe illness in older adults. Generally, these models stress the importance of age as a common predictor of poor clinical outcome but also reinforce the message that age alone is not always predictive of increased mortality. Increasing age often correlates with an increased burden of disease and a decreased life expectancy. Indeed, commonly used ICU-oriented predictive scoring systems, such as the Acute Physiology and Chronic Health Evaluation (APACHE) or Simplified Acute Physiology Score (SAPS), have incorporated age as a predictor of mortality since their development more than 3 decades ago.[8,9] Modern versions of these scoring systems continue to include age as an important covariable.[10] However, many clinicians have recognized the inherent limitation of applying these tools to geriatric populations, as they fail to incorporate physiologic adaptations to aging that may not be present in younger populations (eg, increased systolic pressure due to noncompliant vasculature). For this reason, several scoring tools have been developed to better predict risk of poor outcomes in geriatric patients.

Novel geriatric-specific risk models typically include additional biomarkers or indices of preadmission functional status to improve prediction of in-hospital mortality. Although it is important to note that addition of covariables to any scoring system may increase its predictive capability, the inclusion of targeted geriatric-specific metrics can be important to risk-stratify older adult patients among their age-related peers. These risk models attempt to better incorporate pre-ICU function and comorbidity, highlighting the concept that patients' pre-ICU state may play a significant role in determining or modifying outcomes. Common covariables included in these models that may be absent in other scoring systems include measures of overall functional ability (eg, grip strength, gait speed, the capacity to perform independent activities of daily life),[11,12] biomarkers of heart failure, and measures of overall muscular strength.[13] In the perioperative arena, the National Surgical Quality Improvement Preoperative Mortality Predictor (NSQIP-PMP) score has been found to be especially effective at risk modeling of geriatric surgical outcomes.[13] Like other scoring systems, it takes into account a baseline assessment of functional status to estimate risk.

Uniquely, it accounts for a wide variety of outcomes (eg, surgical site infection, readmission, death, and others), and thus can be an important tool when dealing with perioperative critical illness in older adults.

Global assessment of independence and functional status, such as that incorporated within the NSQIP-PMP and other scoring systems, is perhaps best addressed by measuring preadmission frailty. Briefly, frailty is highly prevalent in geriatric populations[14]; independent of age, increased frailty is associated with higher risk of mortality, functional disability, and reduced quality of life after discharge. These outcomes become apparent within the immediate post-ICU period and continue to persist in the years following.[14–18] Frailty is typically unrecognized with traditional ICU scoring systems such as APACHE or SAPS, and its presence may therefore go unheeded by intensivists. Fortunately, simple screening programs that measure and identify patients at high risk of frailty have been shown to provide meaningful benefit. In fact, compared with traditional risk scoring systems, early recognition of frailty may allow for an improved ability to prognosticate geriatric outcomes after critical illness.[18–20]

As survival after an ICU stay and the ability to sustain patients through use of life-sustaining therapies have both increased, there has been increasing recognition of the importance of "acceptable" survival, and the concept of a "state worse than death." In one study of older adults with serious illness, more than 50% of patients surveyed rated certain states (eg, being ventilator-dependent, having bowel or bladder incontinence) as being worse or equivalent to death.[21] Consequently, there has also been interest in examining prognostication for outcomes other than survival. In one prospective cohort study, physicians' and nurses' ability to prognosticate for functional outcomes (eg, ability to toilet independently) was reasonable, with performance metrics comparable to that of commonly used diagnostic tests.[22] Although patients and families may want information about the likelihood of long-term functional outcomes, certain factors may give clinicians pause. Clinicians should be cognizant of their own beliefs, and the potential for their actions to create "self-fulfilling prophecies" with regard to mortality. Also, surrogates may not truly know patients' preferences for functional outcomes, and they may not take into account patients' abilities to adapt to or cope with new disability. Patients' preferences may also change, particularly in the setting of an acute stressor.[23] Thus, although functional outcomes and quality of life are of paramount importance to older adults, the ability to provide adequate information for these outcomes is limited.

THE ACUTE PHASE OF CRITICAL ILLNESS IN OLDER ADULTS
Decision to Admit to the Intensive Care Unit

Patient autonomy, informed consent, and ethical decision making are hallmarks of all medical care. These principles arise from the reality that although medical care has benefits, which are largely focused on increasing survival, it also comes with substantial risks, and the risk-benefit ratio of undergoing care is a value-based decision that is necessarily individualized. This concept of personalized risk-benefit ratios becomes even more salient when providing critical care to older adults.[20,21] Putatively, young patients are willing to bear the burden of increased risk associated with challenging medical issues, with even slim hopes of functional recovery. In contrast, older patients necessarily have less quantity of life as they age, and quality of life may become increasingly important.[24] As such, older patients may be less willing to accept burdensome risks, or undergo a complex and lengthy recovery for an end-result that leaves them with an unacceptable quality of life. Thus, the decision to admit a patient to the ICU ideally should be contingent on "buy-in" from both the treating clinicians, who must feel that there is realistic benefit to admitting a patient to a high-intensity setting, and from the patient, who believes that undergoing such care is in-line with their preferences.

Clinician "buy-in" for geriatric ICU admissions should not be assumed. Clinicians may hesitate to admit profoundly ill, or very old, patients to ICUs when they deem aggressive medical care to be fruitless.[25] Indeed, in several studies, only 30% to 50% of all older adults with definitive need for ICU admission (ie, those with abnormal vital signs, diagnoses, or conditions mandating high-intensity care as defined by Society of Critical Care Medicine guidelines) were actually admitted to the ICU.[26,27] This reluctance may be a potential barrier to delivering appropriate care, which may affect patient outcomes. This concept was recently explored with a trial that investigated the use of an explicit interventional program designed to promote systematic geriatric ICU admission. Although the intervention did in fact increase ICU utilization, it failed to reduce 6-month mortality rates.[3] It is unclear if this finding suggests that triage providers are able to effectively screen older adults who will not benefit from ICU admission, or if an ICU level of care may not improve mortality in this population.

Patients and their families should also "buy-in" to the choice to pursue care in an ICU. This is a highly individualized process that may change with age. In particular, older adults may be less willing to accept the same components of critical care as their younger counterparts. For example, in well-conducted observational studies, community-dwelling geriatric adults indicate willingness to accept noninvasive ventilation, but reluctance to consent to dialysis.[28] Likewise, compared with their younger peers, many older patients may choose to forgo life-sustaining surgery or invasive mechanical ventilation. Nevertheless, physicians may frequently underestimate elderly patients' desire to pursue life-sustaining interventions.[29] Aggressive medical care should not be withheld solely on the clinician's belief that the patient would not be interested in such advanced measures.

Trial of Intensive Care Unit

Because of the difficulty of determining "benefit" of ICU admission and patients' willingness to undergo care changes with respect to prognosis, the risk-benefit ratio for ICU care changes over time. Consequently, many clinicians advocate for a "trial of ICU" period. This time-limited trial allows for aggressive measures to be instituted with hopes of rapid improvement, while also recognizing the reality that many situations may be futile. The exact duration of these time-limited trials is undetermined, and needs to be tailored to individual diagnoses, clinical goals, and expectations for post-ICU functioning. Indeed, finding the "correct" duration of a time-limited trial is not simple. Trials that are too short may erode patients' and families' trust in providers.[30] Patients who have lower rates of end-organ failure (ie, those who are "healthier") at ICU admission may deserve longer trial periods (on the order of 10–12 days) as opposed to patients with more severe illness, who may benefit from a trial of up to 8 days but see no survival advantage when extending this period further.[31]

There are some ways to implement a time-limited trial of ICU care that may help its efficacy. First, implementation of a time-limited trial necessitates clear and specific communication among ICU providers, patients, family members, and other medical providers. Having explicit goals (eg, ability to recover renal function and avoid dialysis) and the delineation of a specific time frame (eg, 3 days) at which to reevaluate the impact of ICU care help to provide a framework for determining whether the trial has led to improvement in a patient's status.[32] Ultimately, the individual treatment components used during a time-limited trial and its duration should be tailored to specific disease states and patient conditions.[30] Rapid recovery, or less serious initial illness, may warrant extending the trial. Alternatively, failure to progress or profound illness may indicate the need to facilitate end-of-life discussions and/or transition to comfort-based care.

Role of Palliative Care in the Intensive Care Unit

Given the difficulty of determining the risk-benefit ratio of an ICU admission, the use of palliative care has been advocated as a means to mitigate the stress and harm associated with uncertain or unwanted aggressive treatment.[33–35] Palliative care is a multidisciplinary model of care with the overarching goal of improving quality of life for patients with serious illness through pain and symptom management, providing psychosocial support, eliciting personal preferences, and aiding decision making. Use of palliative care may be particularly helpful in critical illness, as the emotional and cognitive stress associated with an ICU stay and potentially terminal condition may hamper decision making for both patients and surrogates. Indeed, in one retrospective analysis, preadmission advance directives indicating patients' desire to avoid aggressive care in terminal situations were not associated with the decision to focus on end-of-life planning (such as withdrawal of aggressive therapies) during an actual period of critical illness.[36] Use of palliative care may improve the decision-making process, as it is associated with an improvement in the perceived quality of communication and families' perceptions of the patient-centeredness of care.[37] Although palliative care is often used to provide support for patients and families, studies have not consistently demonstrated a reduction in psychological symptomatology for surrogates of critically ill patients.[38,39]

Although use of palliative care may be beneficial, it is likely underused and initiated late in the course of illness.[40,41] This reticence is partially due to the misperception that palliative care is equivalent to end-of-life care, or that use of palliative care may hasten mortality.[42] Particularly for patients with surgical critical illness, achieving "buy-in" to initiate palliative care from all treating clinicians is of paramount importance to streamline the decision-making process and reduce conflict.[43,44] The use of formalized criteria, or "triggers," to prompt palliative care consultation has been shown to effectively increase palliative care utilization without increasing health care costs.[45] Certain triggers (eg, age >80 with multiple life-threatening comorbidities) have highlighted the potential need for palliative care in older adult patients. However, triggers based on age alone may not be well-accepted by ICU clinicians.[46]

THE AFTERMATH OF GERIATRIC CRITICAL CARE
Long-Term Outcomes of Critical Illness in Elderly Patients

Although approximately 25% of critically ill older adults will die during their hospital stay, another 25% will die within 1 year of admission.[15] This additional increase in mortality is largely concentrated within the first few months after discharge, and then continues to increase slowly over time.[15] By 3 years after discharge, approximately 40% of all older adult ICU survivors are still alive.[15,47] However, survival may not be the best metric to evaluate the impact of an ICU stay in geriatric populations. Many geriatric patients are not able to return home immediately after their hospital admission, with most requiring short-term rehabilitation. However, at least 20% of those incapable of returning home will require admission to long-term inpatient facilities where the recovery is expected to be prolonged, raising concerns about patients' quality of life during this period.[15] Furthermore, for patients discharged to post-acute care facilities, more than 20% will require readmission to the hospital within 30 days.[48]

The Post Intensive Care Syndrome

Survivors of critical illness are at risk for post intensive care syndrome (PICS), a constellation of symptoms characterized by decreases in physical function, cognitive impairment, psychological symptomatology, and decreased health care–related quality of life.[49,50] Up to 70% of all ICU survivors have difficulty with activities of daily living and 50% require caregiver assistance 1 year after critical illness.[49] With increasing age, functional disability after critical illness becomes increasingly common.[49,51] In fact, only 25% of patients older than 80 return to their preadmission functional status.[15] These functional limitations are particularly detrimental to the aging population, as maintaining independence is of vital importance to older adults.[52,53]

Long-term neurocognitive dysfunction is also a component of PICS. One large prospective study identified a 10% increase in the prevalence of moderate to severe cognitive impairment in older adult survivors of septic shock.[54] In a recent observational study of a heterogeneous group of patients with more diverse causes of critical illness, 20% to 30% of survivors had persistent cognitive impairment 12 months after admission, with deficits comparable to patients with moderate traumatic brain injury or mild Alzheimer disease.[55] Severe cognitive impairment has been associated with a need for an additional 40 hours per week of informal caregiving, increasing the burden on families of affected patients and possibly mandating the need for formalized, inpatient-based living arrangements.[54] ICU survivors are also at risk for other significant symptomatology. As many as 50% of ICU survivors experience depressive or anxiety symptoms.[49] Furthermore, more than 80% of older adults discharged to a post-acute care facility have at least one potential palliative care need.[56]

Efforts to modify PICS-associated outcomes are active and ongoing. Potential interventions include exercise rehabilitation programs,[57] training programs to build or reinforce coping skills,[58,59] meetings with social workers to identify community-based sources of support,[60] and referrals to specialized post-ICU outpatient clinics.[60–64] As of yet, no specific intervention has clearly demonstrated benefit. Despite the absence of definitive anti-PICS therapies, clinicians need not be discouraged about all long-term outcomes of critical illness in older adults. Many older adults do achieve a satisfactory level of functional recovery, even if it is below their preadmission baseline. In one small prospective study, most patients older than 80 years who were alive 1 year after ICU discharge were able to remain self-sufficient, despite some reduction in functional capabilities. Furthermore, these survivors actually had better scores on psychological health evaluations compared with their general population peers, with improvements in social relationship ratings and a reduced fear of dying.[65] These data may give hope to older survivors of critical illness and their families, as they speak to older adults' capacity to adapt to new circumstances and maintain an acceptable quality of life.

SUMMARY

Geriatric admissions to the ICU are common and warrant particular consideration from intensivists. The risks of mortality, prolonged hospital stays, and poor functional outcomes are higher in this group of patients than in their younger peers. However, patients who exhibit a reasonable amount of physiologic reserve (such as those without baseline frailty) often benefit from aggressive medical intervention. During this period of high-acuity illness, clinicians should be aware of issues that are particularly common in older adults, and the need to communicate prognosis in a manner that is meaningful to patients and families. They also should recognize that the need to tailor care toward individualized care plans is paramount, as the risk-to-benefit ratio for intensive care may differ in comparison with younger patients, and also may change over time. With these concepts in mind, clinicians can be assured they are providing high-quality critical care, while respecting patient autonomy and maximizing the value of an ICU admission in these especially vulnerable patients.

REFERENCES

1. Flaatten H, de Lange DW, Artigas A, et al. The status of intensive care medicine research and a future agenda for very old patients in the ICU. Intensive Care Med 2017;43(9):1319–28.
2. Angus DC, Shorr AF, White A, et al. Critical care delivery in the United States: distribution of services and compliance with Leapfrog recommendations. Crit Care Med 2006;34(4):1016–24.
3. Guidet B, Leblanc G, Simon T, et al. Effect of systematic intensive care unit triage on long-term mortality among critically ill elderly patients in France: a randomized clinical trial. JAMA 2017;318(15):1450–9.
4. Sjoding MW, Prescott HC, Wunsch H, et al. Longitudinal changes in ICU admissions among elderly patients in the United States. Crit Care Med 2016;44(7): 1353–60.
5. Angus DC, Kelley MA, Schmitz RJ, et al. Caring for the critically ill patient. Current and projected workforce requirements for care of the critically ill and patients with pulmonary disease: can we meet the requirements of an aging population? JAMA 2000;284(21):2762–70.
6. Becker S, Muller J, de Heer G, et al. Clinical characteristics and outcome of very elderly patients >/=90 years in intensive care: a retrospective observational study. Ann Intensive Care 2015;5(1):53.
7. Teno JM, Gozalo P, Trivedi AN, et al. Site of death, place of care, and health care transitions among US Medicare Beneficiaries, 2000-2015. JAMA 2018;320(3): 264–71.
8. Knaus WA, Zimmerman JE, Wagner DP, et al. APACHE-acute physiology and chronic health evaluation: a physiologically based classification system. Crit Care Med 1981;9(8):591–7.
9. Le Gall JR, Loirat P, Alperovitch A, et al. A simplified acute physiology score for ICU patients. Crit Care Med 1984;12(11):975–7.
10. Vincent JL, Moreno R. Clinical review: scoring systems in the critically ill. Crit Care 2010;14(2):207.
11. Krinsley JS, Wasser T, Kang G, et al. Pre-admission functional status impacts the performance of the APACHE IV model of mortality prediction in critically ill patients. Crit Care 2017;21(1):110.
12. Baldwin MR, Narain WR, Wunsch H, et al. A prognostic model for 6-month mortality in elderly survivors of critical illness. Chest 2013;143(4):910–9.
13. Eamer G, Al-Amoodi MJH, Holroyd-Leduc J, et al. Review of risk assessment tools to predict morbidity and mortality in elderly surgical patients. Am J Surg 2018;216(3):585–94.
14. Brummel NE, Bell SP, Girard TD, et al. Frailty and subsequent disability and mortality among patients with critical illness. Am J Respir Crit Care Med 2017;196(1): 64–72.
15. Heyland DK, Garland A, Bagshaw SM, et al. Recovery after critical illness in patients aged 80 years or older: a multi-center prospective observational cohort study. Intensive Care Med 2015;41(11):1911–20.

16. van der Schaaf M, Dettling DS, Beelen A, et al. Poor functional status immediately after discharge from an intensive care unit. Disabil Rehabil 2008;30(23):1812–8.
17. Muscedere J, Waters B, Varambally A, et al. The impact of frailty on intensive care unit outcomes: a systematic review and meta-analysis. Intensive Care Med 2017; 43(8):1105–22.
18. Hall DE, Arya S, Schmid KK, et al. Association of a frailty screening initiative with postoperative survival at 30, 180, and 365 days. JAMA Surg 2017;152(3):233–40.
19. Le Maguet P, Roquilly A, Lasocki S, et al. Prevalence and impact of frailty on mortality in elderly ICU patients: a prospective, multicenter, observational study. Intensive Care Med 2014;40(5):674–82.
20. Gilbert T, Neuburger J, Kraindler J, et al. Development and validation of a Hospital Frailty Risk Score focusing on older people in acute care settings using electronic hospital records: an observational study. Lancet 2018;391(10132): 1775–82.
21. Rubin EB, Buehler AE, Halpern SD. States worse than death among hospitalized patients with serious illnesses. JAMA Intern Med 2016;176(10):1557–9.
22. Detsky ME, Harhay MO, Bayard DF, et al. Discriminative accuracy of physician and nurse predictions for survival and functional outcomes 6 months after an ICU admission. JAMA 2017;317(21):2187–95.
23. Wilson ME, Hopkins RO, Brown SM. Long-term functional outcome data should not in general be used to guide end-of-life decision-making in the ICU. Crit Care Med 2018;47(2):264–7.
24. Brown GC. Living too long: the current focus of medical research on increasing the quantity, rather than the quality, of life is damaging our health and harming the economy. EMBO Rep 2015;16(2):137–41.
25. Haliko S, Downs J, Mohan D, et al. Hospital-based physicians' intubation decisions and associated mental models when managing a critically and terminally ill older patient. Med Decis Making 2018;38(3):344–54.
26. Garrouste-Orgeas M, Boumendil A, Pateron D, et al. Selection of intensive care unit admission criteria for patients aged 80 years and over and compliance of emergency and intensive care unit physicians with the selected criteria: an observational, multicenter, prospective study. Crit Care Med 2009;37(11):2919–28.
27. Andersen FH, Flaatten H, Klepstad P, et al. Long-term outcomes after ICU admission triage in octogenarians. Crit Care Med 2017;45(4):e363–71.
28. Philippart F, Vesin A, Bruel C, et al. The ETHICA study (part I): elderly's thoughts about intensive care unit admission for life-sustaining treatments. Intensive Care Med 2013;39(9):1565–73.
29. Hamel MB, Teno JM, Goldman L, et al. Patient age and decisions to withhold life-sustaining treatments from seriously ill, hospitalized adults. SUPPORT Investigators. Study to Understand Prognoses and Preferences for Outcomes and Risks of Treatment. Ann Intern Med 1999;130(2):116–25.
30. Vink EE, Azoulay E, Caplan A, et al. Time-limited trial of intensive care treatment: an overview of current literature. Intensive Care Med 2018;44(9):1369–77.
31. Shrime MG, Ferket BS, Scott DJ, et al. Time-limited trials of intensive care for critically ill patients with cancer: how long is long enough? JAMA Oncol 2016;2(1): 76–83.
32. Quill TE, Holloway R. Time-limited trials near the end of life. JAMA 2011;306(13): 1483–4.
33. Institute of Medicine. Dying in America: improving quality and honoring individual preferences near the end of life. Washington, DC: The National Academies Press; 2014.

34. Hua M, Wunsch H. Integrating palliative care in the ICU. Curr Opin Crit Care 2014;20(6):673–80.
35. Critical Care Societies Collaborative. Five things physicians and patients should question. [Choosing Wisely website] 2014. Available at: http://www.choosingwisely.org/doctor-patient-lists/critical-care-societies-collaborative-critical-care/. Accessed June 4, 2014.
36. Wooster M, Stassi A, Hill J, et al. End-of-life decision-making for patients with geriatric trauma cared for in a trauma intensive care unit. Am J Hosp Palliat Care 2018;35(8):1063–8.
37. White DB, Angus DC, Shields AM, et al. A randomized trial of a family-support intervention in intensive care units. N Engl J Med 2018;378(25):2365–75.
38. Carson SS, Cox CE, Wallenstein S, et al. Effect of palliative care-led meetings for families of patients with chronic critical illness: a randomized clinical trial. JAMA 2016;316(1):51–62.
39. Kavalieratos D, Corbelli J, Zhang D, et al. Association between palliative care and patient and caregiver outcomes: a systematic review and meta-analysis. JAMA 2016;316(20):2104–14.
40. Kozlov E, Carpenter BD, Thorsten M, et al. Timing of palliative care consultations and recommendations: understanding the variability. Am J Hosp Palliat Care 2015;32(7):772–5.
41. Rivet EB, Ferrada P, Albrecht T, et al. Characteristics of palliative care consultation at an academic level one trauma center. Am J Surg 2017;214(4):657–60.
42. Hawley P. Barriers to access to palliative care. Palliat Care 2017;10. 1178224216688887.
43. Mosenthal AC, Weissman DE, Curtis JR, et al. Integrating palliative care in the surgical and trauma intensive care unit: a report from the improving palliative care in the Intensive Care Unit (IPAL-ICU) Project Advisory Board and the Center to Advance Palliative Care. Crit Care Med 2012;40(4):1199–206.
44. Norton SA, Powers BA, Schmitt MH, et al. Navigating tensions: integrating palliative care consultation services into an academic medical center setting. J Pain Symptom Manage 2011;42(5):680–90.
45. Nelson JE, Curtis JR, Mulkerin C, et al. Choosing and using screening criteria for palliative care consultation in the ICU: a report from the Improving Palliative Care in the ICU (IPAL-ICU) Advisory Board. Crit Care Med 2013;41(10):2318–27.
46. Wysham NG, Hua M, Hough CL, et al. Improving ICU-based palliative care delivery: a multicenter, multidisciplinary survey of critical care clinician attitudes and beliefs. Crit Care Med 2017;45(4):e372–8.
47. Wunsch H, Guerra C, Barnato AE, et al. Three-year outcomes for Medicare beneficiaries who survive intensive care. JAMA 2010;303(9):849–56.
48. Britton MC, Ouellet GM, Minges KE, et al. Care transitions between hospitals and skilled nursing facilities: perspectives of sending and receiving providers. Jt Comm J Qual Patient Saf 2017;43(11):565–72.
49. Harvey MA. The truth about consequences–post-intensive care syndrome in intensive care unit survivors and their families. Crit Care Med 2012;40(8):2506–7.
50. Hofhuis JG, Spronk PE, van Stel HF, et al. The impact of critical illness on perceived health-related quality of life during ICU treatment, hospital stay, and after hospital discharge: a long-term follow-up study. Chest 2008;133(2):377–85.
51. Herridge MS, Tansey CM, Matte A, et al. Functional disability 5 years after acute respiratory distress syndrome. N Engl J Med 2011;364(14):1293–304.
52. Emory University Division of Geriatric Medicine and Gerontology. Basic principles of geriatrics - "the Big 10" 2008. Available at: http://medicine.emory.edu/divisions/

gen-med-geriatrics/education-geriatrics/big-10.html. Accessed October 10, 2014.

53. Hazzard WR, Halter JB. Hazzard's geriatric medicine and gerontology. 6th edition. New York: McGraw-Hill Medical; 2009.

54. Iwashyna TJ, Ely EW, Smith DM, et al. Long-term cognitive impairment and functional disability among survivors of severe sepsis. JAMA 2010;304(16):1787–94.

55. Pandharipande PP, Girard TD, Jackson JC, et al. Long-term cognitive impairment after critical illness. N Engl J Med 2013;369(14):1306–16.

56. Baldwin MR, Wunsch H, Reyfman PA, et al. High burden of palliative needs among older intensive care unit survivors transferred to post-acute care facilities. A single-center study. Ann Am Thorac Soc 2013;10(5):458–65.

57. Schaller SJ, Anstey M, Blobner M, et al. Early, goal-directed mobilisation in the surgical intensive care unit: a randomised controlled trial. Lancet 2016; 388(10052):1377–88.

58. Cox CE, Hough CL, Carson SS, et al. Effects of a telephone- and web-based coping skills training program compared with an education program for survivors of critical illness and their family members. a randomized clinical trial. Am J Respir Crit Care Med 2018;197(1):66–78.

59. Cox CE, Porter LS, Buck PJ, et al. Development and preliminary evaluation of a telephone-based mindfulness training intervention for survivors of critical illness. Ann Am Thorac Soc 2014;11(2):173–81.

60. McPeake J, Shaw M, Iwashyna TJ, et al. Intensive care syndrome: promoting independence and return to employment (InS:PIRE). Early evaluation of a complex intervention. PLoS One 2017;12(11):e0188028.

61. Connolly B, Salisbury L, O'Neill B, et al. Exercise rehabilitation following intensive care unit discharge for recovery from critical illness. Cochrane Database Syst Rev 2015;(6):CD008632.

62. McPeake J, Hirshberg EL, Christie LM, et al. Models of peer support to remediate post-intensive care syndrome: a report developed by the society of critical care medicine thrive international peer support collaborative. Crit Care Med 2018; 47(1):e21–7.

63. Cuthbertson BH, Rattray J, Campbell MK, et al. The PRaCTICaL study of nurse led, intensive care follow-up programmes for improving long term outcomes from critical illness: a pragmatic randomised controlled trial. BMJ 2009;339: b3723.

64. Schmidt K, Worrack S, Von Korff M, et al. Effect of a primary care management intervention on mental health-related quality of life among survivors of sepsis: a randomized clinical trial. JAMA 2016;315(24):2703–11.

65. Tabah A, Philippart F, Timsit JF, et al. Quality of life in patients aged 80 or over after ICU discharge. Crit Care 2010;14(1):R2.

Chronic Pain Management in the Elderly

Josianna Schwan, MD, Joseph Sclafani, MD, Vivianne L. Tawfik, MD, PhD*

KEYWORDS

- Chronic pain • Polypharmacy • Multidisciplinary treatment • Opioids

KEY POINTS

- Pain management in the elderly should involve a multidisciplinary approach, including multimodal medications, selected interventions, physical therapy, and rehabilitation and psychological treatments.
- There are unique considerations to selecting medications in older adults, including changes in pharmacokinetics, pharmacodynamics, polypharmacy, and likelihood of side effects.
- Physical therapy and psychological approaches should be tailored to the individual and use self-management methods for success.

INTRODUCTION

Chronic pain is one of the most common health conditions among older adults (>65 years) and is associated with significant disability. Chronic pain in the older adult reduces mobility, is associated with depression and anxiety, and can disrupt familial and social relationships.[1] Diagnosis of chronic pain in older adults has significant challenges: patient communication may be difficult due to the presence of a neuromuscular or cognitive disorder, or patients may minimize their symptoms. The treatment of chronic pain in older adults is complex and should involve a multifaceted approach that includes pharmacologic interventions, physical rehabilitation, and interventional procedures to break the pain cycle (**Fig. 1**). It is important for health care providers across all specialties to develop skills to diagnose and manage chronic pain in older patients.

COMMON CAUSES OF CHRONIC PAIN IN OLDER ADULTS

There is a common belief that chronic pain is an unavoidable consequence of getting older.[2,3] Chronic pain does have a high prevalence in the older population, estimated

Disclosure Statement: None.
Department of Anesthesiology, Perioperative & Pain Medicine, Stanford University School of Medicine, 300 Pasteur Drive, Grant Building, Room S007, Stanford, CA 94305, USA
* Corresponding author.
E-mail address: vivianne@stanford.edu

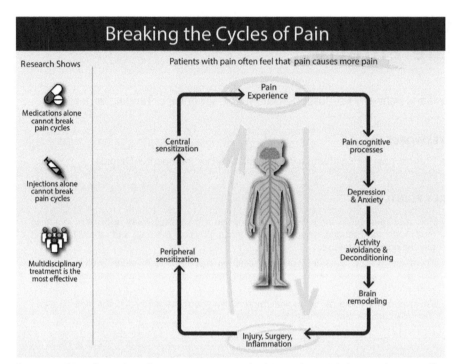

Fig. 1. Breaking the cycles of pain. Pain is a complex biopsychosocial disease that can affect all aspects of life, including mood, sleep, cognition, and function. This is particularly difficult for older adults who may already have comorbid conditions contributing to problems in these areas or who may undergo surgeries that increase their risk of chronic pain. Using a multidisciplinary approach to treat chronic pain is the most likely to be effective and treatment plans should include multimodal medication options, physical therapy, pain psychology, and selected interventions, as appropriate. (*Courtesy of* M.C. Kao, PhD, MD, CIPS, FIPP, Palo Alto, CA.)

to be more than 50%, with 70% of older individuals endorsing pain in multiple sites.[4] The most prevalent painful conditions affecting older adults are arthritis-related, although the incidence of chronic systemic disease that can also result in pain (ie, diabetic complications, cancer-related pain, poststroke pain) is also high among older individuals (**Box 1**).[5]

ASSESSMENT

To treat pain effectively in the older adult, a meaningful assessment of pain is required. In general, a person's self-reported pain level using a pain assessment tool for pain intensity remains the best indicator of pain in older adults[6]; however, there are caveats to using self-reporting in this population. Many older adults will not automatically report pain due to misguided beliefs that pain with aging is expected, fears of diagnostic testing, or concerns regarding the significance of the pain and loss of independence.[7] Furthermore, older adults have an increased number of comorbidities compared with the general population and are more likely to have multiple diagnoses that contribute to pain. As a result, a comprehensive history and physical is recommended, and multiple sources of pain must be considered and addressed. It also should be remembered that older adults have an increased risk of incidental findings

| **Box 1** |
| **Common causes of chronic pain in elderly patients** |
| Cancer-related pain |
| Central poststroke pain |
| Chronic postsurgical pain |
| Diabetic peripheral neuropathy |
| Fibromyalgia |
| Myofascial pain |
| Osteoarthritis |
| Peripheral vascular disease (ischemic pain) |
| Postherpetic neuralgia (shingles) |
| Spinal canal stenosis |
| Trauma-related pain (eg, hip fracture) |

with additional testing and diagnostic imaging, and ancillary tests should be obtained only based on clinical examination findings.[8]

In addition, the assessment of pain in cognitively impaired individuals presents a unique challenge. Studies have estimated that the prevalence of persistent pain in older adults ranges from 24% to 50%, and seniors with and without cognitive impairment had a similar prevalence of conditions that were likely to result in pain.[9] Patients with increasing amounts of cognitive impairment are less likely to self-report pain despite an equal prevalence of painful conditions. As a result, pain issues are often underaddressed among these individuals. Observation of behavior may help determine the incidence of pain in cognitively impaired older adults who are unable to adequately verbalize their symptoms. Pain may be demonstrated in a variety of ways, including changes in functional status, interactions with others, facial expressions, verbalizations, and body movements. Caregivers also may be able to provide additional information that is relevant to the pain assessment.

Tracking functional status as an outcome measure in addition to pain level is important in the treatment of pain in older individuals. This includes mood, mobility, activities of daily living, sleep, appetite, cognitive impairment, and weight changes. Improved management of pain is expected to improve one or more elements of functional status, and untreated pain may result in worsening functional status.[10]

PERIOPERATIVE MANAGEMENT

The older population has unique risks associated with their perioperative management, comprehensively addressed in other sections of this issue.

CHRONIC PAIN MANAGEMENT
General Considerations

Chronic pain management in the older adult can be accomplished through a multidisciplinary approach that includes pharmacologic treatments, physical and psychological rehabilitation, and interventional approaches (see **Fig. 1**). With respect to the selection of pharmacologic agents, multimodal treatment using medications with varying mechanisms of action (**Fig. 2**) may allow for synergistic effects but may also

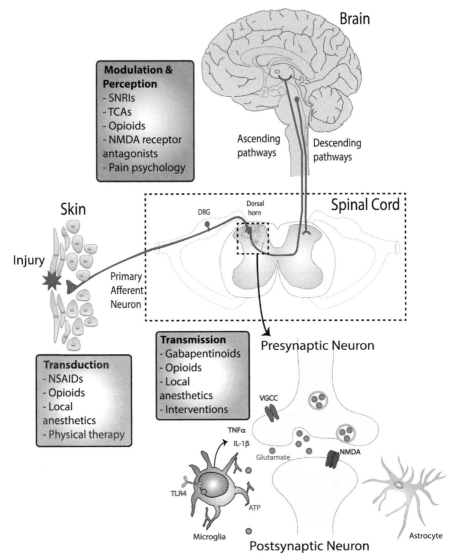

Fig. 2. Sites of action of multidisciplinary treatments for pain management. In most cases, pain is initiated in the periphery where primary afferent neuron terminals may be activated by local inflammatory mediators. Transduction of this signal from the peripheral to the central nervous system can be blocked by certain categories of drugs (NSAIDs, opioids, local anesthetics) and by increasing strength and mobility through physical therapy. Painful signals are then transmitted to the dorsal horn of the spinal cord where the central terminals of the primary afferent neurons form synapses with intrinsic spinal cord neurons. Gabapentinoids, opioids, local anesthetics, and certain interventions can block this peripheral-to-central transmission. Finally, the painful signal is carried to the brain through ascending pathways for perception to occur and descending pathways can also be activated to modulate inputs in the spinal cord. Many medications can act on these systems including SNRIs, TCAs, NMDA receptor antagonists, and opioids. Importantly, psychological interventions can engage descending inhibitory pathways to suppress painful signal transmission. Using multidisciplinary approaches that target different areas of the peripheral and central nervous system may limit side effects and improve efficacy of treatments. DRG, dorsal root ganglion; IL, interleukin; TLR4, Toll-like receptor 4; TNF, tumor necrosis factor; VGCC, voltage-gated calcium channel.

contribute further to polypharmacy and therefore must be undertaken with caution. Prescribers also must account for the narrower therapeutic index of most medications in older adults compared with younger individuals, and advancing age increases the risk of adverse drug reactions.[11] There are both pharmacokinetic and pharmacodynamic considerations for older adults that must be taken into account when prescribing medications for pain. Pharmacokinetic changes include decreased absorption, variability in volume of distribution depending on lipophilicity of the drug, and heightened therapeutic response to protein-bound drugs due to hypo-albuminemia, decreased hepatic metabolism, and decreased renal elimination.[6,12] In terms of pharmacodynamics, changes in the peripheral and central nervous system including pre-existing cognitive deficits, decreased myelination of nerves, and decreased receptor density may all predispose older adults to increased side effects from commonly prescribed medications.[13]

Pharmacologic Agents

Nonsteroidal anti-inflammatory drugs
Mechanism of action and place in therapy Nonsteroidal anti-inflammatory drugs (NSAIDs) are antipyretic and anti-inflammatory medications that function by inhibiting the synthesis of prostaglandins. This inhibition is achieved by blocking the metabolism of arachidonic acid via the cyclo-oxygenase (COX) pathway.[14] Older NSAIDs (aspirin, ibuprofen, naproxen) are nonselective inhibitors of both COX-1 and COX-2. Newer NSAIDs (rofecoxib, celecoxib, and valdecoxib) selectively inhibit COX-2 and have fewer adverse effects. These agents have analgesic, anti-inflammatory, and antipyretic effects, but do not have antiplatelet activity, do not affect bleeding time, and are not as toxic to the gastrointestinal (GI) system. NSAIDs are effective in the treatment of mild-to-moderate chronic pain, particularly in conditions with an inflammatory component. However, side effects must be considered before they are prescribed to an older adult.

Adverse effects and precautions NSAIDs can cause a range of GI toxicities, including nausea, diarrhea, and mucosal damage (GI erosions, ulcers, perforations, bleeding) that are responsible for significant morbidity and mortality in the United States. Thirty percent of patients will complain of dyspepsia on NSAID therapy, and 15% to 30% of NSAID users show evidence of a gastric or duodenal ulcer.[15] Cytoprotective therapy can be initiated with the NSAID (an H2 antagonist or proton pump inhibitor, PPI) to prevent these symptoms, or the use of a COX-2–specific NSAID can reduce the incidence of these side effects. PPIs have been found to be the most effective cytoprotective therapy.[16]

NSAIDs are also associated with renal toxicity, which occurs in 5% of patients taking these agents.[17] Older adults may be at greater risk of renal toxicity than younger patients. Both nonselective and selective COX-2 inhibitors have been shown to cause renal dysfunction,[18] and it is recommended to avoid NSAIDs in patients with a creatinine clearance of less than 30 mL/min.[19]

NSAIDs are also associated with cardiovascular risks. Studies have shown that both selective and nonselective NSAIDs increase the risk of heart failure and exacerbate heart failure symptoms.[20] There is also evidence that COX-2 selective NSAIDs may have prothrombotic activity in patients at risk for major vascular events.[21] There is further evidence that the concomitant administration of either class of NSAID may negate the cardioprotective effects of low-dose aspirin.[22,23] Therefore, the cardiac comorbidities of an older patient must be carefully considered before NSAIDs are initiated.

Antidepressants

Mechanism of action and place in therapy Antidepressants indicated in the use of chronic pain include tricyclic antidepressants (TCAs), and serotonin and norepinephrine reuptake inhibitors (SNRIs) that provide pain relief separate from their antidepressant effects.[24] The mechanism of action of both classes of medications is through inhibiting reuptake of serotonin and norepinephrine resulting in increased amounts of the neurotransmitters in the synaptic cleft. Selective serotonin reuptake inhibitors (SSRIs) have shown limited efficacy in the treatment of pain,[25] suggesting that the synaptic increases in norepinephrine are required for analgesic compared with antidepressant effects. Specifically, the number needed to treat for TCAs is reported as 2 to 3 depending on the pain condition whereas it is >6 for SSRIs. Importantly, however, many patients present to clinic already taking SSRIs. In such cases, discussion with the patient and the patient's prescriber about a potential switch to a TCA or SNRI may be warranted to obtain both analgesic and antidepressant effects with a single agent, thus simplifying medication regimens in a population at high risk of polypharmacy.[26] In addition, it is important to be aware of all serotonergic medications a patient is taking to avoid combination effects leading to serotonin syndrome.[13,27]

Adverse effects and precautions TCAs, SSRIs, and SNRIs have all been known to have increased side effects in older adults. TCAs are highly anticholinergic, and can lead to cognitive dysfunction, sedation, and orthostatic hypotension. All TCAs are included on the Beers list of potentially inappropriate medications in older adults, with the exception of low-dose doxepin.[28] SSRIs and SNRIs have fewer cardiovascular and anticholinergic adverse effects than TCAs, but may be associated with a higher fall risk in older adults.[29]

Anticonvulsants

Mechanism of action and place in therapy Multiple classes of anticonvulsants are commonly used for chronic pain. Older anticonvulsants (carbamazepine, phenytoin, and valproic acid) are sodium channel blockers that suppress nerve hyperexcitability by increasing membrane stability.[14] These are indicated in neuropathic pain, including trigeminal neuralgia in which carbamazepine and oxcarbazepine remain first-line drugs,[30] in spite of only third-tier evidence of efficacy from data involving small numbers of participants with risk of bias according to a recent Cochrane review.[31] Gabapentinoids are alpha-2-delta calcium channel blockers, and also work by modulating primary afferent excitability.[32] Gabapentinoids have become increasingly popular in treating neuropathic pain because they are efficacious with fewer adverse side effects than older anticonvulsants.[33]

Adverse effects and precautions Older anticonvulsants such as carbamazepine should be avoided in older adults because they increase the risk of hyponatremia and SIADH.[19] In cases where it is the first line therapy indicated (ie, for trigeminal neuralgia) the lowest effective dose should be used to decrease the incidence of side effects.

When gabapentinoids are initiated in older adults, they should be started at a low dose (we suggest 100 mg at bedtime with uptitration by 100 mg every 3–4 days as tolerated to standard 3-times-a-day dosing) and monitored carefully for side effects. The most common side effects of gabapentinoids are dizziness, somnolence, fatigue, and weight changes.[34] It should be noted, however, that prescription rates of gabapentinoids have increased threefold between 2002 and 2015 with a particularly skewed increase in use by adults older than 64 and those with multiple comorbidities.[35] This is of particular concern, as new data from the Food and Drug

Administration Adverse Event Reporting System indicates that these medications may have additive effects on respiratory depression when used with other central nervous system depressant drugs, including opioids.[36]

Other analgesics

Cannabinoids Cannabinoids have been found to be effective in a few clinical trials regarding treatment of chronic pain.[37–39] They should be used with caution in older patients, because these patients are at higher risk for a dysphoric response to treatment.[40]

Muscle relaxants Muscle relaxants should be used with caution in adults 65 and older. They are often used in the treatment of acute low back pain, but are associated with side effects such as sedation, dizziness, anticholinergic effects, and weakness.[41]

Low-dose naltrexone Low-dose naltrexone (LDN) has been demonstrated to be effective in chronic pain conditions such as fibromyalgia and complex regional pain syndrome.[42] LDN is thought to be a potent anti-inflammatory agent through antagonism of Toll-like receptor 4 found on myeloid-lineage cells such as microglia (central nervous system immune cells).[43] Although no formal studies have been done on LDN use in the elderly, side effects of LDN are generally very mild, with the most common side effect observed being vivid dreams.[43]

Memantine Memantine is an N-methyl-D-aspartate (NMDA) antagonist that has been found to be effective in treating neuropathic pain,[44] although limited studies evaluated in a recent Cochrane review showed no effect of memantine specifically in phantom limb pain.[45] In general, patients tolerate it well, but it should be used with caution in older patients, as it can cause dizziness.[46]

Opioids

In older adults who are carefully selected and monitored, opioids may help provide effective pain relief as part of a multimodal pain management plan.[47] The effects of opioid medications are mediated through opioid receptors, located in periaqueductal gray as well as throughout the spinal cord, joint synovium, and intestinal mucosa.[14] The analgesic effect is primarily attributed to the μ and κ receptors. It is important to note that there are pharmacokinetic changes relevant to opioid dosing in older adults, with significant variability among patients. This is in part due to an increased fat-to–lean body mass ratio, as well as reduced clearance of renal metabolites.[48] Studies have shown older patients have greater pain relief from opioids for a longer duration compared with younger adults receiving the same dose.[49,50] Central side effects of opioids, including drowsiness and dizziness, may be associated with increased incidence of falls and fractures, so it is recommended that dose titration is done slowly and with caution in older adults.[51]

Tramadol Tramadol is considered a weak opioid agonist as well as a monoamine uptake inhibitor.[27] It reduces the seizure threshold, and should be used cautiously in patients with a history of seizures or those taking other serotonergic drugs.[52] There are few studies on the use of tramadol in older adults, although one study surprisingly showed that its pharmacokinetics are only minimally affected by age, as long as renal and hepatic function are well-maintained.[53]

Oxycodone oral solution In frail older adults, in whom the effects of accidental opioid overdose could be catastrophic, the authors of this article have had success titrating oral oxycodone solution. This formulation is easier for patients with swallowing difficulties and is more amenable to titration when small doses of opioids are preferred (ie, starting dose of <2.5 mg).

Transdermal buprenorphine A longitudinal study of nursing home residents found that the use of long-acting opioids improved functional status and social engagement compared with short-acting opioids.[54] Recently, transdermal buprenorphine has been advocated for use in older adults.[55] Buprenorphine is a partial μ agonist and a κ and δ opioid antagonist.[56] Transdermal buprenorphine is associated with a slow onset and long duration of action (onset of 12–24 hours, duration of action of 3 days).[57] It has a better side-effect profile than most other opioids: there is a ceiling to the side effect of respiratory depression, as well as less profound effect on decreasing gastrointestinal transit times than other opioids.[58] It is also safe for use in renal impairment, which is a major advantage in the elderly.[59]

Opioid addiction in the elderly It is estimated that 6% to 9% of community-dwelling older adults use opioids, and up to 70% of nursing home residents with chronic non-cancer pain receive regularly scheduled opioids.[60–62] Although rates of abuse and misuse are lower than in the younger population, it is estimated that 1% to 3% of older adults use opioids inappropriately.[63] The potential for opioid abuse should be recognized in the older adult population, and screening for abuse and misuse should be done regularly in all older adults who are prescribed opioid medication.

Interventional Therapies

Interventional techniques in pain management offer older adults treatments with fewer systemic side effects than pharmacologic interventions.[64] The most common interventional therapies include epidural steroid injections, lumbar facet injections, percutaneous vertebral augmentation, sacroiliac joint injections, and hip and knee joint injections. In general, these procedures are low risk with few side effects. These procedures can be included as part of a multidisciplinary strategy for chronic pain therapy, and can help reduce pharmacologic interventions (with potentially more systemic side effects) as well as the need for larger surgeries that carry higher risk and have a longer recovery time.[64] It should be noted that many of these procedures are typically performed at an outpatient surgery center, which may not be appropriate for many older adults. The anticoagulation status and comorbidities of each patient must be taken into consideration before performing any interventional therapy, and the procedure should be moved to a hospital setting with appropriate monitoring if the patient is determined to be high risk.[65]

Role of Rehabilitation/Physical Therapy in Managing Pain in Older Adults

The impact of natural senescence on multiple physiologic systems should be considered during the evaluation of older individuals with longstanding chronic pain states. Among the most prominent changes in normal aging is the loss of muscular mass and force generation through the process of sarcopenia.[66] As a result, fast-twitch (2a) fibers disproportionately atrophy secondary to decreased myosin heavy-chain protein synthesis, which results in a 3.5% decrease in muscle power per year after the age of 60.[67,68] Multiple other changes to the musculoskeletal system have been described with aging, including functional decline of the mitochondria (decreased endurance), increased coactivation of agonist-antagonist muscle groups (decreased peak force), decreased motor neuron excitability within the spinal cord, and decreased transmission across the neuromuscular junction.[69] All of these functional declines lead to instability and require compensatory gait adjustments, such as stance-widening, increased double support time, and variability in stride-to-stride distance. Other important physiologic changes to consider with patients of advanced age include decreased joint range of motion from degenerative joint disease, osseous fragility from osteoarthritis, decreased cardiopulmonary compliance, and decreased sensory acuity. Thus, a complete physical evaluation is reasonable to request before initiation of a physical therapy program to rule out contraindications in this population.

The overall therapeutic goal of treatment is an important consideration when caring for patients of advanced age. The primary objective of rehabilitation is to improve impairment (loss of physiologic or anatomic structure or function), which is typically accomplished through modalities that address the underlying pathophysiologic etiology (eg, core strengthening and stabilization exercises for degenerative lumbar spondylosis). However, when improving impairment is unlikely, rehabilitation should focus instead on improving patient disability (restriction in an ability to perform an activity resulting from impairment). Occupational therapists are particularly skilled in recommending adaptations and environmental modifications to decrease patient disability and should be readily consulted to assist in teaching the patient independent living skills when impairments are unlikely to improve.

When impairment is amenable to improvement, multiple modalities of therapy have been shown to improve musculoskeletal function and improve outcomes. Physical therapy programs focused on strength training are particularly effective in improving overall mobility, balance, and physical function in the elderly population.[70–73] For example, resistance-based strengthening therapies have significantly improved patient-reported pain outcomes in older individuals with a primary diagnosis of hip or knee osteoarthritis.[74–76] Similar functional improvement has been reported across a diverse spectrum of active therapeutic modalities in the elderly population. Regimens focused on high-intensity strengthening (8 repetitions at 80% of single repetition maximum) and low-intensity strengthening (13 repetitions at 50% of single repetition maximum) demonstrated similar improvement in endurance and function in one study of individuals 60 years or older.[77] In addition, low-impact modalities such as Tai Chi and aqua-aerobic regimens may modestly improve balance and musculoskeletal function when performed on a regular, consistent basis.[69]

Direct supervision with encouragement to properly increase exercise intensity is a key determinant of program adherence for older individuals, regardless of what type of regimen is recommended. Multiple studies have demonstrated that without supervision, elderly individuals are reluctant to progress their routine and may even exhibit increased confusion or anger.[78,79] Encouraging older patients to attend sessions at an exercise facility or community facility with a qualified and attentive instructor may decrease these unwanted outcomes and simultaneously have a positive effect on mood through the development of positive social interactions.[69]

PSYCHOLOGICAL INTERVENTIONS

Chronic pain is best explained by a biopsychosocial model and its treatment must include interventions aimed at comorbid depression, anxiety, and poor coping skills (see **Fig. 1**). It has been shown, for example, that patients with high levels of catastrophizing, defined as feelings of hopelessness and helplessness with respect to their pain, report higher pain intensity, decreased level of function, and depression.[80] Catastrophizing was also identified as a predictor of persistent pain after total knee replacement.[81] Importantly, participation in just a 1-day perioperative acceptance and commitment therapy workshop results in greater pain reduction at 3 months after orthopedic surgery, and opioid cessation 9 days earlier, compared with patients receiving standard of care.[82] Such studies highlight the importance of psychological management, which carries little risk but high potential for benefit, as part of a multidisciplinary approach to pain management.

COORDINATION OF MULTIDISCIPLINARY CARE AND CONCLUDING REMARKS

The complex medical conditions of older adults puts them at high risk for polypharmacy and medication mismanagement.[83] It is important for primary care physicians, geriatricians, and pain specialists to work together to form a patient-specific health plan that maximizes quality of life while minimizing risks of adverse events and side effects. Because older adults are often not managing their own medications, physicians must also coordinate with patients' caretakers or long-term care facility. Overall, effective pain relief can be obtained for older adults but must involve a multidisciplinary approach that includes physical rehabilitation, occupational therapy, and management of comorbid depression and anxiety through psychological interventions. Finally, self-management strategies that target clearly defined goals for improved function will allow patients to feel engaged in their care and have been shown to improve pain-related disability.[84]

ACKNOWLEDGMENTS

Dr V.L. Tawfik would like to acknowledge funding from the Department of Anesthesiology, Perioperative, and Pain Medicine at Stanford University School of Medicine and the National Institutes of Health Grant K08NS094547.

REFERENCES

1. Gloth FM. Handbook of pain relief in older adults: an evidence-based approach. Totowa (NJ): Humana Press; 2004.

2. Thielke S, Sale J, Reid MC. Aging: are these 4 pain myths complicating care? J Fam Pract 2012;61(11):666–70.

3. Gignac MAM, Davis AM, Hawker G, et al. "What do you expect? You're just getting older": a comparison of perceived osteoarthritis-related and aging-related health experiences in middle- and older-age adults. Arthritis Rheum 2006; 55(6):905–12.

4. Patel KV, Guralnik JM, Dansie EJ, et al. Prevalence and impact of pain among older adults in the United States: findings from the 2011 National Health and Aging Trends Study. Pain 2013;154(12):2649–57.

5. St Sauver JL, Warner DO, Yawn BP, et al. Why patients visit their doctors: assessing the most prevalent conditions in a defined American population. Mayo Clin Proc 2013;88(1):56–67.

6. Bicket MC, Mao J. Chronic pain in older adults. Anesthesiol Clin 2015;33(3): 577–90.

7. Herr KA, Garand L. Assessment and measurement of pain in older adults. Clin Geriatr Med 2001;17(3):457–78, vi.

8. Jensen MC, Brant-Zawadzki MN, Obuchowski N, et al. Magnetic resonance imaging of the lumbar spine in people without back pain. N Engl J Med 1994; 331(2):69–73.

9. Proctor WR, Hirdes JP. Pain and cognitive status among nursing home residents in Canada. Pain Res Manag 2001;6(3):119–25.

10. Hadjistavropoulos T, Herr K, Turk DC, et al. An interdisciplinary expert consensus statement on assessment of pain in older persons. Clin J Pain 2007;23(1 Suppl): S1–43.

11. Beyth RJ, Shorr RI. Epidemiology of adverse drug reactions in the elderly by drug class. Drugs Aging 1999;14(3):231–9.

12. Gagliese L, Melzack R. Chronic pain in elderly people. Pain 1997;70(1):3–14.

13. Spina E, Scordo MG. Clinically significant drug interactions with antidepressants in the elderly. Drugs Aging 2002;19(4):299–320.

14. Goodman LS, Gilman A. Goodman & Gilman's the pharmacological basis of therapeutics. 13th edition. New York: McGraw Hill Medical; 2018.

15. Hawkey CJ. Nonsteroidal anti-inflammatory drug gastropathy. Gastroenterology 2000;119(2):521–35.

16. Yeomans ND, Tulassay Z, Juhász L, et al. A comparison of omeprazole with ranitidine for ulcers associated with nonsteroidal antiinflammatory drugs. Acid suppression trial: ranitidine versus omeprazole for NSAID-associated ulcer treatment (ASTRONAUT) study group. N Engl J Med 1998;338(11):719–26.

17. Shimp LA. Safety issues in the pharmacologic management of chronic pain in the elderly. Pharmacotherapy 1998;18(6):1313–22.

18. Morales E, Mucksavage JJ. Cyclooxygenase-2 inhibitor-associated acute renal failure: case report with rofecoxib and review of the literature. Pharmacotherapy 2002;22(10):1317–21.

19. Gloth FM. Pharmacological management of persistent pain in older persons: focus on opioids and nonopioids. J Pain 2011;12(3 Suppl 1):S14–20.

20. Schmidt M, Lamberts M, Olsen A-MS, et al. Cardiovascular safety of non-aspirin non-steroidal anti-inflammatory drugs: review and position paper by the working group for Cardiovascular Pharmacotherapy of the European Society of Cardiology. Eur Heart J 2016;37(13):1015–23.

21. Coxib and traditional NSAID Trialists' (CNT) Collaboration, Bhala N, Emberson J, Merhi A, et al. Vascular and upper gastrointestinal effects of non-steroidal anti-inflammatory drugs: meta-analyses of individual participant data from randomised trials. Lancet 2013;382(9894):769–79.

22. Etminan M, Samii A. Effect of ibuprofen on cardioprotective effect of aspirin. Lancet 2003;361(9368):1558–9 [author reply: 1559].

23. Burnakis TG. Cyclooxygenase inhibitors and the antiplatelet effects of aspirin. N Engl J Med 2002;346(20):1589–90 [author reply: 1589–90].

24. Saarto T, Wiffen PJ. Antidepressants for neuropathic pain: a Cochrane review. J Neurol Neurosurg Psychiatry 2010;81(12):1372–3.

25. Sindrup SH, Jensen TS. Efficacy of pharmacological treatments of neuropathic pain: an update and effect related to mechanism of drug action. Pain 1999; 83(3):389–400.

26. Mannucci PM, Nobili A, Pasina L, REPOSI Collaborators. Polypharmacy in older people: lessons from 10 years of experience with the REPOSI register. Intern Emerg Med 2018;13(8):1191–200.

27. Beakley BD, Kaye AM, Kaye AD. Tramadol, pharmacology, side effects, and serotonin syndrome: a review. Pain Physician 2015;18(4):395–400.

28. American Geriatrics Society 2015 Beers Criteria Update Expert Panel. American Geriatrics Society 2015 updated Beers criteria for potentially inappropriate medication use in older adults. J Am Ger Soc 2015;2015:1532–5415.

29. Coupland CA, Dhiman P, Barton G, et al. A study of the safety and harms of antidepressant drugs for older people: a cohort study using a large primary care database. Health Technol Assess 2011;15(28):1–202, iii–iv.

30. Di Stefano G, Truini A, Cruccu G. Current and innovative pharmacological options to treat typical and atypical trigeminal neuralgia. Drugs 2018;78(14):1433–42.
31. Wiffen PJ, Derry S, Moore RA, et al. Carbamazepine for chronic neuropathic pain and fibromyalgia in adults. Cochrane Database Syst Rev 2014;(4):CD005451.
32. Tremont-Lukats IW, Megeff C, Backonja MM. Anticonvulsants for neuropathic pain syndromes: mechanisms of action and place in therapy. Drugs 2000; 60(5):1029–52.
33. Ross EL. The evolving role of antiepileptic drugs in treating neuropathic pain. Neurology 2000;55(5 Suppl 1):S41–6 [discussion: S54–8].
34. Straube S, Derry S, Moore RA, et al. Pregabalin in fibromyalgia: meta-analysis of efficacy and safety from company clinical trial reports. Rheumatology (Oxford) 2010;49(4):706–15.
35. Johansen ME. Gabapentinoid use in the United States 2002 through 2015. JAMA Intern Med 2018;178(2):292–4.
36. Throckmorton DC, Gottlieb S, Woodcock J. The FDA and the next wave of drug abuse—proactive pharmacovigilance. N Engl J Med 2018;379(3):205–7.
37. Wilsey B, Marcotte T, Tsodikov A, et al. A randomized, placebo-controlled, cross-over trial of cannabis cigarettes in neuropathic pain. J Pain 2008;9(6):506–21.
38. Karst M, Salim K, Burstein S, et al. Analgesic effect of the synthetic cannabinoid CT-3 on chronic neuropathic pain: a randomized controlled trial. JAMA 2003; 290(13):1757–62.
39. Iskedjian M, Bereza B, Gordon A, et al. Meta-analysis of cannabis based treatments for neuropathic and multiple sclerosis-related pain. Curr Med Res Opin 2007;23(1):17–24.
40. American Geriatrics Society Panel on the Pharmacological Management of Persistent Pain in Older Persons. Pharmacological management of persistent pain in older persons. Pain Med 2009;10(6):1062–83.
41. Billups SJ, Delate T, Hoover B. Injury in an elderly population before and after initiating a skeletal muscle relaxant. Ann Pharmacother 2011;45(4):485–91.
42. Younger J, Noor N, McCue R, et al. Low-dose naltrexone for the treatment of fibromyalgia: findings of a small, randomized, double-blind, placebo-controlled, counterbalanced, crossover trial assessing daily pain levels. Arthritis Rheum 2013;65(2):529–38.
43. Younger J, Parkitny L, McLain D. The use of low-dose naltrexone (LDN) as a novel anti-inflammatory treatment for chronic pain. Clin Rheumatol 2014;33(4):451–9.
44. Pickering G, Morel V. Memantine for the treatment of general neuropathic pain: a narrative review. Fundam Clin Pharmacol 2018;32(1):4–13.
45. Alviar MJM, Hale T, Dungca M. Pharmacologic interventions for treating phantom limb pain. Cochrane Database Syst Rev 2016;(10):CD006380.
46. Olivan-Blázquez B, Herrera-Mercadal P, Puebla-Guedea M, et al. Efficacy of memantine in the treatment of fibromyalgia: a double-blind, randomised, controlled trial with 6-month follow-up. Pain 2014;155(12):2517–25.
47. Opioids for persistent pain: summary of guidance on good practice from the British Pain Society. Br J Pain 2012;6(1):9–10.
48. Cherny NI. Opioid analgesics: comparative features and prescribing guidelines. Drugs 1996;51(5):713–37.
49. Bellville JW, Forrest WH, Miller E, et al. Influence of age on pain relief from analgesics. A study of postoperative patients. JAMA 1971;217(13):1835–41.
50. Kaiko RF, Wallenstein SL, Rogers AG, et al. Narcotics in the elderly. Med Clin North Am 1982;66(5):1079–89.

51. Vestergaard P, Rejnmark L, Mosekilde L. Fracture risk associated with the use of morphine and opiates. J Intern Med 2006;260(1):76–87.
52. Barber JB, Gibson SJ. Treatment of chronic non-malignant pain in the elderly: safety considerations. Drug Saf 2009;32(6):457–74.
53. Likar R, Wittels M, Molnar M, et al. Pharmacokinetic and pharmacodynamic properties of tramadol IR and SR in elderly patients: a prospective, age-group-controlled study. Clin Ther 2006;28(12):2022–39.
54. Won A, Lapane KL, Vallow S, et al. Long-term effects of analgesics in a population of elderly nursing home residents with persistent nonmalignant pain. J Gerontol A Biol Sci Med Sci 2006;61(2):165–9.
55. Vadivelu N, Hines RL. Management of chronic pain in the elderly: focus on transdermal buprenorphine. Clin Interv Aging 2008;3(3):421–30.
56. Negus SS, Mello NK, Linsenmayer DC, et al. Kappa opioid antagonist effects of the novel kappa antagonist 5'-guanidinonaltrindole (GNTI) in an assay of schedule-controlled behavior in rhesus monkeys. Psychopharmacology 2002; 163(3–4):412–9.
57. Sorge J, Sittl R. Transdermal buprenorphine in the treatment of chronic pain: results of a phase III, multicenter, randomized, double-blind, placebo-controlled study. Clin Ther 2004;26(11):1808–20.
58. Griessinger N, Sittl R, Likar R. Transdermal buprenorphine in clinical practice—a post-marketing surveillance study in 13,179 patients. Curr Med Res Opin 2005; 21(8):1147–56.
59. Filitz J, Griessinger N, Sittl R, et al. Effects of intermittent hemodialysis on buprenorphine and norbuprenorphine plasma concentrations in chronic pain patients treated with transdermal buprenorphine. Eur J Pain 2006;10(8):743–8.
60. Campbell CI, Weisner C, Leresche L, et al. Age and gender trends in long-term opioid analgesic use for noncancer pain. Am J Public Health 2010;100(12): 2541–7.
61. Marcum ZA, Perera S, Donohue JM, et al. Analgesic use for knee and hip osteoarthritis in community-dwelling elders. Pain Med 2011;12(11):1628–36.
62. Lapane KL, Quilliam BJ, Chow W, et al. Pharmacologic management of noncancer pain among nursing home residents. J Pain Symptom Manage 2013; 45(1):33–42.
63. Papaleontiou M, Henderson CR, Turner BJ, et al. Outcomes associated with opioid use in the treatment of chronic noncancer pain in older adults: a systematic review and meta-analysis. J Am Geriatr Soc 2010;58(7):1353–69.
64. Brooks AK, Udoji MA. Interventional techniques for management of pain in older adults. Clin Geriatr Med 2016;32(4):773–85.
65. Mathis MR, Naughton NN, Shanks AM, et al. Patient selection for day case-eligible surgery: identifying those at high risk for major complications. Anesthesiology 2013;119(6):1310–21.
66. Janssen I, Heymsfield SB, Ross R. Low relative skeletal muscle mass (sarcopenia) in older persons is associated with functional impairment and physical disability. J Am Geriatr Soc 2002;50(5):889–96.
67. Barry BK, Carson RG. The consequences of resistance training for movement control in older adults. J Gerontol A Biol Sci Med Sci 2004;59(7):730–54.
68. Morley JE, Baumgartner RN, Roubenoff R, et al. Sarcopenia. J Lab Clin Med 2001;137(4):231–43.
69. Braddom's physical medicine & rehabilitation. 5th edition. Philadelphia: Elsevier; 2016.

70. de Vries NM, van Ravensberg CD, Hobbelen JSM, et al. Effects of physical exercise therapy on mobility, physical functioning, physical activity and quality of life in community-dwelling older adults with impaired mobility, physical disability and/or multi-morbidity: a meta-analysis. Ageing Res Rev 2012;11(1):136–49.
71. Gill TM, Baker DI, Gottschalk M, et al. A program to prevent functional decline in physically frail, elderly persons who live at home. N Engl J Med 2002;347(14): 1068–74.
72. Fiatarone MA, Marks EC, Ryan ND, et al. High-intensity strength training in nonagenarians. Effects on skeletal muscle. JAMA 1990;263(22):3029–34.
73. Frontera WR, Hughes VA, Krivickas LS, et al. Strength training in older women: early and late changes in whole muscle and single cells. Muscle Nerve 2003; 28(5):601–8.
74. Ettinger WH, Burns R, Messier SP, et al. A randomized trial comparing aerobic exercise and resistance exercise with a health education program in older adults with knee osteoarthritis. The Fitness Arthritis and Seniors Trial (FAST). JAMA 1997;277(1):25–31.
75. Kovar PA, Allegrante JP, MacKenzie CR, et al. Supervised fitness walking in patients with osteoarthritis of the knee. A randomized, controlled trial. Ann Intern Med 1992;116(7):529–34.
76. van Baar ME, Dekker J, Oostendorp RA, et al. The effectiveness of exercise therapy in patients with osteoarthritis of the hip or knee: a randomized clinical trial. J Rheumatol 1998;25(12):2432–9.
77. Vincent KR, Braith RW, Feldman RA, et al. Resistance exercise and physical performance in adults aged 60 to 83. J Am Geriatr Soc 2002;50(6):1100–7.
78. Jette AM, Rooks D, Lachman M, et al. Home-based resistance training: predictors of participation and adherence. Gerontologist 1998;38(4):412–21.
79. Nelson ME, Layne JE, Bernstein MJ, et al. The effects of multidimensional home-based exercise on functional performance in elderly people. J Gerontol A Biol Sci Med Sci 2004;59(2):154–60.
80. Keefe FJ, Brown GK, Wallston KA, et al. Coping with rheumatoid arthritis pain: catastrophizing as a maladaptive strategy. Pain 1989;37(1):51–6.
81. Burns LC, Ritvo SE, Ferguson MK, et al. Pain catastrophizing as a risk factor for chronic pain after total knee arthroplasty: a systematic review. J Pain Res 2015;8: 21–32.
82. Dindo L, Zimmerman MB, Hadlandsmyth K, et al. Acceptance and commitment therapy for prevention of chronic postsurgical pain and opioid use in at-risk veterans: a Pilot Randomized Controlled Study. J Pain 2018;19(10):1211–21.
83. Maher RL, Hanlon J, Hajjar ER. Clinical consequences of polypharmacy in elderly. Expert Opin Drug Saf 2014;13(1):57–65.
84. Nicholas MK, Asghari A, Blyth FM, et al. Long-term outcomes from training in self-management of chronic pain in an elderly population: a randomized controlled trial. Pain 2017;158(1):86–95.

The Ethics of Surgery at End of Life

Michael C. Lewis, MD[a], Nicholas S. Yeldo, MD[b],*

KEYWORDS

- Ethics • End-of-life • Anesthesiology • Geriatrics • Autonomy • DNR

KEY POINTS

- In making decisions, anesthesiologists must respect and incorporate basic medical ethical principles. Professional groups in anesthesiology have encouraged anesthesiologists to become leaders in the medical decision-making process as perspectives and laws on ethics continue to evolve.
- There is a societal mandate that attention be paid to a patient's values and wishes. Informed consent allows patients to gain clear understanding of their conditions and all available treatment options. To facilitate this process an understanding of the principles and process of decision-making capacity is essential.
- Anesthesiologists often face ethical challenges concerning care issues at the end of life.
- A previously common practice of suspending DNR orders is no longer mandatory and should be addressed in a patient-centered, goal-directed approach.
- Futility and inadvisable care are defined differently and have different implications on clinical practice.

INTRODUCTION

Anesthesiology practice in the twenty-first century demands a great deal more of physicians than just perioperative supervision, pain medicine, and intensive care management. Anesthesiologists, like all physicians, are frequently faced with ethically challenging clinical situations in which we are obligated and empowered to appropriately influence medical decision-making.

During our medical training we are socialized to "do everything we can," to "save" our patients, and to "fight our hardest" for those under our care. However, this approach is currently being questioned with increasing frequency. In juxtaposition,

Disclosure Statement: No disclosures.
[a] Department of Anesthesiology, Pain Management & Perioperative Medicine, Henry Ford Health System, 2799 West Grand Boulevard, CFP 343, Detroit, MI 48202, USA; [b] Educational Programs, Anesthesiology Residency, Henry Ford Health System, 2799 West Grand Boulevard, CFP 343, Detroit, MI 48202, USA
* Corresponding author.
E-mail address: NYeldo1@HFHS.ORG

many now push back with the question: "when do these efforts go too far?" With our present technical and clinical capabilities, it is progressively becoming clearer that the rigid application of the "do all to save all" principle does not always benefit those we serve.

From *Quinlan* in 1976, to *Cruzan* in 1990, to *Schiavo* in 2005 there have been vast philosophic and, subsequently, legal debates around end-of-life decisions and practices. The previously mentioned cases, and more, have focused attention on the core ethical value of self-determination, which underlies the tenet of autonomy. As such, we have been forced to more closely scrutinize our medical decision-making processes to include clarity of, and respect for, the overall wishes of the patient, which it is hoped have been previously stated or implied. This approach evokes a myriad of ethical, legal, and personal considerations that can create complex challenges for the care team, patients, and their families.[1–5] Regardless of the perceived progress made to date, physicians continue to struggle with how to reconcile the rift between ethical theory and the clinical care of patients who are near the end-of-life.

Unfortunately, well into the twenty-first century, aggressive interventions remain the default treatment in American medicine with attention to palliation still falling far short.[6] Physicians still generally lack proper education on ethical and legal principles regarding end-of-life care and, as such, are often unable to incorporate these principles into practice.[7,8]

THE ROLE OF THE ANESTHESIOLOGIST

Practitioners may often be faced with difficult situations when they are consulted to provide anesthesia for technical interventions or surgical procedures on patients for whom there is questionable clinical benefit. Obviously, in the practice of anesthesiology, like in the rest of medicine, conflict may arise among physicians, patients, and/or family members regarding goals of care. This is a source of great internal moral conflict for the anesthesia provider. Moreover, patients and family members may disagree with treatment options presented or denied. Complicating some situations further, family members often disagree with each other about treatment decisions that must be made in the presence of a patient who lacks proper decision-making capacity. At the extreme, patients and family members may put excessive pressure on care teams to provide clinical interventions that are not medically indicated.

It is not uncommon for anesthesiologists to feel pressured to acquiesce to decisions made by surgical and procedural colleagues in the face of questionable benefit. Such factors as production pressure, damaged professional relationships, loss of income to the health care system or a surgical colleague, complacency, and desire for conflict avoidance are only a few of the factors that may deter an anesthesiologist from expressing concern about treatment plans. One may even question if it is even our role, as consultants, to express our concerns to colleagues and patients. Are we simply being disruptive when we to step in and challenge a decision already agreed on by a surgeon and patient? In doing this, are we undermining the relationship built among a surgeon, a patient, and/or their family? Dr Carl Hug, in the 1999 E. A. Rovenstine Memorial Lecture at the American Society of Anesthesiologists annual meeting, forcefully encouraged anesthesiologists to become leaders in ethical decision-making.[9]

This article arms the reader with an understanding of the basic and current ethical and legal principles surrounding controversies in care of patients at the end-of-life. This discussion should serve to empower the anesthesiologist with the necessary language and understanding to assume an active role in ethical advocacy for their patients.

BASIC PRINCIPLES OF MEDICAL ETHICS

Table 1 highlights the basic principles of medical ethics and includes the negative impact these principles may create and examples of each principle in practice. It is important for clinicians to remind themselves of these principles in their daily practice.

Informed Consent

Informed consent is defined as an agreement or permission to proceed, accompanied by full notice about the care, treatment, or service that is the subject of the consent. Informed consent is rooted in the fundamental ethical principle of the right of self-determination and recognizes that patients are autonomous; that is, that they are independent agents with the capacity to make decisions regarding their well-being without coercion. A patient must be provided an understanding of the nature, risks, and alternatives of a medical procedure or treatment before the physician or other health care professional begins any such course. After receiving this information, the patient then either consents to or refuses such a procedure or treatment.[10]

Process of informed consent

In contrast to what is commonly believed, informed consent is a communication process rather than merely obtaining a signed consent document. This process occurs when communication between a patient and physician results in the patient's authorization or agreement to undergo a specific medical intervention.

Table 1 Basic principles of medical ethics		
Ethical Principle	**Definition**	**Downside**
Autonomy	"Self-rule," promotes patients to act as their own agent, free will with informed consent.	Consumerism: Commitment to noninvolvement in client decision making. The act of noncaring.
Beneficence	To do good or "provide benefit." The basic principle of "caring" requires one to act in accordance with a patient's welfare.	Paternalism: Health care provider makes decision for the patient based on provider's values more than patient's values.
Nonmaleficence	To do no harm. Involves careful calculation of risk in medical decision making and determining risk/benefit ratio. The balance of benefit and harm, also known as utility.	Nonaction or unwillingness to offer treatments with questionable benefit.
Justice	To be fair. This principle is guided by favoring distributive justice over entitlement and requires the appropriate distribution of limited resources.	Restriction of higher end resources from those who could afford it.
Veracity	"Truth-telling," defined as full, honest disclosure.	Assaulting patients with "the truth."
Fidelity	The capable patient must be provided with the complete truth about his or her medical condition.	Confidentiality can impede quality and efficiency of care.

In seeking a patient's informed consent, or the consent of the patient's surrogate if the patient lacks decision-making capacity or declines to participate in making decisions, physicians should:

a. Assess the patient's ability to understand relevant medical information and the implications of treatment alternatives and to make an independent, voluntary decision.
b. Present relevant information accurately and sensitively, in keeping with the patient's preferences for receiving medical information. The physician should include information about:
   i. The diagnosis (when known);
   ii. The nature and purpose of recommended interventions;
   iii. The burdens, risks, and expected benefits of all options, including forgoing treatment.
c. Document the informed consent conversation and the patient's (or surrogate's) decision in the medical record in some manner. When the patient/surrogate has provided specific written consent, the consent form should be included in the record.[11]

Emergency Situations

The common expression goes that "Man plans and God laughs." Our reality is not solely built in the world of predictable elective procedures; often, the unexpected happens. In emergencies, when a decision must be made urgently, the patient is often not able to participate in decision-making and the patient's surrogate is not available, physicians may initiate treatment without prior informed consent. This is justified based on implied consent, a situation wherein the patient implicitly grants consent simply by their presentation for care and the facts or circumstances surrounding the event. In such situations, the physician should inform the patient/surrogate at the earliest opportunity and obtain consent for ongoing treatment in keeping with these guidelines.[11]

Given that the justification for obtaining informed consent is to respect the individual patient's right to determine what happens to their bodies, difficulties sometimes surround situations where the patient cannot make these decisions for themselves. A requirement of autonomous choice is that patients actually make a decision that incapacitated patients cannot. In situations where there has been no prior written or verbal advance directive communicated, surrogates and clinicians must recall the patient's previous conversations, values, and beliefs to then make a decision that best represents the patient's most likely wishes. This substituted judgment does not actually constitute an autonomous choice by the patient, but rather attempts to make decisions that are authentic to the patient' beliefs and desires.[12] Importantly, evidence suggests that more than 90% of patients prefer family members to work with the clinician to make medical decisions for them if they are incapacitated.[13]

Decision-Making Capacity

In Western societies patients older than 18 years of age are generally considered adults and presumed legally competent to make health care decisions unless otherwise determined by a court. Consent to treat a minor must be given by a parent or legal guardian unless state law recognizes certain conditions that may qualify as an exception to the general requirement for parental or guardian consent. For example, depending on the state law, minors may be legally authorized to consent to their own health care if they are: married; pregnant and consenting for prenatal care; already a parent; otherwise emancipated; or in active military service.

The terms "capacity" and "competence" are sometimes used interchangeably, but historically they have held separate, although overlapping, meanings. Capacity is most often used to denote an individual's decision-making abilities in the context of a specific choice, such as medical treatment. Medically speaking, capacity refers to the ability to understand and use information about an illness and proposed treatment options to make a choice that is consistent with one's own values and preferences. Clinicians assess capacity to decide whether patients can make their own decisions. By contrast, competence refers to a legal judgment, informed by an assessment of capacity, relating to whether individuals have the legal right to make their own decisions.[14]

The law and ethics have settled on four decision-making abilities that constitute capacity: (1) understanding, (2) appreciation, (3) expressing a choice, and (4) reasoning (**Table 2**). A formal assessment of an individual's decision-making abilities in the context of a medical decision constitutes an assessment of capacity.

Advance Directives

The US Supreme Court has adjudicated and codified the virtually unlimited right of a competent patient to refuse treatment. This decision is rooted in the liberty interest of the Fourteenth Amendment, which states: "No State shall make or enforce any law which shall abridge the privileges or immunities of citizens of the United States; nor shall any State deprive any person of life, liberty or property."[15]

For the incompetent patient, formal written or oral directives are the preferred methods of directing end-of-life care.[16] These advance directives are the documents a person completes while still in possession of decisional capacity and define how treatment decisions should be made, on her or his behalf, in the event she or he loses the capacity to make such decisions. They are legal tools directing treatment, decision-making, and/or appointment of surrogate decision makers.

It is important to remember that advance directives are only acted on when the patient has lost the capacity to make decisions for himself. It is also important to remember that advance directives can be revoked orally or in writing by the patient at any time, so long as he or she has maintained decisional capacity.

The two main forms of advance directive documents are the:

1. Durable power of attorney for health care or health care proxy
2. Living will

In situations where an incompetent patient has not documented their wishes, their surrogates are charged with directing medical care based on what the patient would have wanted were they able to decide for themselves. Presumably, a surrogate is

Table 2	
Decision-making abilities that constitute capacity	
Decision-Making Ability	**Definition**
Understanding	The ability to state the meaning of the relevant information (eg, diagnosis, risks and benefits of a treatment or procedure, indications, and options of care)
Appreciation	The ability to explain how information applies to oneself
Expressing a choice	The ability to state a decision
Reasoning	The ability to compare information and infer consequences of choices

someone who has had a close and personal relationship with the patient and has the best understanding of the patient's values, goals of care, and wishes. This principle is known as substituted judgment. Commonly, the pressures placed on surrogates as medical decision-makers can create a great deal of anxiety, fear, and guilt. A newer principle, called substituted interest, helps to alleviate this burden. This model suggests that surrogates communicate to physicians the values, beliefs, and goals of the patient, rather than frankly making concrete decisions for treatment plans. The physician can then direct care based on a combination of these communicated values and beliefs and what actions are considered to be in the best interest of the patient. This model serves to ameliorate the potential anguish and guilt commonly experienced by surrogates.[17]

GUIDELINES FOR CARE OF PATIENTS WITH DO-NOT-RESUSCITATE ORDERS OR DIRECTIVES THAT LIMIT TREATMENT

Professional bodies in the disciplines of anesthesiology and surgery have revisited and revised their recommendations on treatment of patients with do-not-resuscitate (DNR) orders or directives limiting certain treatments. We are no longer in an era where DNR orders must, by law, be fully reversed before proceeding with surgical or procedural care, yet many clinicians continue to believe this to be true. The American Society of Anesthesiologists, in a guideline statement on patients with DNR orders or other limiting directives, warns against hospital policies that automatically suspend DNR orders stating that these policies "may not sufficiently address a patient's rights to self-determination in a responsible and ethical manner."[18] This statement insists on physicians revisiting and reviewing these orders with patients and surrogates at the time of the procedure with the intent of clarifying or modifying the directives based on patient wishes. Waisel and colleagues,[18–20] describe the essential components of a perioperative DNR discussion (**Box 1**).

Box 1
Essential components of a perioperative do-not-resuscitate discussion

1. Planned procedure and anticipated benefit.
2. Advantages and opportunities of having specific, identified clinicians providing therapy for a defined period.
3. Likelihood of requiring resuscitation.
4. Reversibility of likely causes requiring resuscitation.
5. Description of potential interventions and their consequences.
6. Chances of successful resuscitation including improved outcomes of witnessed arrests compared with unwitnessed arrests.
7. Ranges of outcomes with and without resuscitation.
8. Responses to iatrogenic events.
9. Intended and possible venues and types of postoperative care.
10. Postoperative timing and mechanisms for reevaluation of the DNR order.
11. Establishment of an agreement through a goal-directed approach or revocation of the DNR order for the perioperative period.
12. Documentation.

Once this discussion takes place, the American Society of Anesthesiologists statement on ethical guidelines for the anesthesia care of patients with DNR orders or other directives that limit treatment suggests three possibilities for a favorable outcome:

A. Full attempt at resuscitation: The patient or designated surrogate may request the full suspension of existing directives during the anesthetic and immediate postoperative period; thereby, consenting to the use of any resuscitation procedures that may be appropriate to treat clinical events that occur during this time.[18]
B. Limited attempt at resuscitation defined with regard to specific procedures: The patient or designated surrogate may elect to continue refusal of certain specific resuscitation procedures (eg, chest compressions, defibrillation or tracheal intubation). The anesthesiologist should inform the patient or designated surrogate about which procedures are essential to the success of the anesthetic and the proposed procedure, and which procedures are not essential and may be refused.[18]
C. Limited attempt at resuscitation defined with regard to the patient's goals and values: The patient or designated surrogate may allow the anesthesiologist and surgical/procedural team to use clinical judgment in determining which resuscitation procedures are appropriate in the context of the situation and the patient's stated goals and values. For example, some patients may want full resuscitation procedures to be used to manage adverse clinical events that are believed to be quickly and easily reversible, but may want to refrain from treatment of conditions that are likely to result in permanent sequelae, such as neurologic impairment or unwanted dependence on life-sustaining technology.[18]

One cannot underestimate the importance of documentation. All communication and modifications must be clearly documented in the patient's medical record. Plans for reinstatement of directives should also be clarified and documented with attention paid to when, in the postoperative period, the orders should resume. These discussions may include members from other pertinent specialties and all modifications should be communicated to the entire care team. The more detailed the documentation and communication, the greater the chance at a satisfactory outcome.

THE GOAL-DIRECTED APPROACH TO DO-NOT-RESUSCITATE ORDER ASSESSMENT AND MODIFICATION

Truog and colleagues[21] suggest approaching clarification and documentation of perioperative DNR orders through a goal-directed approach. This approach goes much further than typical procedure-directed approaches, which list specific allowable interventions in the event of cardiac arrest or other acute catastrophic events. These inflexible, procedure-directed approaches fail to address the highly complex, dynamic nature of anesthesia practice and leave room for a great deal of confusion for physicians faced with these acute, catastrophic events.

The goal-directed approach begins with the anesthesiologist communicating, to the patient, the possible physiologic impacts that anesthesia may have on them, including their specific disease processes, which usually differs greatly from their experiences in other medical settings. It is then important to elicit, from the patient, their goals for the surgery or procedure and to ask them to recommunicate their goals and wishes in the event of a catastrophic event (eg, cardiac arrest) and also for end-of-life care.

At this point, the patient authorizes the anesthesiologist to use their best clinical judgment to decide how certain interventions will impact the patient's personal desires and to act in accordance with the stated goals and wishes. The anesthesiologist may use their judgment to predict likely outcomes from the surgical and anesthetic process to create a personalized resuscitation plan consistent with the stated desires of their patients.[20,21] This goal-directed approach allows for trials of therapy to treat easily reversible events to achieve patient's goals. Examples include chest tube placement for pneumothorax, intubation for bronchoscopy in event of mucous plugging, cardioversion for witnessed arrest, or limited vasopressor use to counteract anesthetic effects.[18–22]

Waisel[20] states the temporary and reversible goal-directed perioperative DNR order can be documented as: "The patient desires resuscitative efforts during surgery and in the PACU only if the adverse events are believed to be both temporary and reversible, in the clinical judgment of the attending anesthesiologists and surgeons."

With thorough explanation and detailed documentation by the anesthesiologist, patients and physicians can feel comfortable adhering to patients' wishes, which usually permit temporary therapy for reversible insults, but also reject any intervention that will likely result in long-term deficits or dependence on artificial medical support.[18]

Iatrogenic factors leading to cardiac arrest should have no influence on the decision-making process for physicians.[19,20] The patient does not care about the cause, they care about the outcome. As difficult as it may be to exercise restraint in the face of iatrogenic causes of arrest, we must respect the patient's wishes and goals of care and withhold therapy if indicated.

FUTILITY AND INADVISABLE CARE IN THE PERIOPERATIVE PERIOD

Medical futility is challenging to define; however, futility is broadly conceptualized as therapies that will not accomplish their intended goal. Three types of futility are briefly defined next:

Physiologic futility: Describes medical interventions that could not possibly result in a physiologic goal (eg, treating a bacterial infection with an antibiotic known to be resistant to the specific bacteria).[23,24]

Quantitative futility: Focuses on the numeric probability of achieving the intended goal of therapy, which is generally presumed to be cure and survival.[25]

Qualitative futility: Shifts the focus from achieving a level of certainty to a focus on the quality of the potential benefits.[26]

There is a great deal of debate regarding these definitions and their applications to medical practice that go beyond the scope of this article. It is important, however, for the anesthesiologist to have a basic understanding of futility and inadvisable care and how to approach the conflict surrounding these situations. For purposes of this discussion, futility should be viewed as a treatment that cannot, in any likelihood, achieve the desired goal. These specific measures are easier to accept by patients and families because the lack of effect is often clear.

However, treatments that are extremely unlikely to be beneficial, are extremely costly, or carry an uncertain benefit-to-risk ratio to a patient, may be considered inappropriate and, hence, inadvisable. Inadvisable care should not be labeled as futile because the distinction is not clear-cut. Sources of conflict surround the definition of inadvisable care, such as different opinions about the goals of treatment, different views about how to interpret the likelihood of the treatment success, and problems in the patient-caregiver relationship. These can create significant dilemmas in the decision-making process and should be explored and addressed. A judgment that a treatment is inadvisable should occur only after completing a detailed process that ensures respect and consideration of all relevant viewpoints.[27]

Texas state law, in 1999, addressed this issue and paved the way for a legal due process to resolve questions of inadvisable care.[28] In the event of conflicts regarding the withdrawal or withholding of inadvisable care, physicians were able to request an ethics and peer committee review of the treatments in question. If the committee concurred with the physician, that the care proposed was inadvisable, the physician then had the right to withdraw and/or withhold treatment, but only after a 10-day period that allows for surrogates to arrange patient transfer to another health care facility.[28]

In 2004, the impact of the law was reviewed in a survey sent to Texas hospitals. The results of the survey seemed to favor a more structured, legal process for dealing with these conflicts. It remains to be seen whether this example will set the stage for future policy change.[29]

THE ROLE OF ANESTHESIOLOGISTS IN THE QUALITY OF END-OF-LIFE CARE

The American Society of Anesthesiologists has created and reaffirmed a statement pertaining to the impact of the anesthesiologist on quality end-of-life care of our patients. The statement stresses the importance of the anesthesiologist in improving the quality of patient care in this period. The statement encourages the furthering of education of our patients, families, health care workers, and physicians to promote "available, compassionate, comprehensive and interdisciplinary end-of-life care."[30]

SUMMARY

The role of the anesthesiologist cannot be understated when it comes to ethical decision making, and this is especially true at end-of-life. To best serve our patients within the limits of the law, the anesthesiologist must arm themselves with an understanding of how the laws surrounding ethical decision-making impact our daily practices. It is also important to know what rights and duties a patient or surrogate has in the decision-making process. With the proper understanding of our responsibilities and the tools available to us, anesthesiologists can fulfill their roles as leaders and advocates for their patients as we continue to evolve our approaches to ethical decision-making at the end of life.

REFERENCES

1. President's commission on ethical problems in medicine and in biomedical behavioral research. Deciding to forego life-sustaining treatment. Washington, DC: Government Printing Office; 1983. Available at: http://www.bioethics.gov/reports/past_commissions/deciding_to_forego_tx.pdf.
2. Hastings Center. Guidelines on the termination of life-sustaining treatment and the care of the dying. Bloomington (IN): Indiana University Press; 1987.
3. New York State Task Force on Life and the Law. When others must choose: deciding for patients without capacity. Albany (NY): New York Department of Health; 1992.
4. National Center for State Courts. Guidelines for state court decision making in life-sustaining medical treatment cases. Revised 2nd edition. St. Paul (MN): West Publishing Company; 1993.
5. Meisel A. Forgoing life-sustaining treatment: the legal consensus. Kennedy Inst Ethics J 1992;2(4):309–45.
6. Field MJ, Cassel CK, editors. Approaching death: improving care at the end of life. Washington, DC: National Academy Press; 1997.

7. Downing MT, Way DP, Caniano DA, et al. Result of a national survey on ethics education in general surgery residency programs. Am J Surg 1997;174(3):364–8.

8. Webb M. The good death: the New American search to reshape the end of life. New York: Bantam Books; 1997.

9. Hoey j. Foreword. In: Singer P, editor. Bioethics at the bedside: a clinician's guide. Ottawa (Canada): Canadian Medical Association; 1999:vii–viii.

10. American Society of Anesthesiologists syllabus on ethics 1999: introduction to informed consent. Park Ridge (IL): American Society of Anesthesiologists; 1999. p. A-1. Available at: http://www.asahq.org/publicationsAndServices/EthicsSyllabus. pdf. Accessed April 4, 2008.

11. AMA Principles of Medical Ethics: I,II,V,VIII.

12. Brudney D. Choosing for another: beyond autonomy and best interests. Hastings Cent Rep 2009;39:31.

13. Puchalski CM, Zhong Z, Jacobs MM, et al. Patients who want their family and physician to make resuscitation decisions for them: observations from SUPPORT and HELP. Study to understand prognoses and preferences for outcomes and risks of treatment. Hospitalized Elderly Longitudinal Project. J Am Geriatr Soc 2000;48:S84.

14. Siegel AM, Barnwell AS, Sisti DA. Assessing decision-making capacity: a primer for the development of hospital practice guidelines. HEC Forum 2014;26:159.

15. Emanuel EJ. Securing patients' right to refuse medical care: in praise of the Cruzan decision. Am J Med 1992;92:307–12.

16. Paola FA, Anderson JA. The process of dying. In: Sanbar SS, Gibofsky A, Firestone MH, et al, editors. Legal medicine. 3rd edition. St. Louis (MO): Mosby-Year Book; 1995. p. 404–23.

17. Sulmasy DP, Snyder L. Substituted interests and best judgments: an integrated model of surrogate decision making. JAMA 2010;304:1946–7.

18. American Society of Anesthesiologists. Ethical guidelines for the anesthesia care of patients with do not resuscitate orders or other directives that limit treatment. Available at: http://www.asahq.org/For-Members/ClinicalInformation/~/media/ For%2520Members/documents/Standards%2520Guidelines%2520Stmts/Ethical %2520Guidelines%2520for%2520the%2520Anesthesia%2520Ca. Accessed September 5, 2011.

19. Waisel DB, Burns JP, Johnson JA, et al. Guidelines for perioperative do-not-resuscitate policies. J Clin Anesth 2002;14:467–73.

20. Waisel DB. Chapter 5. Ethics and conflicts of interest in anesthesia practice. In: Longnecker DE, Brown DL, Newman MF, et al, editors. Anesthesiology. 2nd edition. New York: McGraw-Hill; 2012. Available at: http://accessanesthesiology. mhmedical.com/content.aspx?bookid=490&sectionid=40114684. Accessed December 05, 2018.

21. Truog RD, Waisel DB, Burns JP. DNR in the OR: a goal-directed approach. Anesthesiology 1999;90:289–95.

22. Casarett DJ, Stocking CB, Siegler M. Would physicians override a do-not-resuscitate order when a cardiac arrest is iatrogenic? J Gen Intern Med 1999;35–8.

23. Brody BA, Halevy A. Is futility a futile concept? J Med Philos 1995;20:123.

24. Jones JW, McCullough LB. Extending life or prolonging death: when is enough actually too much? J Vasc Surg 2014;60:521.

25. Schneiderman LJ, Jecker NS, Jonsen AR. Medical futility: its meaning and ethical implications. Ann Intern Med 1990;112:949.

26. Bernat JL. Medical futility: definition, determination, and disputes in critical care. Neurocrit Care 2005;2:198.
27. The Ethics Committee of the Society of Critical Care Medicine. Consensus statement of the Society of Critical Care Medicine's Ethics Committee regarding futile and other possibly inadvisable treatments. Crit Care Med 1997;25:887–91.
28. Texas Advance Directive Act. Texas Health & Safety Code Section 166.046. Procedure if not effectuating a directive or treatment decision.
29. Smith ML, Gremillion G, Slomka J, et al. Texas hospitals' experience with the Texas Advance Directives Act. Crit Care Med 2007;35(5):1271–6.
30. American Society of Anesthesiologists. Statement of quality end-of-life care. Available at: https://www.asahq.org/standards-and-guidelines/statement-on-quality-of-end-of-life-care. Accessed November 10, 2018.

Shared Decision-Making

Allen N. Gustin Jr, MD[a,b,c],*

KEYWORDS

- Shared decision-making • Decision aids • Risk calculators • Anesthesiology
- Surgery • Patient-centered care

KEY POINTS

- Shared decision-making is a component of patient-centered care.
- Patients do not want invasive procedures when the outcome likely results in severe disability.
- Shared decision-making engages the patient's core values and goals, allowing clinicians to guide patients with health care choices.
- Shared decision-making increases the chances a patient will seek less aggressive care.
- Decision aids and risk calculators improve patient knowledge, reduce patient anxiety, and improve interactions with clinicians.

INTRODUCTION

Older adults are the fastest growing segment of the US population, and patients older than 80 years have the highest rates of multimorbidity.[1] One-third of older Americans undergo surgery in the last 12 months of their life, most of them within the last month.[2] Data show that 1 in every 150 hospitalized patients dies from a complication, with 40% of those complications occurring in surgical patients,[2] and half of surgical complications are considered preventable.[3] These combined statistics demonstrate that our aging population has a high frequency of surgical care in the last year of life, despite high rates of perioperative complications and mortality.

Importantly, three-quarters of seriously ill patients say they would not choose life sustaining treatments if they knew the outcome would be survival with severe cognitive or functional impairment.[2] In an attempt to reconcile these points, questions immediately come to mind:

Disclosure Statement: No financial relationships to disclose.
[a] Stritch School of Medicine, Maywood, IL, USA; [b] Anesthesiology, Critical Care Medicine, Hospice/Palliative Medicine, Maywood, IL, USA; [c] Department of Anesthesiology and Perioperative Medicine, Loyola University Medical Center, 2160 South First Avenue, Building 103 Room 3113, Maywood, IL 60153, USA
* Loyola University Medical Center, 2160 South First Avenue, Building 103 Room 3113, Maywood, IL 60153.
E-mail address: allen.gustin@lumc.edu

Anesthesiology Clin 37 (2019) 573–580
https://doi.org/10.1016/j.anclin.2019.05.001
1932-2275/19/© 2019 Elsevier Inc. All rights reserved.
anesthesiology.theclinics.com

1. How many patients are offered less invasive options?
2. How should patients be counseled about the risk of functional and cognitive impairment after major surgery? and
3. Who is best suited to help patients weigh the risks and benefits of surgical procedures?[2]

Shared decision-making with patients, as opposed to clinicians making decisions on behalf of patients, has been gaining increasing momentum in health care policy.[4] The Institute of Medicine's (IOM) report in 2001, "Crossing the Chasm," set the stage for further patient engagement in health care decisions and highlighted "shared decision-making" as a new paradigm for consideration by clinicians.[5] The IOM's report advocates that all patient care decisions be based on the patient's goals and values.[6] A lack of guidance exists on how to accomplish shared decision-making in clinical practice.[4] Furthermore, the definitions of shared decision-making can be varied and confusing.[7]

HISTORY OF SHARED DECISION-MAKING

In 1988, the Picker Commonwealth Program for Patient-Centered Care (now called the Picker Institute) coined the term "patient-centered care" to highlight the need for the US health care system to shift focus from disease processes back to the individual patient.[6] "Patient-centered care" stressed the importance of understanding the patients' experience of illness and addressing the patients' needs within our complex and fragmented health care system.[6] The Picker Institute identified the 8 characteristics (**Box 1**) that are considered the most important indicators of quality and safety of US health care.[6] The concept of "patient-centered care" was expanded further in the IOM's report "Crossing the Quality Chasm" as one of the fundamental approaches to improving the quality of the US health care system.[5] The IOM's report focused on the patient as the locus of control, envisioning a health care system that encourages shared decision-making and accommodating the patient's preferences.[8] The IOM's report stated that if patients were truly informed of the risks and benefits of health care options (ie, shared decision-making using decision aids), then patients may not seek aggressive procedures not in line with their care goals. Given the impact of the IOM's report, shared decision-making was further adopted into the Affordable Care

---

Box 1
The Picker Institute's characteristics considered the most important indicators of quality and safety of US health care

1. Respect for the patient's values, preferences, and expressed needs.

2. Coordinated integrated care.

3. Clear, high-quality information and education for the patient and family.

4. Physical comfort including pain management.

5. Emotional support and alleviation of fear and anxiety.

6. Involvement of family members and friends as appropriate.

7. Continuity, including care site transitions.

8. Access to care.

Data from Barry MJ, Edgman-Levitan S. Shared decision making–pinnacle of patient-centered care. N Engl J Med 2012;366(9):780–1.

Act (ACA).[9] The ACA mandated that health care programs develop, evaluate, and disseminate decision aids that enhance shared decision-making among patients and their clinicians.[9]

WHAT IS SHARED DECISION-MAKING?

Definitions vary as to what clinicians consider shared decision-making vary, which has led to problems reliably measuring its occurrence.[10] Is it explaining the clinical situation to the patient and recommending options that the patient can accept or reject or outlining the treatment options and leaving the final decision to the patient?[7] The leeway and the responsibility given to the patient for making the decision can vary widely.[7] The greater the uncertainty of the options and the greater the clinician's ambivalence about the right choice, the greater the likelihood that the patient will be asked to make the decision.[7]

One formal definition of shared decision-making is "an approach where clinicians and patient share the best available evidence when faced with the tasks of making decisions, and where patients are supported to consider options to achieve informed preferences."[4,11] Importantly, decisions based solely on risk and benefit assessment (as determined by risk calculations) often do not take into account the patient's concerns and values.[7] A "sweet spot" for shared decision-making may require clinicians to work against their natural impulses to tell the patient what to do when they are certain of what's best and to leave the patient to decide when the clinician is not so sure.[7]

Unfortunately, despite clinicians believing that they are sharing in decisions with the patient, the care being provided does not always align with the patient's preferences.[8] In one study where more than 3500 medical decisions were made, less than 10% met the minimal standard for informed decision-making.[8] In another study, only 41% of Medicare patients believed that their treatment plan reflected their preferences for palliative care over more aggressive interventions.[8] Variation in the utilization of surgical procedures suggests that patients may receive care aligned not with their values and preferences but with their clinician's payment incentives.[8]

Surgical decisions have evolved little toward an ideal of shared decision-making.[2] The conversation continues to focus on the surgeon assuming the conventional role as patient protector.[12] Patients may not be presented with all the treatment options, which could include waiting for a period of time, consideration of medical treatments, less invasive surgical options, or percutaneous approaches.[2] For patients at high risk of adverse events after surgery or in cases in which the balance of risk and benefits may be equivocal, the traditional surgical model falls far short of the ideal situation for the patient.[2] Striving to make perioperative care more patient centered should be the goal. Anesthesiologists have a unique position in the perioperative care team and can participate in some of these discussions.[2]

DECISION MAKING: A MODEL

Shared decision-making involves a 3-step model:

1. Choice talk (introducing reasonable options),
2. Option talk (providing more details), and
3. Decision talk (making a decision).[4]

This model outlined in **Fig. 1** is not prescriptive, which means that a clinician's interactions with patients are, by necessity, characterized as fluid.[4] Decision support tools (2 forms being represented as the decision aid and the risk calculator) provide crucial

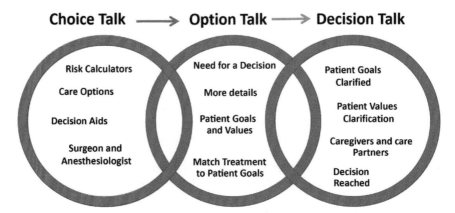

Fig. 1. Conceptual framework for shared decision-making.

input into this process. Patients will want time to study new information and consider their personal preferences, particularly for the future that is unknown to them, to think about outcome states that they have never experienced or considered.[4] If the patient desires to make decisions with other friends and family, then the clinician should attempt to make sure the information is provided to everyone for deliberation.[4]

ANESTHESIOLOGY AS AN OPPORTUNITY FOR SHARED DECISION-MAKING

How does the anesthesiologist engage patients in shared decision-making? Anesthesia treatment options for patients should include any care partners, caregivers, plans for medications, methods of administration, cost, and side-effect profiles. The anesthesiologist elicits each patient's values and goals, targets discussions to clinical options based on those values and goals, and should partner with the surgeon and the patient in order to help the patient make the best individual decisions. Patient-centered care is respectful and responsive to individual preferences, needs, and values; the patient's values should guide all the clinical anesthetic decisions.[9]

As an anesthesiologist, engaging a patient in shared decision-making can be challenging when one meets the patient for the first time in the preoperative area or when the patient needs an urgent or emergent procedure. Time may not allow for a full discussion of the patient's goals and values. As for elective procedures, time may be available for an anesthesiologist to discuss all aspects of the procedure and how the anesthesia plan can meet the goals and values of the patients while providing the best control of perioperative symptoms of the patient.

And finally, what about the patient who presents to the operating room with active treatment-limiting advanced directives (eg, a do not resuscitate or do not intubate preference)?[13] The American Society of Anesthesiologists' (ASA) ethical practice guidelines discourage the automatic rescission of advanced directives.[14] Rather, the ASA advocates for the anesthesiologist to determine which aspects of the advanced directive (if any) will remain active for the anesthetic.[14] A basic tenet of shared decision-making is that clinicians are the experts in the evidence and patients are the experts in what matters most to them.[15] Each patient may require an in-depth conversation to ensure the goals of the patient are in line with and parallel with the goals of the anesthetic care.

Currently, no published studies on the use of shared decision-making within anesthesiology practice exist; rather, studies have focused solely on surgical care. Shared decision moves away from the paternalistic approach toward a clinical interaction eliciting patient's values and goals and then, through informed consent discussion, to present the patient with a rigorous overview of potential therapeutic benefits and harms in relation to practices.[10] Numerous studies show the difficulty of adapting shared decision-making to surgical practice.[10] Informed consent, as it is currently practiced, may not necessarily be an effective mechanism for enhancing patient involvement in preoperative decision-making; it more often functions as an institutional and legal requirement lending little opportunity for patients to exercise autonomy.[10] Overall, informed consent is nonetheless necessary, as it serves as a legal document meant to avoid the legal tort of battery.[16]

BARRIERS AND FACILITATORS TO SHARED DECISION-MAKING

Many facilitators and barriers to shared decision-making exist. Facilitators for shared decision-making are few as outlined in **Box 2**.[17] Many more barriers to shared decision-making exist as outlined in **Box 3**.[4,9,17,18] Some clinicians feel patients lack health literacy and find sharing in decision-making sometimes impossible. Some patients may come from cultural backgrounds that lack a tradition of individuals making autonomous decisions.[4] Although time constraint is a perceived clinician barrier to shared decision-making, a Cochrane Collaboration review found that shared decision-making increased time by only 3 minutes per patient encounter.[9,18] Other studies showed no increase in time.[9]

DECISION AIDS AND RISK CALCULATORS

Decision aids familiarize patients with treatment options.[19] A decision aid states the decision, presents evidence about benefits and risks, and provides their probability with different options for treatment, while guiding the individual through various values that inform the decision.[9] Clinicians, patients, and policy makers need to be assured that the decision aids that are adopted into routine clinical care are evidence-based, balanced, and able to meet patients' information needs.[15]

Decision aids serve different purposes for patients and for physicians. For clinicians, decision aids can provide a framework to help guide patients through decision-making.[9] For patients, decision aids are designed to empower their participation in decision-making by expanding their knowledge and promoting their engagement with their clinician.[19] These tools go beyond simple risk presentation and aim to educate patients about their options, outcomes, and tradeoffs.[19] Misconceptions

---

Box 2
Facilitators to shared decision-making

Clinician Factor:

Use of decision aids.

Institutional Factor:

Decision aids implemented into computerized records.

Data from Dobler CC, Sanchez M, Gionfriddo MR, et al. Impact of decision aids used during clinical encounters on clinician outcomes and consultation length: a systematic review. BMJ Qual Saf 2018.

Box 3
Barriers to shared decision-making

Clinician Factors:

1. Lack of familiarity of what shared decision-making should be

2. Clinician attitudes to shared decision-making with the patient

3. Clinician knowledge regarding evidence and value of shared decision-making

4. Lack of resources

5. Time commitment

6. Health literacy of the patient

7. Competing priorities

8. Clinician needing to step out of his/her comfort zone when using new decision aids

Institutional Factor:

Lack of resources

Patient Factors:

1. Health literacy

2. Patient attitudes to shared decision-making

3. Patient's cultural background

Data from Refs.[4,9,17,18]

---

exist and some clinicians hesitate to make a recommendation because it feels like a violation of a patient's autonomy,[19] whereas other clinicians are under the impression that shared decision-making requires that patients make the decision. If the surgeon and anesthesiologist have learned enough about the patient, then they may offer an informed recommendation. Potential language to initiate this conversation is, "I would like to make a recommendation, but I need to know more about what is important to you first."[19]

Shared decision-making is also supported by risk calculators. The American College of Surgeons' (ACS) National Surgical Quality Improvement Program Surgical Calculator provides empirically derived, patient-specific risks for common adverse perioperative outcomes.[20] It serves as a tool to improve shared decision-making and informed consent for patients undergoing elective surgical procedures. In one study, 90% of patients desired a review of their ACS Calculator report before future surgical consents.[20] High-risk patients were 3 times more likely to underestimate their risk of any complication, serious complication, and length of stay as compared with low-risk patients.[20] The ACS calculator decreased anxiety levels in 71% of participants.[20] This risk calculator can aid the surgeon (and potentially the anesthesiologist) in discussing the risks with patients.

Decision aids and risk calculators are effective in promoting patient engagement in health care choices.[18,21,22] Benefits include increased patient knowledge, less anxiety of the care process, improved health care outcomes, reductions in unwarranted variation in care and costs, and greater alignment of care with patients values.[8] Recognition that informed patients often choose more conservative and hence less expensive medical options has made shared decision-making a focus of value-based care.[15] Barriers to the implementation of decision aids in clinical practice exist, but time may, surprisingly, not be one of them: decision aids only added 2.6 minutes longer to each patient visit, while generating a trend toward a reduction in major elective invasive surgery in favor of more conservative options.[18] In 2008, the Lewin Group estimated that implementation of shared decision-making for just 11 procedures would yield more than 9 billion in savings nationally over 10 years.[8]

MEDICAL PATERNALISM IS NOT DEAD

True consent is the informed exercise of a choice, which requires knowledgeable evaluation of the options available and the risks that depend on each option.[23] Consent is not merely the granting of permission but an exercise in choosing, and choice requires disclosure of certain information.[23] The spirit of informed decision-making reflects the recognition that only patients are experts on their own values.[23] But the resultant approach ironically assumes a value framework that not all patients possess. What if, for instance, the patient's preference is to know less?[23] Do situations exist when some degree of medical paternalism is appropriate? Are there circumstances where medical paternalism should supersede shared decision-making? Some patients want to share in decision-making and some patients may want more medical paternalism, letting the surgeon or anesthesiologist make all the decisions. In years past, medical paternalism was common and clinicians would tell their patients what to do, less frequently giving the patient a choice.[23] Sometimes when discussing treatment options, clinicians cover all information for consent.[23] Times do occur when patients want the physician to decide everything. Seeing the terror of uncertainty in a patient's face, clinicians need to make their best recommendation and say "I don't know how things are going to turn out, but I promise I'll be there with you the whole way."[23] In these situations, the best option for the patient may be for the clinician to take control of the clinical situation and make the choices for the patient.[23]

SUMMARY

Shared decision-making has arrived, too late and too early—too late for the need and too early for the level of preparation among clinicians and their clinical practice.[15] Turning shared decision-making from words on paper to actual patient engagement takes a great deal of effort. Decision aids do have a role in shared decision-making, have been shown to reduce the use of surgical resources, and should be used more in clinical practice. Clinicians must learn to be less medically paternalistic and become more effective coaches or partners, learning how to ask what matters most to the patient.[6] Shared decision-making should be adopted into all clinical practices, as it is the cornerstone of patient-centered care and value-based care.

REFERENCES

1. Ryan BL, Bray Jenkyn K, Shariff SZ, et al. Beyond the grey tsunami: a cross-sectional population-based study of multimorbidity in Ontario. Can J Public Health 2018;109(5-6):845–54.

2. Glance LG, Osler TM, Neuman MD. Redesigning surgical decision making for high-risk patients. N Engl J Med 2014;370(15):1379–81.

3. Gawande AA, Thomas EJ, Zinner MJ, et al. The incidence and nature of surgical adverse events in Colorado and Utah in 1992. Surgery 1999;126(1):66–75.

4. Elwyn G, Frosch D, Thomson R, et al. Shared decision making: a model for clinical practice. J Gen Intern Med 2012;27(10):1361–7.

5. Institute of Medicine (US) Committee on Quality of Health Care in America. Crossing the quality chasm: a new health system for the 21st century. Washington (DC): National Academies Press (US); 2001.
6. Barry MJ, Edgman-Levitan S. Shared decision making–pinnacle of patient-centered care. N Engl J Med 2012;366(9):780–1.
7. Fried TR. Shared decision making–finding the sweet spot. N Engl J Med 2016; 374(2):104–6.
8. Oshima Lee E, Emanuel EJ. Shared decision making to improve care and reduce costs. N Engl J Med 2013;368(1):6–8.
9. Armstrong MJ, Shulman LM, Vandigo J, et al. Patient engagement and shared decision-making: What do they look like in neurology practice? Neurol Clin Pract 2016;6(2):190–7.
10. Clapp JT, Arriaga AF, Murthy S, et al. Surgical consultation as social process: implications for shared decision making. Ann Surg 2019;269(3):446–52.
11. Elwyn G, Laitner S, Coulter A, et al. Implementing shared decision making in the NHS. BMJ 2010;341:c5146.
12. Gustin AN Jr, Aslakson RA. Palliative care for the geriatric anesthesiologist. Anesthesiol Clin 2015;33(3):591–605.
13. Errando CL. Anaesthesia for the professional singer. Eur J Anaesthesiol 2002; 19(9):687.
14. Craig DB. Do not resuscitate orders in the operating room. Can J Anaesth 1996; 43(8):840–51.
15. Spatz ES, Krumholz HM, Moulton BW. Prime time for shared decision making. JAMA 2017;317(13):1309–10.
16. Jones JW, McCullough LB, Richman BW. A comprehensive primer of surgical informed consent. Surg Clin North Am 2007;87(4):903–18, viii.
17. Dobler CC, Sanchez M, Gionfriddo MR, et al. Impact of decision aids used during clinical encounters on clinician outcomes and consultation length: a systematic review. BMJ Qual Saf 2019;28(6):499–510.
18. Stacey D, Légaré F, Lewis K, et al. Decision aids for people facing health treatment or screening decisions. Cochrane Database Syst Rev 2017;(4):CD001431.
19. Kopecky KE, Urbach D, Schwarze ML. Risk calculators and decision aids are not enough for shared decision making. JAMA Surg 2019;154(1):3–4.
20. Raymond BL, Wanderer JP, Hawkins AT, et al. Use of the American College of Surgeons national surgical quality improvement program surgical risk calculator during preoperative risk discussion: the patient perspective. Anesth Analg 2018.
21. Sepucha K, Atlas SJ, Chang Y, et al. Patient decision aids improve decision quality and patient experience and reduce surgical rates in routine orthopaedic care: a prospective cohort study. J Bone Joint Surg Am 2017;99(15):1253–60.
22. Nicholas Z, Butow P, Tesson S, et al. A systematic review of decision aids for patients making a decision about treatment for early breast cancer. Breast 2016;26: 31–45.
23. Rosenbaum L. The paternalism preference–choosing unshared decision making. N Engl J Med 2015;373(7):589–92.

Future Directions for Geriatric Anesthesiology

Philippe Desmarais, MD, MHSc, FRCPC[a,b,c], Nathan Herrmann, MD, FRCPC[d],
Fahad Alam, MD, MHSc, FRCPC[e,f], Stephen Choi, MD, MSc, FRCPC[e,f],
Sinziana Avramescu, MD, FRCPC, PhD[e,f,g],*

KEYWORDS

- Anesthesia • Evidence-based medicine • Geriatrics • Innovation
- Interdisciplinary care • Medical technology • Patient-centered outcomes
- Precision medicine

KEY POINTS

- Perioperative care will become increasingly patient centered, with older adults and their caregivers taking a bigger role in the decision-making process.
- Interdisciplinary and multidisciplinary collaborations in the perioperative setting will become the norm as they ensure the delivery of holistic and personalized care to older patients.
- Age-friendly and dementia-friendly initiatives will change the way programs and interventions are elaborated and delivered at all levels of the health care system.
- Fast-evolving technologies, such as immersive reality and machine learning, will drastically change how we teach and practice medicine, as well as educate patients and caregivers.
- Precision medicine will permit the creation and utilization of new and better pharmacologic agents, which may improve outcomes in the postoperative setting and enhance recovery after surgery.

Disclosure Statement: S.Avramescu and S.Choi receive "in-kind" cognitive assessment tools from Cogstate LTD. for research studies.
[a] Cognitive & Movement Disorders Clinic, Sunnybrook Health Sciences Centre, 2075 Bayview Avenue, Room A455, Toronto, Ontario M4N 3M5, Canada; [b] L.C. Campbell Cognitive Neurology Research Unit, Sunnybrook Health Sciences Centre, 2075 Bayview Avenue, Toronto, Ontario M4N 3M5, Canada; [c] Hurvitz Brain Sciences Program, Sunnybrook Research Institute, University of Toronto, 2075 Bayview Avenue, Toronto, Ontario M4N 3M5, Canada; [d] Department of Psychiatry, University of Toronto, Sunnybrook Health Sciences Centre, 2075 Bayview Avenue, Room FG19, Toronto, Ontario M4N 3M5, Canada; [e] Department of Anesthesia, University of Toronto, 123 Edward Street, Toronto, Ontario M5G 1E2, Canada; [f] Department of Anesthesia, Sunnybrook Health Sciences Centre, 2075 Bayview Avenue, Room M3200, Toronto, Ontario M4N 3M5, Canada; [g] Department of Anesthesia, Humber River Hospital, 1235 Wilson Avenue, Toronto, Ontario M3M 0B2, Canada
* Corresponding author. Department of Anesthesia, Humber River Hospital, 1235 Wilson Avenue, Toronto. Ontario M3M 0B2, Canada.
E-mail address: sinziana.avramescu@utoronto.ca

Anesthesiology Clin 37 (2019) 581–592
https://doi.org/10.1016/j.anclin.2019.05.002
1932-2275/19/© 2019 Elsevier Inc. All rights reserved.

INTRODUCTION

The demographics of populations around the world have changed considerably in the past decades and they will continue to change rapidly. Life expectancy at birth continues to increase progressively, now estimated to be at 72 years of age for those born in 2016.[1] The World Health Organization predicts that the 600 million people aged 60 years and older in 2000 will grow to an estimated 1.2 billion in the year 2025 and to 2 billion by the year 2050.[2] Unfortunately, parallel to increasing life expectancy, years of life with illness or disability are also increasing, partly attributable to the increased prevalence of chronic conditions and frailty with aging.[3] The world population is aging rapidly, and older adults now constitute the major portion of health care users. The US National Hospital Discharge Survey reported that older adults (≥65 years) represented 33% of hospital discharges and 44% of days of inpatient care in 2010.[4] Furthermore, the number of surgeries performed in older patients is increasing at a rate greater than the aging of the population. In order to meet the different needs of the aging population, physicians of every specialty will have to adapt the ways they provide medical and surgical care. When trying to envision the future of geriatric anesthesia specifically, one would have to consider how the future would look like at different levels: the Patient, the Environment, and the Anesthesia Specialty. The authors discuss each of these points separately (**Box 1**).

THE PATIENT

The relationship between patients and physicians has greatly changed in the past century with physicians taking less a paternalistic approach in their delivery of care and with patients and families becoming increasingly involved in the decision-making

---

Box 1
Future directions in geriatric anesthesia

At the level of the patient
- Patient-centered care and personalized care
- Shared decision-making
- Communication aids and tools
- Involvement of older patients and their families in the administration of interventions
- Interdisciplinary and multidisciplinary teams

At the level of the environment
- Age-friendly and dementia-friendly programs, services, and facilities
- Geriatric approaches implemented at all levels of the health care system
- Postanesthesia and post-ICU follow-up clinics
- New technologies for training future surgeons and anesthesiologists
- New technologies to assist surgeons and anesthesiologists
- New technologies to inform, prepare, and treat older adults

At the level of the specialty
- Engagement of older adults in clinical research
- Redefining outcomes; patient-centered and caregiver-centered outcomes
- Enhanced recovery after surgery; more regional anesthetic approaches
- New drugs with better target engagement
- Opioids and derivatives
- Cannabinoids and derivatives
- International collaborations and initiatives in geriatric anesthesia
- Mandatory training in geriatric medicine for medical students
- Expanded training in geriatric anesthesia for anesthesiology residents

process. Decisions, such as determining what investigations should be undertaken, what drugs or surgical procedures should be used, and whether resuscitation should be attempted, no longer depend solely on the expertise and experience of physicians. The authors envision that perioperative care will become gradually more centered on the older patient; decisions regarding surgical and anesthetic options will be shared with capable patients and their families, and patients will be surrounded by comprehensive interdisciplinary (ie, multiple specialties focused on a single common goal) and multidisciplinary (ie, where each member focuses on their own goals as they relate to patient care) teams throughout their surgical journey.

Patient-Centered Care

In the health care system, care is currently being reframed around the patient as opposed to being previously centered on a disease or a condition (eg, heart failure clinics, anticoagulation clinics). The perspectives, preferences, and the everyday lifestyle of patients are now considered when planning an intervention such as a surgical procedure or a pain management plan. More than ever before, physicians are expected to provide medical and surgical care aligned with patients' goals, which are often related to quality of life and maintenance of independent living. Indeed, medicine is becoming increasingly more personalized, and quality of care is now measured according to how successful patients' expectations and needs are met.[5,6] This is a paradigm shift from assessing quality of care based on availability of new technologies, operational facilities, or level of specialization of health care workers.[5] Hence, physicians have to be cognizant of the patient's personal goals at every assessment, explore their understanding of the intervention's risks and benefits, and evaluate whether the proposed interventions really meet patients' expectations.

Shared Decision-Making

Although all patients coming for anesthesia and surgery today give informed consent for the procedure, this process is rarely the result of a truly shared decision. The rapidly increasing population of older adults has very different life experiences, expectations, and values. Patients may have treatment preferences influenced not only by the risk of mortality and likelihood of potential benefits from the procedure but also by the burden of treatment, the risk of postoperative cognitive and functional impairment, and the access to postoperative support, home care, and rehabilitation.[7] Consequently, a "one size fits all" informed consent for various procedures and interventions may not be appropriate anymore and will have to be personalized for each patient. Shared decision-making allows both the clinician and the patient to have input in the decision-making process. Lilley and colleagues have developed a conceptual framework whereby an appropriate decision about whether to pursue surgery requires the best clinical evidence, qualified health care providers, a health care facility capable of managing the perioperative care, and well-informed patients involved in the surgical decision-making process.[8] Shared decision-making involves 3 basic steps:

1. Patients must be informed; specifically, they must be given an objective presentation of reasonable options and be told the risks and benefits of those options;
2. Patients should consider their own values, goals, and fears, and reflect on the impact of each option presented;
3. Finally, patients must communicate their goals and concerns to their health care provider, so they can be incorporated into the decision at hand.[9]

Considering that older patients are more likely to have sensory deficits, such as hearing and vision impairment,[10] and multiple medical conditions[3] and that postintervention recovery trajectories are less predictable than in younger patients,[11] the shared decision-making process cannot be a rushed conversation. Discussions on goals of care should occur early in the surgical journey of patients, and the decisions should be reassessed whenever important changes in health status occur. Postoperative brain health risks should be addressed explicitly with older patients.[12] Recently published best practices for postoperative brain health recommend that all patients older than 65 years of age be informed of the risk of postoperative delirium and cognitive dysfunction.[13] The possibility to forego surgery should be presented as a viable and acceptable alternative in certain situations.

Effective communication tools and techniques will have to be elaborated in the near future in order to ensure meaningful and productive discussions with older adults in the perioperative setting. An interesting idea includes the development of decision aids for certain discrete scenarios, similar to those elaborated for the treatment of hyperlipidemia,[14] breast cancer treatment,[15] or knee replacements.[16] Decision aids have been shown to improve patients' knowledge about their options and reduce their choice conflict related to feeling unclear about their values.[17,18] However, some have argued that shared decision-making may confuse patients, particularly in the setting of complex medical situations that can be overwhelming[19] or when patients have cognitive deficits. Nonetheless, engaging capable older patients and their families in care planning, despite the complexity of the decisions to make, is essential in order to provide the appropriate and desired treatments.[20,21]

The involvement of patients and their families in the perioperative setting will not stop at making decisions preoperatively but will also include involving them in the delivery of care throughout their surgical journey, such as potentially administering screening tools for common perioperative complications. For instance, family members may help the medical and surgical team detect the emergence of delirium in their loved ones by administering the Family Confusion Assessment Method.[20] In the near future, other caregiver-administered tools and self-administered tools may prove to be clinically beneficial and increase the team's efficiency. In addition, by learning self-management skills, patients can improve their health and reduce their needs for formal care.

Interdisciplinary and Multidisciplinary Perioperative Care

Older surgical patients may benefit from interdisciplinary and multidisciplinary approaches to care that involve not only their anesthesiologists and surgeons but also consultation from other specialists, rehabilitation medicine, nutrition, social work, and their longitudinal primary care provider. Geriatric specialists can be particularly helpful in managing older patients. They often lead training of various health care providers in geriatric principles related to common health care conditions observed in older adults and are often the best informed on models of care that are more effective and efficient in delivering services specific to older adults' needs. The preoperative Comprehensive Geriatric Assessment performed by geriatricians has previously been demonstrated to effectively identify older patients at high risk of postoperative complications and death,[22,23]whereas comprehensive geriatric care has been shown to reduce the incidence and severity of delirium[24] and improve mobility outcomes after surgery.[25] Work remains to be done to define and optimize the role of each care provider in assessment of risk, communication of risk, and decision-making with patients.

THE ENVIRONMENT

Although the partnership between patients and physicians will continue to evolve, with roles and responsibilities shifting between them, the setting where these interactions will occur will also change considerably. Innovations in engineering, technology, as well as in the design and implementation of age-friendly services will all reshape the work environment and processes.

Innovative and Optimized Infrastructures, Units, and Programs

Previous studies have revealed how current models of providing care, institutions, and facilities are not always age-friendly and may be in fact hazardous to older adults who are more prone to iatrogenic complications.[26] Some of the most frequently reported obstacles include the following:

1. Accessibility to programs and services secondary to mobility difficulties;
2. Bed rest in the context of hospitalization that can be particularly deleterious to older patients; and
3. Reliance of health care providers on patients' intact sensory modalities and cognitive functions to provide information and obtain consent.

Fortunately, solutions exist to some of these barriers that have been shown to improve the quality of care when they are applied.[27] Age-friendly and dementia-friendly initiatives have been developed and implemented around the world, such as the Age-Friendly Hospital Initiative[28] and the Hospital Elder Life Program.[29] These initiatives involve multipronged strategies aimed at preventing functional and cognitive decline in hospitalized older individuals, such as avoiding constipation and dehydration, encouraging early mobilization, and ensuring use of hearing and visual aids. Many of these simple recommendations have in fact been included in the Best Practices Guideline for the Optimal Perioperative Management of the Geriatric Patient of the American College of Surgeons.[30] It is expected that other similar geriatric approaches will permeate into the perioperative setting and ultimately become the standard of care across all units and services. Another noteworthy initiative is the International Perioperative Neurotoxicity Working Group that has recently published recommendations pertaining to the best practices for postoperative brain health, which will surely guide future endeavors to improve care in the perioperative setting.[13]

Although more studies are required, "virtual medical units" are an interesting concept to potentially reduce the number of postoperative complications. The virtual ward care model involves discharging patients at high risk of readmission sooner from the hospital and having a mobile multidisciplinary team monitoring and managing the patients in the community.[31–33] This model could be used in the perioperative setting where anesthesiologists would play a greater role in monitoring the recovery of patients and treating them in the community instead of in a hospital bed. Although whether these new models of providing care are clinically beneficial based on patient-centered outcomes remains to be determined, anesthesiologists will likely play an important role in delivering this type of care.

Technology

The arrival of new technologies, such as immersive realities, is currently transforming the landscape of medical education and health care. Fast-evolving technologies are changing the practice of medicine in general and will likely assist anesthesiologists in their work. Potential applications include diagnosing specific conditions more accurately, assessing complex anatomy more precisely, monitoring patients more optimally, and performing technical tasks with higher accuracy, just to name a few. Furthermore, to maximize the efficient use of resources for geriatric patients, technological advancements could also enhance health care providers' capacity to deliver care to older adults. This includes the use of assistive and health information technologies that improve both the communication among all caregivers and the efficient use of professionals.[34] Although there may be some concerns related to the adoption of technology by seniors, in fact, our means of interfacing with digital information will likely change from screens and hardware to gestures, emotions, and gazes. Immersive reality technologies, such as multitouch displays, telepresence (an immersive meeting experience that offers high video and audio clarity), 3-dimensional environments, natural language processing, intelligent software, and simulation, will transform not only health care and medical education but also teaching and learning in general.[35] Time will tell if these new technologies will have a positive impact on the care of older patients specifically, but they will certainly be an integral part of the work environment in the near future.

THE ANESTHESIA SPECIALTY

Delivering anesthesia care has never been safer. The mortality rate after general anesthesia was approximately 1 in 1000 in the 1940s,[36] and it is now less than 1 in 100,000 cases.[37] Therefore, it is anticipated that the authors' specialty will move away from survival outcomes and more toward quality of life outcomes, particularly when it comes to the care we provide for older patients. In order to make this shift possible, we must change the way we conduct research, we must partner with our patients to develop patient-centered outcome measures, and we must broaden the scope of our practice outside of the operating room. At a higher level, we predict that the field as a whole will move in the direction of precision medicine, with growing emphasis on drug discovery and design, new methods of patient phenotyping, and an expanded focus on novel ways of tailoring anesthesia care decisions to patients' unique features. However, we cannot ignore still commonly used drugs such as opioids, which are causing a public health crisis, or cannabis, which is legalized in Canada and several US states and may significantly affect anesthesia care of the elderly. It is our responsibility to educate our trainees and other health care providers about the basic concepts of geriatric anesthesiology and about how the evolution our specialty is currently undergoing may particularly affect the older adult population.

Review How We Conduct Research

There are few specific interventions for older patients that are evidence based. Historically, older adults have been underrepresented in clinical trials because of eligibility criteria such as age, windows for inclusion, and extensive exclusion criteria that may disproportionately affect them. Studies have reported arbitrary upper age limits in up to 42% of clinical trials.[38,39] Several reasons have been stated for justifying the exclusion of older adults from clinical research, such as logistical factors (eg, cannot drive to the research site), presence of cognitive impairment (eg, difficulties following instructions, consent issues), higher attrition rate, and a higher pathology heterogeneity causing differential responses to investigated interventions. Nonetheless, the systematic exclusion of older adults has contributed to important knowledge gaps in geriatric anesthesia. Fortunately, research practices are evolving and the representation of older adults in clinical trials is improving.[40] Because of pharmacodynamic and pharmacokinetic changes associated with aging, more studies conducted in older surgical populations are needed in order to provide evidence-based care. Similarly, since the world population is aging and age is the major risk factor for dementia, more rigorous studies involving older patients with cognitive impairment will have to be conducted and will have to include cognitive outcomes.

For future perioperative clinical trials investigating changes in cognitive outcomes to be clinically informative, they will have to include neuropsychological assessments performed before and after surgical interventions, assess return to baseline, and evaluate functional implications of cognitive change. As well, successful implementation of research findings into clinical practice will necessitate routine use of cognitive testing in the perioperative period, which is currently difficult for numerous logistic reasons. Computer-based cognitive assessment tools may be one answer to screening more frequently older patients before and after surgery because they are fast, they can be administered remotely and repetitively, and results can be compared with age-matched controls. However, they are less accurate than office-based assessments that use specialized assessments of multiple cognitive domains. Older individuals may be less at ease with computer-based assessments and may prefer paper-based tests. Although a tool with perfect psychometric properties that can be administered quickly and can provide extensive information on all cognitive domains is utopic, the development of innovative, valid, and practical neuropsychological assessment tools will likely involve new technologies. Routine neuropsychological testing implemented in perioperative practice will also permit the assessment of prospective interventions to prevent and mitigate postoperative cognitive dysfunction in older surgical patients at high risk. Indeed, a growing and promising new area of research is cognitive prehabilitation before necessary semielective surgeries for the prevention of postoperative cognitive dysfunction and delirium.[41,42]

Finally, to close the knowledge gaps in geriatric anesthesia, patients and their caregivers will have to be engaged more in clinical research, not only as participants but also as collaborators. They can help select meaningful objectives for future studies.[43] It can be hypothesized that the high attrition rates of elderly participants reported in clinical trials are partly a result of participants' unmet expectations by trial objectives. Present outcomes of clinical trials will probably be redefined in the collaborative process, with a greater importance given to functional and cognitive outcomes than to survival. Patient-centered outcome measures, such as quality of life scores, functional scales, and mobility scores, and caregiver-centered outcome measures, such as burden on caregiver and quality of life scores, will inevitably have to be part of future clinical trials.

Precision Anesthesia

The significantly increased safety in anesthesia has been the result, at least in part, of standardization of practice, which has recently evolved into innovative programs such as the Perioperative Surgical Home[44] or Enhanced Recovery Programs.[45] The pitfall of these population-based practices is a potential rigidity that diminishes the importance of individual patient variability, which is significant in the case of older patients. The authors and other investigators[46] anticipate that the future of geriatric anesthesia will move toward precision medicine, based on individualized care that takes into account the heterogeneity of the elderly. Several centers have already implemented pre-emptive pharmacogenetic testing programs[47] and more than 10% of FDA-approved drugs already contain pharmacogenomic information on their labels.[48] Anesthesia has been a slow adopter of precision medicine advancements. There are still many gaps and barriers to the wide adoption and implementation of pharmacogenomics and biology-focused care in the perioperative setting. It is thought that precision anesthesia is more than genes and small molecules and begins with leveraging minimally invasive surgical techniques, regional anesthesia, opioid-sparing regimens, and neuroprotection. For example, in geriatric medicine minimizing general anesthetics and opioids can improve functional recovery and decrease postoperative complications.[49]

Older patients are also at high risk of developing delirium and postoperative cognitive dysfunction,[50,51] and there is active and robust study into anesthesiologist-led interventions hypothesized to reduce the incidence of delirium or diminish other cognitive consequences of the perioperative setting. For instance, dexmedetomidine, a highly potent and selective α2-adrenoceptor agonist has been shown to reduce the occurrence of intensive care unit (ICU) delirium in the postoperative period,[52] although its role for postoperative delirium outside the ICU setting is unclear. Nonetheless, because of its opioid- and anesthetic-sparing effects as well as its direct antiinflammatory properties, dexmedetomidine is now being trialed for long-term neuroprotection after high-risk surgery in geriatric patients.[53]

New Drugs with Better Target Engagement

Recent advances in genomics, proteomics, and metabolomics will enable the identification of new drug targets and the development of better drugs, thus moving pharmacology into the age of precision medicine. The "Holy Grail" in anesthesia will be the creation of drugs with maximal anesthetic, analgesic, and amnestic properties with virtually no side effects (eg, hemodynamic instability, cognitive impairment, postoperative nausea, and vomiting). Perhaps a single drug will have all those properties, reducing the significant polypharmacy today's "balanced anesthetic" typically requires. In the meantime, drug innovations are primarily focused on modifying the chemical structures of existing drugs in order to improve their pharmacologic profile and diminish side effects. Such novel drugs include midazolam derivatives such as remimazolam and ADV6209[54,55]; etomidate derivatives such as methoxycarbonyl-etomidate, carboetomidate, and cyclopropyl-methoxycarbonyl metomidate[56,57]; and propofolalternatives.[58]

Although still anecdotal, studies on opioid-free anesthesia are gaining relevance in the context of the opioid crisis and may represent interesting avenues to pursue in the future.[59,60] Opioids contribute to sedation, constipation, nausea, vomiting, and pruritus, all side effects that older patients are more prone to experience. In addition, cannabinoids and their derivatives will most likely have clinical utilities in the near future in the perioperative setting, possibly for treating postoperative nausea and vomiting, to stimulate appetite, as well as to alleviate pain, depression, and anxiety.[61] However, before these new molecules can be widely prescribed and administered to older patients, their adverse effect profile will have to be better defined in this patient population.

Collaborations and Initiatives in Geriatric Anesthesiology

With the broadened understanding of older patients' particularities and needs, guidelines have been developed in the past few years to summarize current evidence in regard to perioperative care of the older patients as well as to highlight some of the many existing gaps that will have to be addressed in future studies. The Best Practices Guideline for the Optimal Perioperative Management of the Geriatric Patient of the American College of Surgeons represented the first collaborative initiative on the matter.[29] Similarly, with the increased appreciation of the importance of postoperative delirium and cognitive dysfunction, groups of experts around the world have assembled to create brain health programs and initiatives, such as the Perioperative Brain Health Initiative of the American Society of Anesthesiologists. The International Perioperative Neurotoxicity Working Group, with their recently published recommendations on postoperative brain health risks, represents another concrete example of a collaborative process aimed at improving the care of older patients.[13] The expert opinions and scientific evidence included in these guidelines will serve as the basis for approaching anesthesia care for older adults and optimizing their perioperative care.

Geriatric Education

As scientific knowledge will continue to increase exponentially in the near future, catalyzed by new technologies, successful translation into clinical practice of new discoveries will require enhanced training of all health care providers in geriatric principles. As previously mentioned, principles of the comprehensive geriatric assessment are beneficial not only to older patients but to all patients, including the surgical patient. Ideally, this may take the form of mandatory training in geriatric medicine for medical students and expanded training in geriatric anesthesia for anesthesiology residents. As well, the prospective development of fellowship training programs in geriatric anesthesia will certainly help to address the need for increased expertise and specialized care for this growing population of health care users.

SUMMARY

Geriatric anesthesia is a new subspecialty where much has to be built from the ground up. In the context of an aging world population, providing optimal care in the perioperative setting is an urgent matter but also a great opportunity to improve the standard of care. Innovations at all levels of the health care system will drastically change how we practice geriatric anesthesia.

REFERENCES

1. World Health Organization. World Health Statistics 2018: monitoring health for the SDGs, sustainable development goals. Available at: http://www.who.int/gho/publications/world_health_statistics/2018/en/. Accessed September 3, 2018.
2. World Health Organization. Ageing and health.key facts. Available at: http://www.who.int/news-room/fact-sheets/detail/ageing-and-health. Accessed September 3, 2018.
3. Barnett K, Mercer SW, Norbury M, et al. Epidemiology of multimorbidity and implications for health care, research, and medical education: a cross-sectional study. Lancet 2012;380:37–43.
4. CDC/NCHS National Hospital Discharge Survey. Available at: https://www.cdc.gov/nchs/nhds/index.htm. Accessed September 3, 2018.
5. Hanefeld J, Powell-Jackson T, Balabanova D. Understanding and measuring quality of care: dealing with complexity. Bull World Health Organ 2017;95:368–74.
6. World Health Organization. WHO global strategy on people-centred and integrated health services. 2015. Available at: http://apps.who.int/iris/bitstream/10665/155002/1/WHO_HIS_SDS_2015.6_eng.pdf. Accessed September 3, 2018.
7. Fried TR, Bradley EH, Towle VR, et al. Understanding the treatment preferences of seriously ill patients. N Engl J Med 2002;346:1061–6.
8. Lilley EJ, Bader AM, Cooper Z. A values-based conceptual framework for surgical appropriateness: an illustrative case report. Ann Palliat Med 2015;4:54–7.
9. Elwyn G, Durand MA, Song J, et al. A three-talk model for shared decision making: multistage consultation process. BMJ 2017;359:j4891.
10. Correia C, Lopez KJ, Wroblewski KE, et al. Global sensory impairment among older adults in the United States. J Am Geriatr Soc 2016;64:306–13.
11. de Rooij SE, Govers AC, Korevaar JC, et al. Cognitive, functional, and quality-of-life outcomes of patients aged 80 and older who survived at least 1 year after

planned or unplanned surgery or medical intensive care treatment. J Am Geriatr Soc 2008;56:816–22.

12. Hogan KJ, Bratzke LC, Hogan KL. Informed consent and cognitive dysfunction after noncardiac surgery in the elderly. Anesth Analg 2018;126:629–31.

13. Berger M, Schenning KJ, Borwn CH, et al. Best practices for postoperative brain health: recommendations from the fifth international perioperative neurotoxicity working group. Anesth Analg 2018;127:1406–13.

14. Shared Decision Making National Resource Center of Mayo Clinic. Statin Decision Aid. Available at: https://statindecisionaid.mayoclinic.org. Accessed September 3, 2018.

15. Savelberg W, van der Weijden T, Boersma L, et al. Developing a patient decision aid for the treatment of women with early stage breast cancer: the struggle between simplicity and complexity. BMC Med Inform Decis Mak 2017;17:112.

16. Jayadev C, Khan T, Coulter A, et al. Patient decision aids in knee replacement surgery. Knee 2012;19:746–50.

17. Fowler FJ Jr, Levin CA, Sepucha KR. Informing and involving patients to improve the quality of medical decisions. Health Aff (Millwood) 2011;30:699–706.

18. Stacey D, Légaré F, Col NF, et al. Decision aids for people facing health treatment or screening decisions. Cochrane Database Syst Rev 2014;(28):CD001431.

19. Rosenbaum L. The paternalism preference –choosing unshared decision making. N Engl J Med 2015;373:589–92.

20. Heyland DK, Barwich D, Pichora D, et al. Failure to engage hospitalized elderly patients and their family in advance care planning. JAMA Intern Med 2013; 173:778–87.

21. Steis MR, Evans L, Hirschman KB, et al. Screening for delirium using family caregivers: Convergent validity of the family confusion assessment method and interviewer-rated confusion assessment method. J Am Geriatr Soc 2012;60: 2121–6.

22. Kim KI, Park KH, Koo KH, et al. Comprehensive geriatric assessment can predict postoperative morbidity and mortality in elderly patients undergoing elective surgery. Arch Gerontol Geriatr 2013;56:507–12.

23. Kristjansson SR, Nesbakken A, Jordhoy MS, et al. Comprehensive geriatric assessment can predict complications in elderly patients after elective surgery for colorectal cancer: a prospective observational cohort study. Crit Rev Oncol Hematol 2010;76:208–17.

24. Marcantonio ER, Flacker JM, Wright RJ, et al. Reducing delirium after hip fracture: a randomized trial. J Am Geriatr Soc 2001;49:516–22.

25. Prestmo A, Hagen G, Sletvold O, et al. Comprehensive geriatric care for patients with hip fractures: a prospective, randomised, controlled trial. Lancet 2015;385: 1623–33.

26. Creditor MC. Hazards of hospitalization of the elderly. Ann Intern Med 1993;188: 219–23.

27. Landefeld CS, Palmer RM, Kresevic DM, et al. A randomized trial of care in a hospital medical unit especially designed to improve the functional outcomes of acutely ill older patients. N Engl J Med 1995;332:1338–44.

28. Huang AR, Larente N, Morais JA. Moving towards the age-friendly hospital: a paradigm shift for the hospital-based care of the elderly. Can Geriatr J 2011; 14:100–3.

29. Yue J, Tabloski P, Dowal SL, et al. NICE to HELP: operationalizing National Institute for Health and Clinical Excellence guidelines to improve clinical practice. J Am Geriatr Soc 2014;62:754–61.

30. Mohanty S, Rosenthal RA, Russell MM, et al. Optimal perioperative management of the geriatric patient: a best practices guideline from the American College of Surgeons NSQIP and the American Geriatrics Society. J Am Coll Surg 2016; 222:930–47.

31. Dhalla IA, O'Brien T, Morra D, et al. Effect of a postdischarge virtual ward on re-admission or death for high-risk patients: a randomized clinical trial. JAMA 2014; 312:1305–12.

32. Low LL, Tan SY, Ng MJM, et al. Applying the integrated practice unit concept to a modified virtual ward model of care for patients at highest risk of readmission: a randomized controlled trial. PLoS One 2017;12:e0168757.

33. Lewis C, Moore Z, Doyle F, et al. A community virtual ward model to support older persons with complex health care and social care needs. Clin Interv Aging 2017; 12:985–93.

34. Stabile M, Cooper L. Review article: the evolving role of information technology in perioperative patient safety. Can J Anaesth 2013;60:119–26.

35. Huff G, Saxberg B. Full immersion 2025: how will 10-year-olds learn? Education Next Summer 2009;9:79–82.

36. Dripps RD, Lamont A, Eckenhoff JE. The role of anesthesia in surgical mortality. JAMA 1961;178:261–6.

37. Li G, Warner M, Lang BH, et al. Epidemiology of anesthesia-related mortality in the United States, 1999-2005. Anesthesiology 2009;110:759–65.

38. Beers E, Moerkerken DC, Leufkens HGM, et al. Participation of older people in preauthorization trials of recently approved medicines. J Am Geriatr Soc 2014; 62:1883–90.

39. Zulman DM, Sussman JB, Chen X, et al. Examining the evidence: a systematic review of the inclusion and analysis of older adults in randomized controlled trials. J Gen Intern Med 2011;26:783–90.

40. Desmarais P, Miville C, Milán-Tomás Á, et al. Age representation in antiepileptic drug trials: a systematic review and meta-analysis. Epilepsy Res 2018;142:9–15.

41. Culley DJ, Crosby G. Prehabilitation for prevention of postoperative cognitive dysfunction? Anesthesiology 2015;123:7–9.

42. Humeidan ML, Otey A, Zuleta-Alarcon A, et al. Perioperative cognitive protection-cognitive exercise and cognitive reserve (The Neurobics Trial): a single-blind randomized trial. Clin Ther 2015;37:2641–50.

43. Sacristán JA, Aguarón A, Avendaño-Solá C, et al. Patient involvement in clinical research: Why, when, and how. Patient Prefer Adherence 2016;10:631–40.

44. Vetter TR, Boudreaux AM, Jones KA, et al. The perioperative surgical home: how anesthesiology can collaboratively achieve and leverage the triple aim in health care. Anesth Analg 2014;118:1131–6.

45. Miller T, Thacker JK, White WD, et al. Reduced length of hospital stay in colorectal surgery after implementation of an enhanced recovery protocol. Anesth Analg 2014;118:1052–61.

46. Iravani M, Lee LK, Cannesson M. Standardized care versus precision medicine in the perioperative setting: can point-of-care testing help bridge the gap? Anesth Analg 2017;124:1347–53.

47. Dunnenberger HM, Crews KR, Hoffman JM, et al. Preemptive clinical pharmacogenetics implementation: current programs in five US medical centers. Annu Rev Pharmacol Toxicol 2015;55:89–106.

48. Frueh FW, Amur S, Mummaneni P, et al. Pharmacogenomic biomarker information in drug labels approved by the United States Food and Drug Administration: prevalence of related drug use. Pharmacotherapy 2008;28:992–8.

49. Luger TJ, Kammerlander C, Gosch M, et al. Neuroaxial versus general anaesthesia in geriatric patients for hip fracture surgery: does it matter? OsteoporosInt 2010;21(Suppl 4):S555–72.

50. Williams-Russo P, Urquhart BL, Sharrock NE, et al. Postoperative delirium: predictors and prognosis in elderly orthopedic patients. J Am Geriatr Soc 1992; 40:759–67.

51. Mason SE, Noel-Storr A, Ritchie CW. The impact of general and regional anesthesia on the incidence of post-operative cognitive dysfunction and post-operative delirium: a systematic review and meta-analysis. J Alzheimers Dis 2010;22(Suppl 3):S67–79.

52. Su X, Meng ZT, Wu XH, et al. Dexmedetomidine for prevention of delirium in elderly patients after non-cardiac surgery: a randomised, double-blind, placebo-controlled trial. Lancet 2016;388:1893–902.

53. Choi S, Avramescu S. Dexmedetomidine to reduce the incidence of POCD after open cardiac surgery. Available at: https://clinicaltrials.gov/ct2/show/ NCT03480061. Accessed October 1, 2018.

54. Rogers WK, McDowell TS. Remimazolam, a short-acting GABA(A) receptor agonist for intravenous sedation and/or anesthesia in day-case surgical and non-surgical procedures. IDrugs 2010;13:929–37.

55. Marçon F, Guittet C, Manso MA, et al. Population pharmacokinetic evaluation of ADV6209, an innovative oral solution of midazolam containing cyclodextrin. Eur J Pharm Sci 2018;114:46–54.

56. Pejo E, Liu J, Lin X, et al. Distinct hypnotic recoveries after infusions of methoxycarbonyletomidate and cyclopropylmethoxycarbonylmetomidate: the role of the metabolite. Anesth Analg 2016;122:1008–14.

57. Pejo E, Cotten JF, Kelly EW, et al. In vivo and in vitro pharmacological studies of methoxycarbonyl-carboetomidate. Anesth Analg 2012;115:297–304.

58. Egan TD, Obara S, Jenkins TE, et al. AZD-3043: a novel, metabolically labile sedative–hypnotic agent with rapid and predictable emergence from hypnosis. Anesthesiology 2012;116:1267–77.

59. Ziemann-Gimmel P, Goldfarb AA, Kooppman J, et al. Opioid-free total intravenous anaesthesia reduces postoperative nausea and vomiting in bariatric surgery beyond triple prophylaxis. Br J Anaesth 2014;112:906–11.

60. Horlocker TT, Hebl JR, Kinney MA, et al. Opioid-free analgesia following total knee arthroplasty–a multimodal approach using continuous lumbar plexus (psoas compartment) block, acetaminophen, and ketorolac. Reg Anesth Pain Med 2002;27:105–8.

61. Whiting PF, Wolff RF, Deshpande S, et al. Cannabinoids for medical use: a systematic review and meta-analysis. JAMA 2015;313:2456–73.

Printed and bound by CPI Group (UK) Ltd, Croydon, CR0 4YY

08/05/2025

01864746-0007